The SAGES Manual

Springer
New York
Berlin
Heidelberg
Barcelona
Budapest
Hong Kong
London
Milan
Paris
Singapore
Tokyo

Carol E.H. Scott-Conner, M.D., Ph.D.
Department of Surgery
University of Iowa Hospitals and Clinic
Editor

The SAGES Manual

Fundamentals of Laparoscopy and
GI Endoscopy

With a Foreword by Desmond H. Birkett, M.D.

With 273 Figures

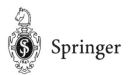 Springer

Carol E.H. Scott-Conner, M.D., Ph.D.
Department of Surgery
University of Iowa Hospitals and Clinic
200 Hawkins Drive, 1516 JCP
Iowa City, IA 52242-1086, USA

The SAGES manual: fundamentals of laparoscopy and GI endoscopy/
    Carol E.H. Scott-Conner, editor: with a foreword by Desmond H. Birkett.
        p. cm.
    Includes bibliographical references and index.
    ISBN 0-387-98496-8 (softcover: alk. paper)
    1.   Abdomen—Endoscopic surgery—Handbooks, manuals, etc.
2. Laparoscopy—Handbooks, manuals, etc. 3. Laparoscopic surgery—
Handbooks, manuals, etc. 4. Gastroscopy—Handbooks, manuals, etc.
I. Scott-Conner, Carol E.H.
[DNLM: 1. Laparoscopy handbooks. 2. Endoscopy, Gastrointestinal
handbooks. WI 39S129 1998]
RD540.S24 1998
617.5'5059—dc21   98-29512

Printed on acid-free paper.

Production managed by Lesley Poliner; manufacturing supervised by Joe Quatela.
Camera-ready copy prepared using Microsoft Word.
Printed and bound by Edwards Brothers, Inc., Ann Arbor, MI.
Printed in the United States of America.

9 8 7 6 5 4 3 2 1

ISBN 0-387-98496-8 Springer-Verlag New York Berlin Heidelberg   SPIN 10660242

Foreword

The practice patterns of general surgery have changed significantly in the last decade as a result of the increasing use of flexible endoscopy, both diagnostic and therapeutic, and also the introduction of laparoscopic endoscopy as a therapeutic technique. These changes have occurred over a short period of time and continue rapidly with the increasing use of advanced laparoscopic procedures. Residents who have completed their training and are entering the practice of general surgery must be very familiar with, and must be well educated in, these two areas. Flexible endoscopy and laparoscopy will be a significant part of their practice and with time will become more important and more widely used.

Residency programs are struggling to develop educational programs that will adequately prepare residents for the future of endoscopy and laparoscopy. This is difficult in some programs because of the lack of clinical endoscopic material, the lack of understanding of the importance of endoscopic techniques in their medical communities, and a lack of interest and training of their staff. There is also a lack of good textbooks or educational tools aimed directly at residents to help these programs. There is a definitive need for a comprehensive textbook directed at the education of residents.

SAGES (Society of American Gastrointestinal Endoscopic Surgeons) has for many years made resident education a priority. The society runs basic and advanced laparoscopic courses for residents and is developing tools to aid residency programs with their responsibility of providing an adequate educational environment. Now that the dust has had time to settle, and procedures have been standardized and refined, complications understood, and the rationale for the use of the procedures defined, there is a need for a good textbook for residents. SAGES has undertaken this important step in residency education by producing this pocket-sized manual of flexible endoscopy and laparoscopy, which is a quick and complete reference guide for surgical residents. The editor, Carol Scott-Conner, M.D., is to be commended for an extremely thorough job in the selection of chapter titles and members of the society, who are experts in their fields, to write these chapters. The manual is written in a notebook style, with liberal use of headings to facilitate the use of the manual as a quick reference tool. It is liberally illustrated with line drawings that significantly enhance the text. It deals with all aspects of diagnostic flexible endoscopy, including endoscopic retrograde cholangiopancreatography. It includes significant detail on therapeutic flexible endoscopy, and guides to the management of patients undergoing these procedures. There is a comprehensive coverage of laparoscopy from the understanding of the equipment and its workings, through the basic physiological changes during laparoscopy, to the practical side of the laparoscopic procedures. There is an extensive description of the management of patients undergoing these procedures. The manual is so complete that it is a little larger than was originally intended; this is not a deficiency but an advantage to the reader, as the information is thorough, comprehensive, and at the fingertips. These features make the manual an excellent companion and quick reference tool to which residents can refer when treating all aspects of flexible endoscopy or laparoscopy that they might encounter.

The scope, detail, and quality of the contents confirm and demonstrate the SAGES commitment to residency education. This manual is a must for all general surgical residents and should be considered by any resident entering a discipline that treats patients with videoscopic minimally invasive procedures.

Desmond H. Birkett, M.D.
Burlington, Massachusetts
August 20, 1998

Preface

This manual has been a true labor of love. Many skilled surgical endoscopists and laparoscopists contributed untold time, effort, and expertise to this project. Think of it as a way to take SAGES experts with you, in your pocket, your briefcase, or your OR locker. The manual is organized into two sections: Laparoscopy and Gastrointestinal Endoscopy. Each section begins with general information and progresses to specific procedures. While each chapter builds the foundation for the next, we have also tried to make each chapter stand alone, to serve the needs of the reader who turns to it for specific instructions on a particular procedure.

The laparoscopic revolution took many of us by surprise and introduced all of us to the concept of the learning curve. Patience and practice, hours reviewing videotapes, suturing with simulators, and box trainers are necessary to master the skills needed for these procedures. While this book cannot substitute for that investment of personal time, it can smooth the way by passing along pearls and technical tips from experienced laparoscopic and endoscopic surgeons.

Innumerable individuals deserve my profound thanks. I will name just a few here. First, I extend my sincere appreciation to all those authors who were patient with me through the editing process. Next, I remain grateful for the residents and students who continue to teach and inspire all of us. Thanks go also to my husband, for his unswerving support; Laura Gillan, the editor who first conceived this project and guided it through to completion; the SAGES Editorial Advisory Board, Desmond Birkett, M.D., Jeffrey Ponsky, M.D., and Gregory Van Stiegmann, M.D.; and Mary Shirazi, the talented and responsive medical illustrator who did the majority of the artwork. Finally, I wish to give thanks to SAGES, an organization that epitomizes surgeons working together to share and increase surgical knowledge.

Carol E.H. Scott-Conner, M.D., Ph.D.
Iowa City, Iowa
April 10, 1998

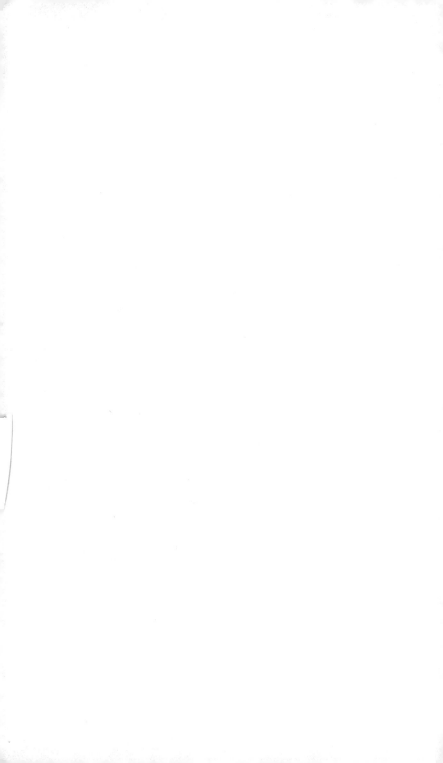

Contents

Foreword v

Desmond H. Birkett

Preface.. vii

Carol E.H. Scott-Conner

Contributors... xv

Part 1: Laparoscopy

I. General Principles

1. Equipment Setup and Troubleshooting 1

Mohan C. Airan

2. Patient Preparation 12

Mohan C. Airan

3. Anesthesia and Monitoring.. 15

Mazen A. Maktabi, Mohan C. Airan, and Carol E.H. Scott-Conner

4. Access to Abdomen... 22

Nathaniel J. Soper

5.1. Pneumoperitoneum.. 37

Claudia L. Corwin

5.2. Abdominal Wall Lift Devices.. 43

Edmund K.M. Tsoi, Albert K. Chin, and Claude H. Organ, Jr.

5.3. Generation of Working Space: Extraperitoneal Approaches 52

David M. Brams

6. Principles of Laparoscopic Hemostasis 57

Richard M. Newman and L. William Traverso

7. Principles of Tissue Approximation 69

Zoltan Szabo

8. Principles of Specimen Removal.. 82

Daniel J. Deziel

9. Documentation 88

Daniel J. Deziel

10.1. Special Problems: Massive Obesity 94
Cornelius Doherty

10.2. Laparoscopy During Pregnancy 98
Myriam J. Curet

10.3. Previous Abdominal Surgery 104
Norman B. Halpern

II. Diagnostic Laparoscopy and Biopsy

11. Emergency Laparoscopy 109
Jonathan M. Sackier

12. Elective Diagnostic Laparoscopy and Cancer Staging 115
Frederick L. Greene

III. Laparoscopic Cholecystectomy and Common Duct Exploration

13.1. Laparoscopic Cholecystectomy 128
Karen Deveney

13.2. Laparoscopic Cholecystectomy: Avoiding Complications 137
Joseph Cullen

13.3. Laparoscopic Cholecystectomy: Cholangiography 143
George Berci

13.4. Laparoscopic Cholecystectomy: Ultrasound and Doppler 162
Maurice E. Arregui

14.1. Laparoscopic Common Bile Duct Exploration: Transcystic
     Duct Approach 167
Joseph B. Petelin

14.2. Common Bile Duct Exploration via
     Laparoscopic Choledochotomy 178
Alfred Cuschieri and Chris Kimber

15. Complications of Laparoscopic Cholecystectomy and Laparoscopic
     Common Duct Exploration 188
Mark A. Talamini, Joseph Petelin, and Alfred Cuschieri

IV. Hiatal Hernia and Heller Myotomy

16. Laparoscopic Treatment of Gastroesophageal Reflux and
     Hiatal Hernia 196
Jeffrey H. Peters

17. Laparoscopic Cardiomyotomy (Heller Myotomy) 213
Margret Oddsdottir

V. Laparoscopic Gastric Surgery

18. Laparoscopic Gastrostomy 221
Thomas R. Gadacz

19. Laparoscopic Vagotomy... 227
Thomas R. Gadacz

20. Laparoscopic Plication of Perforated Ulcer.. 233
Thomas R. Gadacz

21. Gastric Resections 236
Alfred Cuschieri

22. Laparoscopic Bariatric Surgery 247
James W. Maher and Cornelius Doherty

VI. Laparoscopic Procedures on the Small Intestine, Appendix, and Colon

23. Small Bowel Resection, Enterolysis,
      and Enteroenterostomy 254
Bruce David Schirmer

24. Placement of Jejunostomy Tube... 267
Bruce David Schirmer

25. Laparoscopic Appendectomy 275
Keith N. Apelgren

26. Laparoscopic Colostomy 281
Anne T. Mancino

27. Laparoscopic Segmental Colectomies, Anterior Resection, and
      Abdominopereneal Resection 286
Eric G. Weiss and Steven D. Wexner

28. Laparoscopic-Assisted Proctocolectomy
      with Ileal-Pouch-Anal Anastamosis... 300
Amanda Metcalf

VII. Laparoscopic Approaches to the Pancreas, Spleen, and Retroperitoneum

29. Distal Pancreatectomy 307
Barry Salky

30. Laparoscopic Cholecystojejunostomy
    and Laparoscopic Gastrojejunostomy 314
Carol E.H. Scott-Conner

31. Laparoscopic Splenectomy 326
Robert V. Rege

32. Lymph Node Biopsy, Dissection, and Staging Laparoscopy 336
Lee L. Swanstrom

33. Laparoscopic Adrenalectomy 353
Marjorie J. Arca and Michel Gagner

VIII. Hernia Repair

34. Laparoscopic Inguinal Hernia Repair: Transabdominal Preperitoneal
    (TAPP) and Totally Extraperitoneal (TEP) 364
Muhammed Ashraf Memon and Robert J. Fitzgibbons, Jr.

35. Laparoscopic Repair of Ventral Hernia 379
Gerald M. Larson

IX. Pediatric Laparoscopy

36. Pediatric Laparoscopy: General Considerations 386
Thom E. Lobe

37.1. Pediatric Laparoscopy: Specific Surgical Procedures I 389
Anthony Sandler

37.2. Pediatric Laparoscopy: Specific Surgical Procedures II 396
Thom E. Lobe

38. Pediatric Laparoscopy: Complications 399
Thom E. Lobe

Part 2: Flexible Endoscopy

I. Flexible Endoscopy: General Principles

39. Characteristics of Flexible Endoscopes, Troubleshooting and
    Equipment Care 407
Jeffrey L. Ponsky and Carol E.H. Scott-Conner

40. Endoscope Handling 415
Jeffrey L. Ponsky

41. Monitoring, Sedation, and Recovery 419
Jeffrey L. Ponsky

II. Upper Gastrointestinal Endoscopy

42. Diagnostic Upper Gastrointestinal Endoscopy 422
John D. Mellinger

43.1.1. Variceal Banding 438
Gregory Van Stiegmann

43.1.2. Sclerotherapy of Variceal Bleeding 442
Choichi Sugawa

43.2.1. Control of Nonvariceal Upper GI Bleeding 448
Choichi Sugawa

43.2.2-5. Upper Gastrointestinal Endoscopy—Therapeutic 457
Timothy M. Farrell and John G. Hunter

43.2.6. Percutaneous Endoscopic Feeding Tube Placement 462
Carol E.H. Scott-Conner and Jeffrey Ponsky

44. Complications of Upper Gastrointestinal Endoscopy 470
Brian J. Dunkin

III. Small Bowel Enteroscopy

45. Small Bowel Enteroscopy 480
Charles H. Andrus and Scott H. Miller

IV. Endoscopic Retrograde Cholangiopancreatography

46.1. Endoscopic Retrograde Cholangiopancreatography 485
Harry S. Himal

46.2. Surgically Altered Anatomy and Special Considerations 496
Maurice E. Arregui

47. Cannulation and Cholangiopancreatography 502
David Duppler

48. Therapeutic ERCP 508
Gary C. Vitale

49. Complications of ERCP 516
Morris Washington and Ali Ghazi

V. Choledochostomy

50. Diagnostic Choledochoscopy 523
Bruce V. MacFadyen, Jr.

51. Therapeutic Choledochoscopy and Its Complications............................ 529
Raymond P. Onders and Thomas S. Stellato

VI. Flexible Sigmoidoscopy

52. Flexible Sigmoidoscopy 534
John A. Coller

53. Therapeutic Flexible Sigmoidoscopy 543
Irwin B. Simon

VII. Colonoscopy

54. Diagnostic Colonoscopy.. 551
Bassem Y. Safadi and Jeffrey M. Marks

55. Therapeutic Colonoscopy, Complications of Colonoscopy.................... 565
C. Daniel Smith, Aaron S. Fink, Gregory Van Stiegmann, and
David W. Easter

VIII. Pediatric Endoscopy

56. Pediatric Gastrointestinal Endoscopy 577
Thom E. Lobe

Appendix: SAGES Publications.. 586

Index 589

Contributors

Mohan C. Airan, M.D., Department of Surgery, The Chicago Medical School, 2340 Highland Avenue, Suite 250, Lombard IL 60148, USA

Charles H. Andrus, M.D., Department of Surgery, Loyola University, Stritch School of Medicine, 2160 South First Avenue, Maywood IL 60153, USA

Keith N. Apelgren, M.D., Department of Surgery, Michigan State University, B424 Clinical Center, East Lansing MI 48824, USA

Marjorie J. Arca, M.D., Department of Pediatric Surgery, University of Michigan Hospitals, 1500 East Medical Center Drive, Ann Arbor MI 48109, USA

Maurice E. Arregui, M.D., St. Vincent's Hospital and Health Center, 8402 Harcourt Road, Suite 811, Indianapolis IN 46260, USA

George Berci, M.D., Department of Surgery, Suite 8215, Cedars Sinai Medical Centers, 8700 Beverly Boulevard, Los Angeles CA 90048, USA

David M. Brams, M.D., Department of General Surgery, Lahey Hitchcock Medical Center, 41 Mall Road, Burlington MA 01805, USA

Albert K. Chin, M.D., Origin Medsystems Inc., Menlo Park CA 94025, USA

John A. Coller, M.D., Department of Colon & Rectal Surgery, Lahey Hitchcock Medical Center, 41 Mall Road, Burlington MA 01805, USA

Claudia L. Corwin, M.D., Department of Surgery, University of Iowa Hospitals and Clinics, 200 Hawkins Drive, 1521 JCP, Iowa City IA 52242-1086, USA

Joseph Cullen, M.D., Department of Surgery, University of Iowa, 4622 JCP, Iowa City IA 52242-1086, USA

Myriam J. Curet, M.D., Center for Minimally Invasive Surgery, University of New Mexico Health Sciences Center, 2211 Lomas Boulevard NE, Albuquerque NM 87106, USA

Sir Alfred Cuschieri, M.D., Department of Surgery, Ninewells Hospital & Medical School, Dundee, Scotland, DD1 9SY, UK

Karen E. Deveney, M.D., Department of Surgery, Oregon Health Sciences University, 3181 SW Sam Jackson Park Road, Portland OR 97201-3098, USA

Daniel J. Deziel, M.D., Department of General Surgery, Rush Medical College, 1653 West Congress Parkway, Chicago IL 60612, USA

Cornelius Doherty, M.D., Department of Surgery, University of Iowa, 200 Hawkins Drive, 4628 JCP, Iowa City IA 52242-1086, USA

Brian J. Dunkin, M.D., Department of Surgery, University of Maryland School of Medicine, 22 South Greene Street, Room N4E35, Baltimore, M.D. 21201, USA

David W. Duppler, M.D., Fox Valley Surgical Associates, 1818 N Meade Street, Appleton WI 54911, USA

David W. Easter, M.D., Department of Surgery 8891, University of California San Diego, 225 Dickenson, San Diego CA 92103, USA

Timothy M. Farrell, M.D., Department of Surgery, H124C, Emory University Hospital, 1364 Clifton Road, NE, Atlanta GA 30322, USA

Aaron S. Fink, M.D., Atlanta Veterans Administration Medical Center (112), 1670 Clairmont Road, Decatur GA 30033, USA

Robert J. Fitzgibbons, Jr., M.D., Creighton/St. Joseph, Department of Surgery, 601 North 30th Street, Suite 3704, Omaha NE 68131, USA

Thomas R. Gadacz, M.D., Department of Surgery, Medical College of Georgia, 1120 15th Street, Augusta GA 30912, USA

Michel Gagner, M.D., Department of Laparoscopic Surgery, Mount Sinai Medical Center, 5 East 98th Street, Box 1103, New York NY 10029-6574, USA

Ali Ghazi, M.D., Beth Israel Medical Center, 1st Avenue and 16th Street, New York NY 10003, USA

Frederick L. Greene, M.D., Department of Surgery, Carolinas Medical Center, PO Box 32861, Charlotte NC 28232-2861, USA

Norman B. Halpern, M.D., Department of Surgery, University of Alabama, University Station, Birmingham AL 35294, USA

Harry S. Himal, M.D., Toronto Hospital, Western Division, University of Toronto, West Wing, 3rd Floor, Rm 3-801, 399 Bathurst Street, Toronto, Ontario M5T 2S8, Canada

John G. Hunter, M.D., Department of Surgery, H124C, Emory University Hospital, 1364 Clifton Road NE, Atlanta GA 30322, USA

Chris Kimber, M.D., Department of Surgery, Ninewells Hospital & Medical School, Dundee, Scotland DD1 9SY, UK

Gerald M. Larson, M.D., Department of Surgery, University of Louisville, 550 South Jackson Street, Louisville KY 40292, USA

Thom E. Lobe, M.D., 777 Washington Avenue, Suite P210, Memphis TN 38105, USA

Bruce V. MacFadyen, Jr., M.D., Department of Surgery, University of Texas Medical School, 6431 Fannin Street, Rm 4292, Houston TX 77030, USA

James W. Maher, M.D., Department of Surgery, University of Iowa, 200 Hawkins Drive, 4601 JCP, Iowa City IA 52242-1086, USA

Mazen A. Maktabi, M.D., University of Iowa School of Medicine, 6540 JCP, 200 Hawkins Drive, Iowa City IA 52242, USA

Anne T. Mancino, M.D., University of Arkansas for Medical Sciences, 4301 W Markham, Slot 725, Little Rock AR 72205, USA

Jeffrey M. Marks, M.D., Department of Surgery, Mt. Sinai Medical Center, Case Western Reserve University School of Medicine, One Mount Sinai Drive, Cleveland OH 44106, USA

John D. Mellinger, M.D., West Michigan Surgical Specialists, PC, 245 Cherry Street SE, Grand Rapids MI 49503-4597, USA

Muhammed Ashraf Memon, M.D., Department of Transplant Surgery, St. Louis University Hospital, 3635 Vista Avenue at Grand Boulevard, St. Louis MO 63110, USA

Amanda M. Metcalf, M.D., Department of Surgery, University of Iowa, 200 Hawkins Drive, 4605 JCP, Iowa City IA 52242-1086, USA

Scott H. Miller, M.D., Department of Surgery, Loyola University, Chicago, Stritch School of Medicine, 2160 South First Avenue, Maywood IL 60153, USA

Richard M. Newman, M.D., Department of Surgery, New York University School of Medicine, Bellevue Hospital Center, 27th Street and 1st Avenue, New York NY 10016, USA

Margret Oddsdottir, M.D., Department of Surgery, Landspitalinn University Hospital, Hringbraut, IS-101 Reykjavik, Iceland

Raymond P. Onders, M.D., University Hospitals of Cleveland, 11100 Euclid Avenue, Cleveland OH 44106-1350, USA

Claude H. Organ, Jr., M.D., Department of Surgery, University of California Davis-East Bay, 1411 East 31st Street, Oakland CA 94602, USA

Joseph B. Petelin, M.D., 9119 West 74th Street, Suite 355, Shawnee Mission KS 66204, USA

Jeffrey H. Peters, M.D., Department of Surgery, University of Southern California Healthcare Consulation, 1510 San Pablo Street, Los Angeles CA 90033, USA

Jeffrey L. Ponsky, M.D., Department of Surgery, Cleveland Clinic Foundation, 9500 Euclid Avenue, Desk A80, Cleveland OH 44195, USA

Robert V. Rege, M.D., 250 East Superior Street, Suite 201, Chicago IL 60611, USA

Jonathan M. Sackier, M.D., Department of Surgery, George Washington University, 2150 Pennsylvania Avenue NW 415, Washington DC 20037, USA

Bassem Y. Safadi, M.D., Department of Surgery, Mt. Sinai Medical Center, One Mount Sinai Drive, Cleveland OH 44106, USA

Barry A. Salky, M.D., Division of Laparoscopic Surgery, Mt. Sinai Hospital, 1 Gustav Levy Place, New York NY 10029, USA

Anthony Sandler, M.D., Department of Surgery, University of Iowa Hospitals and Clinics, 200 Hawkins Drive, 1565 JCP, Iowa City IA 52242-1086, USA

Bruce David Schirmer, M.D., Department of Surgery, University of Virginia Health Science Center, Box 10005, Charlottesville VA 22906-0005, USA

Carol E.H. Scott-Conner, M.D. Ph.D., Department of Surgery, University of Iowa, 200 Hawkins Drive, 1516 JCP, Iowa City IA 52242-1086, USA

Irwin B. Simon, M.D., Department of Surgery, University of Nevada School of Medicine, 3196 Maryland Parkway, Suite 303, Las Vegas NV 89109, USA

C. Daniel Smith, M.D., Department of General Surgery, Emory University School of Medicine, 25 Prescott Street, Suite 5430, Atlanta GA 30308, USA

Nathaniel J. Soper, M.D., Washington University School of Medicine, One Barnes Hospital Plaza, Box 8109, St. Louis MO 63110, USA

Thomas A. Stellato, M.D., Case Western Reserve University, University Hospitals of Cleveland, University Surgeons, Inc., 1100 Euclid Avenue, Cleveland OH 44106-1350, USA

Gregory Van Stiegmann, M.D., Department of Surgery, University of Colorado Health Sciences Center, 4200 E 9th Avenue, C-313, Denver CO 80262, USA

Choichi Sugawa, M.D., Department of Surgery, Wayne State University School of Medicine, 6-C, University Health Center, 4201 St. Antoine, Detroit MI 48201, USA

Lee L. Swanstrom, M.D., Department of Surgery, Legacy Portland Hospitals, 501 North Graham Street #120, Portland OR 97227-1604, USA

Zoltan Szabo, Ph.D., MOET Institute, Microsurgery & Operative Endoscopy Training, 153 States Street, San Francisco CA 94114, USA

Mark A. Talamini, M.D., Johns Hopkins Hospital, 600 North Wolfe Street, Blalock 665, Baltimore, M.D. 21287, USA

L. William Traverso, M.D., Department of General, Thoracic & Vascular Surgery, Virginia Mason Medical Center, 1100 Ninth Avenue, C6-GSUR, Seattle WA 98111, USA

Edmund K.M. Tsoi, M.D., Department of Surgery, University of California, Davis-East Bay, 1411 East 31st Street, Oakland CA 94602, USA

Gary C. Vitale, M.D., Department of Surgery, University of Louisville, Ambulatory Care Building, 550 South Jackson Street, Louisville KY 40292, USA

Morris Washington, M.D., Beth Israel Hospital, 1st Avenue and 16th Street, New York NY 10003, USA

Eric G. Weiss, M.D., Department of Colorectal Surgery, Cleveland Clinic Florida, 3000 West Cypress Creek Road, Fort Lauderdale FL 33309, USA

Steven D. Wexner, M.D., Department of Surgery, Cleveland Clinic Florida, Desk W30, 3000 West Cypress Creek Road, Fort Lauderdale FL 33309, USA

1. Equipment Setup and Troubleshooting

Mohan C. Airan, M.D., F.A.C.S.

A. Room Layout and Equipment Position

1. **General considerations** include the size of the operating room, location of doors, outlets for electrical and anesthetic equipment, and the procedure to be performed. Time spent in positioning the equipment and operating table is well spent. Come to the operating room sufficiently early to assure proper setup, and to ascertain that all instruments are available and in good working order. This is particularly important when a procedure is being done in an operating room not normally used for laparoscopic operations, or when the operating room personnel are unfamiliar with the equipment (for example, an operation performed after hours).

2. **Determine the optimum position and orientation for the operating table.** If the room is large, the normal position for the operating table will work well for laparoscopy.

3. **Small operating rooms** will require diagonal placement of the operating table and proper positioning of the laparoscopic accessory instrumentation around the operating table.

4. **An equipment checklist** helps to ensure that all items are available and minimizes delays once the patient has arrived in the operating room. Here is an example of such a checklist. Most of the equipment and instruments listed here will be needed for operative laparoscopy. Additional equipment may be needed for advanced procedures. This will be discussed in subsequent sections.

   a. Anesthesia equipment
   b. Electric operating table with remote control if available
   c. Two video monitors
   d. Suction irrigator
   e. Electrosurgical unit, with grounding pad equipped with current monitoring system
   f. Ultrasonically activated scissors, scalpel, or other specialized unit if needed
   g. Laparoscopic equipment, generally housed in a cart on wheels:
      i. Light source
      ii. Insufflator
      iii. Video cassette recorder (VCR), other recording system, tapes

       iv.   Color printer (optional)
       v.   Monitor on articulating arm
       vi.   Camera – processor unit

h. C-arm x-ray unit (if cholangiography is planned) with remote monitor

i. Mayo stand or table with the following laparoscopic instrumentation:

       i.   #11, #15 scalpel blades and handles
       ii.   Towel clips
       iii.   Veress needle or Hasson cannula
       iv.   Gas insufflation tubes with micropore filter, if desired
       v.   Fiberoptic cable to connect laparoscope with light source
       vi.   Video camera with cord
       vii.   Cords to connect laparoscopic instruments to the electrosurgical unit, with various adapters for all instruments needed
       viii.   6″ curved hemostatic forceps
       ix.   Small retractors (Army-Navy or similar pattern) for umbilical incision
       x.   Trocar cannulae (size and numbers depend on the planned operation, with extras available in case of accidental contamination)
       xi.   Laparoscopic instruments

            Atraumatic graspers
            Locking toothed jawed graspers
            Needle holders
            Dissectors – curved, straight, right-angle
            Bowel grasping forceps
            Babcock clamp
            Scissors – Metzenbaum, hook, microtip
            Fan retractors – 10 mm, 5 mm
            Specialized retractors, such as endoscopic curved retractors
            Biopsy forceps
            Tru-cut biopsy – core needle

       xii.   Monopolar electrocautery dissection tools
            L-shaped hook
            Spade-type dissector/coagulator

       xiii.   Ultrasonically activated scalpel (optional)
            Scalpel
            Ball coagulator
            Hook dissector
            Scissors dissector/coagulator/transector

       xiv.   Endocoagulator probe (optional)
       xv.   Basket containing:
            Clip appliers
            Endoscopic stapling devices
            Pretied suture ligatures
            Endoscopic suture materials

Extra trocars
j.   Robot holder if available

B. Room and Equipment Setup

1. **With the** operating **table positioned**, and all equipment in the room, reassess the configuration. Once the patient is anesthetized and draped, it is difficult to reposition equipment. Consider the room size (as previously discussed), location of doors (particularly if a C-arm is to be used), and the quadrant of the abdomen in which the procedure will be performed. Figure 1.1 shows a typical setup for a laparoscopic cholecystectomy or other procedure in the upper abdomen.
2. **Set up the equipment** before bringing the patient into the operating room. A systematic approach, starting at the head of the table, is useful.
    a.   There should be sufficient space to allow the anesthesiologist to position the anesthesia equipment and work safely.
    b.   Next, consider the position of the monitors and the paths that connecting cables will take. Try to avoid "fencing in" the surgeon and assistants. This is particularly important if surgeon and assistant need to change places or move (for example, during cholangiography).
    c.   The precise setup must be appropriate to the planned procedure. The setup shown is for laparoscopic cholecystectomy or other upper abdominal procedures. Room and equipment setups for other laparoscopic operatings are discussed with each individual procedure in the sections that follow (Sections II to IX). A useful principle to remember is that the laparoscope must point toward the quadrant of the abdomen with the pathology, and the surgeon generally stands opposite the pathology and looks directly at the main monitor.
    d.   If a C-arm or other equipment will need to be brought in during the procedure, plan the path from the door to the operating table in such a manner that the equipment can be positioned with minimal disruption. This will generally require that the cabinet containing the light source, VCR, insufflator, and other electronics be placed at the side of the patient farthest from the door. Consider bringing the C-arm into the room before the procedure begins.
    e.   Additional tables should be available so that water, irrigating solutions, and other items are not placed on any electrical units where spillage could cause short circuits, electrical burns, or fires.

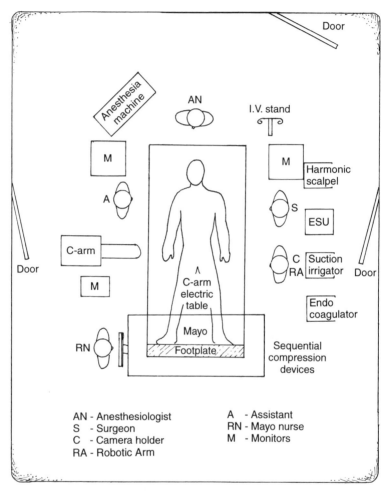

Figure 1.1. **Basic room setup**. This is the typical setup for laparoscopic chole-cystectomy. The room must be sufficiently large to accommodate all of the equipment (see Fig. 1.2 for setup for smaller room). A similar setup can be used for hiatus hernia repair or other upper abdominal surgery. In these cases, one 21″ or larger monitor can be used in the center where the anesthesiologist usually sits, with the anesthesiologist positioned to the side. The position of the surgeon (S), camera holder (C), and the assistant (A) depends on the procedure that is planned. The best position for the monitor is opposite the surgeon in his line of sight. A C-arm, if used, should be placed perpendicular to the operating table. A clear pathway to the door facilitates placement of the C-arm, and should be planned when the room is set up.

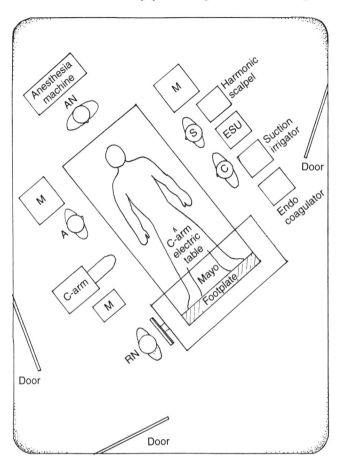

Figure 1.2. **Laparoscopic cholecystectomy, small operating room.** The monitors, anesthesia machine, and relative position of surgeon and first assistant have been adapted to the diagonal operating table placement.

3. **Check the equipment** and ascertain the following:
   a. There should be two full carbon dioxide cylinders in the room. One will be used for the procedure, and the second is a spare in case the pressure in the first cylinder becomes low. The cylinder should be hooked up to the insufflator and the valve turned on. The pressure gauge should indicate that there is adequate gas in the cylinder. If the cylinder does not appear to fit properly, **do not force it**. Each type of gas cylinder has a unique kind of fitting, and failure to fit properly may indicate that the cylinder contains a different kind of gas (for example, oxygen).

b. If the carbon dioxide cylinder needs to be changed during a procedure:
   i. Close the valve body with the proper handle to shut off the gas (old cylinder)
   ii. Unscrew the head fitting
   iii. Replace the gasket in the head fitting with a new gasket, which is always provided with a new tank of gas
   iv. Re-attach the head fitting so that the two prongs of the fitting are seated in the two holes in the carbon dioxide gas tank valve body
   v. Firmly align and tighten the head fitting with the integral pointed screw fisture
   vi. Open the carbon dioxide gas tank valve body, and pressure should be restored to the insufflator.
c. Look inside the back of the cabinet housing the laparoscopic equipment. Check to be certain that the connections on the back of the units are tightly plugged in (Fig. 1.3).

4. **Attention to detail** is important. The following additional items need careful consideration, and can be checked as the patient is brought into the room and prepared for surgery:
   a. Assure table tilt mechanism is functional, and that the table and joints are level and the kidney rest down.
   b. Consider using a footboard and extra safety strap for large patients.
   c. Position patient and cassette properly on operating table for cholangiography.
   d. Notify the radiology technologist with time estimate.
   e. Assure proper mixing and dilution of cholangiogram contrast solution for adequate image.
   f. Assure availability of Foley catheter and nasogastric tube, if desired.
   g. Assure all power sources are connected and appropriate units are switched on. Avoid using multiple sockets or extension cords plugged into a single source, as circuits may overload.
   h. Check the insufflator (see Chapter 4, Access to Abdomen). Assure insufflator alarm is set appropriately.
   i. Assure full volume in the irrigation fluid container (recheck during case).
   j. Assure adequate printer film and video tape if documentation is desired.
   k. Check the electrosurgical unit; make sure the auditory alarm of the machine is functioning properly and the grounding pad is appropriate for the patient, properly placed, and functioning.

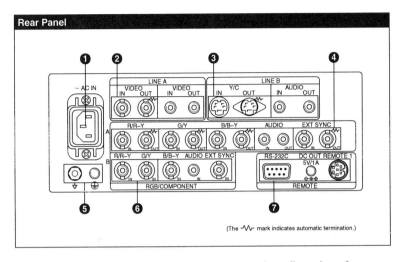

Figure 1.3. **Connections on rear panel.** The actual configuration of connections on the rear panels varies, but there are some general principles that will help when tracing the connections. The video signal is generated by the camera box. A cable plugs into the "video out" port of the camera box and takes the video signal to the VCR or monitor by plugging into a "video in" port. A common arrangement takes the signal first to the VCR, and then from the "video out" port of the VCR to the "video in" port of the monitor. (see Chapter 9, Documentation). Some cameras have split connectors that must be connected to the proper ports. Once connected, these should not be disturbed. The surgeon should be familiar with the instrumentation as connections frequently are loose or disconnected. The last monitor plugged in should have an automatic termination of signal port to avoid deterioration of the picture quality.

5. **Once you are gowned and gloved**, connect the light cable and camera to the laparoscope. Focus the laparoscope and white balance it. Place the laparoscope in warmed saline or electrical warmer. Verify the following:

   a. Check Veress needle for proper plunger/spring action and assure easy flushing through stopcock and/or needle channel.

   b. Assure closed stopcocks on all ports.

   c. Check sealing caps for cracked rubber and stretched openings.

   d. Check to assure instrument cleaning channel screw caps are in place.

   e. Assure free movements of instrument handles and jaws.

f.   If Hasson cannula to be used, assure availability of stay sutures and retractors.

C. Troubleshooting

Laparoscopic procedures are inherently complex. Many things can go wrong. The surgeon must be sufficiently familiar with the equipment to troubleshoot and solve problems. Table 1.1 gives an outline of the common problems, their cause, and suggested solutions.

Table 1.1

Problem	Cause	Solution
1. Poor insufflation/ loss of pneumo- peritoneum	CO_2 tank empty	Change tank
	Open accessory port stopcock(s)	Inspect all accessory ports—close stop- cock(s)
	Leak in sealing cap or stopcock	Change cap or cannula
	Excessive suctioning	Allow abdomen to re- insufflate
	Instrument cleaning channel screw cap missing	Replace screw cap
	Loose connection of insufflator tubing at Source or at port	Tighten connection
	Hasson stay sutures loose	Replace or secure su- tures
2. Excessive pressure required for insuf- flation (initial or subsequent)	Veress needle or can- nula tip not in free peritoneal cavity	Reinsert needle or can- nula
	Occlusion of tubing (kinking, table wheel, inadequate size tubing, etc.)	Inspect full length of tubing, replace with proper size as neces- sary
	Port stopcock turned off	Assure stopcock is opened
	Patient is "light"	More muscle relaxant
3. Inadequate lighting (partial/complete loss)	Loose connection at source or at scope	Adjust connector

Table 1.1. continued

Problem	Cause	Solution
	Light is on "manual-minimum"	Go to "automatic"
	Bulb is burned out	Replace bulb
	Fiberoptics are damaged	Replace light cable
	Automatic iris adjusting to bright reflection from instrument	Reposition instruments, or switch to "manual"
	Monitor brightness turned down	Readjust setting
4. Lighting too bright	Light is on "manual-maximum"	Go to "automatic"
	"Boost" on light source activated.	Deactivate "boost"
	Monitor brightness turned up	Readjust setting
5. No picture on monitor(s)	Camera control unit or other components (VCR, printer, light source, monitor) not on	Make sure all power sources are plugged in and turned on
	Cable connector between camera control unit and/or monitors not attached properly	Cable should run from "video out" on camera control unit to "video in" on primary monitor; use compatible cables for camera unit and light source Cable should run from "video out" on primary monitor to "video in" on secondary monitor

Table 1.1. continued

Problem	Cause	Solution
6. Poor-quality picture: a. Fogging, haze	Condensation on lens of cold scope entering warm abdomen.	Gently wipe lens on viscera; use anti-fog solution, or warm water; it is preferred not to wipe the lens on the viscera or the end of the telescope may get hot; gently wiping on liver or uterine surface is preferable
	Condensation on scope eyepiece, camera lens, coupler lens	Detach camera from scope (or camera from coupler), inspect and clean lens as needed
b. Flickering electrical interference	Moisture in camera cable connecting plug	Use compressed air to dry out moisture (don't use cotton-tip applicators on multiprong plug)
	Poor cable shielding	Replace video cable between monitors
	Insecure connection of video cable between monitors	Reattach video cable at each monitor
c. Blurring, distortion	Incorrect focus	Adjust camera focus ring
	Cracked lens, internal moisture	Inspect scope and camera, replace as needed
7. Inadequate suction/irrigation	Occlusion of tubing (kinking, blood clot, etc.)	Inspect full length of tubing; if necessary, detach from instrument and flush tubing with sterile saline
	Occlusion of valves in suction/irrigator device	Detach tubing, flush device with sterile saline

Table 1.1. continued

Problem	Cause	Solution
	Not attached to wall suction	Inspect and secure suction canister connectors, wall source connector
	Irrigation fluid container not pressurized	Inspect compressed gas source, connector, pressure dial setting
8. Absent/inadequate cauterization	Patient not grounded properly	Assure adequate patient grounding pad contact, and pad cable-electro-surgical unit connection
	Connection between electrosurgical unit and pencil not secure	Inspect both connecting points
	Foot pedal or hand-switch not connected to electrosurgical unit	Make connection

D. Selected References

SAGES Continuing Education Committee. Laparoscopy Troubleshooting Guide. SAGES, 1993.

Sony Corporation. Rear panel diagram for Trinitron Color Video Monitor, 1995.

2. Patient Preparation

Mohan C. Airan, M.D., F.A.C.S.

A. Preparation for Surgery

Patient preparation, like much of surgery, must be individualized based upon the procedure planned and the physiologic status of the patient. Special considerations for particular procedures are given in Sections II to IX.

1. **All patients** undergoing **elective laparoscopy** should be NPO (nothing per mouth) after midnight.

2. A minimal **bowel preparation** is desirable to ensure that the gas in the gastrointestinal tract has been evacuated. A preoperative enema is advised for laparoscopic cholecystectomy.

3. If the patient has undergone preoperative gastrointestinal endoscopy, such as endoscopic retrograde cholangiopancreatography (ERCP), significant distention of small and large intestine may hamper laparoscopy. A more vigorous bowel preparation may be required to thoroughly evacuate this gas. An abdominal radiograph is a useful adjunct to physical examination and serves to confirm adequacy of bowel preparation. Nasogastric suction may be needed if ileus is a factor.

4. In patients with **inadequate motility**, 10 mg of Reglam followed by a rectal suppository may help ensure evacuation of gas. Occasionally it is necessary to leave a rectal tube in place, and allow the pressure of the pneumoperitoneum to assist in pushing gas out of the colon. If distention persists, consider using an open (Hasson) technique for access (see Chapter 4, section C, "Open" Technique with Hasson Cannula).

5. **Inform the patient** about the planned procedure, potential complications, and alternatives.

6. **Obtain informed consent** not only for the proposed procedure but also for laparotomy and any open surgical procedure that may be required. Document the patient's understanding of and consent to the planned procedure and the possible open operation, as well as clear understanding of potential complications and alternative methods of treatment.

7. Laboratory studies, electrocardiogram, and other **preoperative workup** should be performed on an individualized basis.

8. For many laparoscopic surgical procedures, a **type and screen** specimen should be sent to the blood bank so that blood is readily available in the rare event it should be needed.

9. Elective laparoscopic procedures are most commonly performed as short stay or ambulatory surgical procedures. **Patient education** is

critically important and should begin in the office or clinic when the patient is scheduled for surgery.

B. Patient Preparation in the Operating Room

When the patient has gone into the operating room and is placed on the operating table, take care to pad all the nerve compression points. Make certain that the sheets are not bunched up underneath the back or in the gluteal area, which may compress the skin and produce pressure ulcerations. Untie any knots in the gown, and remove anything that could produce a lump or bump under the patient. Additional items to attend to include:

1. **Sequential compression devices** are applied to the lower limbs.
2. Place a **foot board**, if reverse Trendelenburg position is planned (for example, for laparoscopic cholecystectomy), with adequate padding to prevent pressure on the feet.
3. Place an **egg-crate mattress** or other padding device underneath the heels to prevent compression changes in the heel area.
4. Place the **grounding plate** (patient return electrode) away from any plates and screws in the lower limbs.
5. Properly **pad all bony points**.
6. Place a **Foley catheter** to evacuate the bladder, if desired.
7. Place a **retaining strap** around the abdomen.
8. Consider **arm position**. Depending upon the procedure, the size of the patient, and the needs of the anesthesia team, one or both arms may need to be extended on arm boards. For laparoscopic cholecystectomy, the left arm may be extended and instruments placed on top of the sheets over the left arm. In general, access is better if the arms are tucked. This is crucial for procedures in the mid- or lower abdomen.
9. For some procedures, such as laparoscopic hiatal hernia repair, some surgeons prefer the so-called European position (where the patient is placed in a **semi-lithotomy position** (frog position) and the surgeon stands between the legs. In this case, the legs must be carefully positioned and padded to avoid pressure complications.
10. Similarly, for procedures requiring a combined **lithotomy-Trendelenburg position** with elevation of the legs into stirrups, such as laparoscopic proctectomy, it is extremely important to pad and protect the lower extremities. Check and recheck the adequacy of this padding. Sometimes shoulder restraints may be needed.
11. Place a nasogastric or orogastric tube to deflate the stomach before Veress needle puncture.

C. Selected References

Ko ST, Airan M. Review of 300 consecutive laparoscopic cholecystectomies: development, evolution and results. Surg Endosc (1991)5:104.

Olsen DO. Cholecystectomy for Acute Cholecystitis. In: MacFadyen B, Pnasky J (eds) Operative Laparoscopy and Thoracoscopy. Philadelphia: Lippincott-Raven; 1996:233.

Cuschieri AE. Hiatal hernia and reflux esophagitis. In Hunter JG, Sackier JM eds. Minimally Invasive Surgery. New York: McGraw-Hill; 1993: 99.

Berci G. Technique of Laparoscopic Cholecystectomy. In: Cuschieri A, Berci G, eds. Laparoscopic Biliary Surgery. Boston: Blackwell Scientific; 1992: 69-71.

Airan MC. Basic Techniques. In: MacFadyen B, Ponsky J (eds) Operative Laparoscopy and Thoracoscopy. Philadelphia: Lippincott-Raven; (1996): 93-123.

3. Anesthesia and Monitoring

Mazen A. Maktabi, M.D.
Mohan C. Airan, M.D., F.A.C.S.
Carol E.H. Scott-Conner, M.D., Ph.D., F.A.C.S.

A. Preoperative Considerations

Before surgery, patients should be evaluated by a qualified anesthesia provider (Table 3.1).

Table 3.1. Preoperative evaluation for laparoscopic surgery

Systems affected by pneumoperitoneum
• Airway
• Respiratory system
• Cardiovascular system
Other relevant systems
• Central nervous system
• Endocrine system
• Gastrointestinal system
Other relevant history
• Past anesthetic experience
• Past anesthetic family history
• Allergies (particularly to local anesthetics)
• Medications

Patients with compromised cardiac and respiratory systems present a particular challenge. The mechanical effect of pneumoperitoneum, neuroendocrine changes, and absorbed CO_2 all influence the physiologic response (see Section 5.1.2, Physiologic Changes). The advantages and disadvantages of laparoscopic versus an open procedure should be assessed with specific reference to the condition of the heart and lungs.

Most laparoscopic surgery is done on a **short-stay** or outpatient basis. These specific goals should be kept in mind:

1. **Prevent postoperative nausea and vomiting (PONV).** Prophylactic antiemetics such as droperidol, metoclopramide, or ondansetron are effective. Timing of administration is crucial for success. For example, ondansetron (4 mg i.v.) is most effective when administered immediately before the end of laparoscopic surgery.
2. **Rapid emergence from anesthesia.**
3. **Minimal postoperative pain.**

B. Choice of Anesthetic and Specific Considerations

Laparoscopic surgery may be done with general, regional, or even local anesthesia. The choice of anesthesic and specific anesthesia considerations for each modality are briefly discussed here.

1. **General anesthesia with endotracheal (ET) tube** allows excellent airway protection and compensation for hypercarbia. Specific considerations when laparoscopy is performed under general anesthesia include:

   a. **Airway protection with an ET tube** is important because high intra-abdominal pressure may cause reflux of gastric contents and lead to aspiration. A face mask or laryngeal mask airway may be adequate for short diagnostic procedures (low insufflation pressures) by surgeons with considerable experience. A history of hiatus hernia or gastroesophageal reflux is an absolute contraindication to performing a general anesthetic without protecting the airway with a cuffed endotracheal tube.

   b. **Increase ventilation** to maintain normocapnia in the presence of increased CO_2 absorption from peritoneal surfaces.

   c. **Muscle relaxation** is obtained by the use of nondepolarizing agents in addition to adequate depth of anesthesia. The choice of muscle relaxants depends on the length of surgery and the medical condition of the patient. Inadequate muscle relaxation is one of the major causes of inability to attain adequate pneumoperitoneum within the pressure set-point of the insufflator.

   d. The use of **nitrous oxide** is controversial. Recent blinded studies suggest no difference in bowel distention with and without nitrous oxide. However, it is reasonable to discontinue nitrous oxide if the intra-abdominal viscera are noted to be distended. Nitrous oxide may reach concentrations that support combustion within the bowel lumen; this is a potential explosion hazard.

2. **Regional anesthesia** may be an appropriate technique for brief procedures that can be performed with lower insufflation pressures. **Numerous difficulties can occur with regional anesthesia** for laparoscopy. First, interventional laparoscopy requires a high level of sensory block (T4-T5). Regional anesthesia to this level also produces significant sympathetic blockade, causing hypotension. Breathing difficulties due to a high block may cause considerable discomfort and breathing difficulties in an awake patient whose diaphragm is already stretched and elevated because of the pneumoperitoneum. Laparoscopic procedures require several changes of patient position during the procedure. This may cause cardiovascular instability in a patient whose hemodynamic compensatory mechanisms have been limited by the sympathectomy of regional anesthesia. The **successful use of a regional anesthetic** (spinal or epidural anesthesia) depends on:

    a.   **Patient acceptance**.

    b.   The **absence of contraindications**, which include:
- i.   hypovolemia
- ii.   bleeding disorders
- iii.   infection that is close to the lumbar puncture site
- iv.   peripheral neurological disease
- v.   allergy to the local anesthetic agent

    c.   The **duration** of the procedure.

    d.   The **skill and expertise** of the surgeon and anesthesiologist.

3.   **Local anesthesia**—Simple diagnostic laparoscopy and some brief laparoscopic procedures may be performed under local anesthesia. Attention to some technical points are important for this to be successful. Local anesthesia is contraindicated in the uncooperative patient, when a prolonged procedure is planned, or when the patient is allergic to local anesthetics.

    a.   Raise a **skin wheal** at the initial puncture site.

    b.   **Infiltrate a cone** down to the peritoneal level, including generous infiltration of the peritoneum.

    c.   Ask the patient to tense up the abdominal wall, to provide resistance to the Veress needle. Alternatively, use an open technique with a Hasson cannula.

    d.   **Insufflate slowly** and **limit insufflation pressure** to less than 10 to 12 mm if possible.

    e.   **Reflex bradycardia** may occur, necessitating release of pneumoperitoneum or treatment with atropine.

    f.   Infiltrate the **second and any additional puncture sites** to the peritoneal level under direct vision. Raise a wheal above the peritoneum by injecting local anesthesia into the preperitoneal space.

C. Monitoring and Safety Considerations

Basic ASA (American Society of Anesthesiologists) monitors include:
1.   Breath sounds (precordial or esophageal stethoscope)
2.   Electrocardiogram (continuous)
3.   Blood pressure, pulse (continuous, noninvasive)
4.   Continuous oxygen saturation (pulse oximeter)
5.   Expired carbon dioxide (capnograph)
6.   Temperature

Additional monitoring depends on the general condition of the patient and the complexity of the procedure, and invasive monitoring may be used for sicker patients and complex procedures. An indwelling bladder catheter and a nasogastric tube are important to decrease the chances of injury to the urinary bladder and stomach.

Fire prevention is a crucial safety consideration. The operating room is an oxygen-rich environment. The ends of fiberoptic light cables become extremely hot and can ignite drapes. This is particularly prone to happen at the beginning or end of the surgical procedure, when everyone is occupied with getting the case started or the room turned around. Simple preventive measures include never leaving the light source turned on unless a laparoscope is connected to the light cable.

D. Intraoperative Considerations

1. **Physiologic changes** associated with pneumoperitoneum are summarized in Table 3.2 and discussed in greater detail in Section 5.1.2 (Physiologic Changes).
2. **Signs of deteriorating cardiopulmonary function** include:
   a. gradual or sudden drop in systemic blood pressure or increasing difficulty in maintaining a normal blood pressure
   b. decreased percent oxygen saturation
   c. pulse rate may increase, decrease, or remain the same
3. The differential diagnosis of some important clinical findings during laparoscopic surgery:
   a. **Hypercapnia** is usually due to venous absorption of CO_2. However, this condition may also be due to pneumothorax or right main stem intubation if the peak airway pressure is also increased.
   b. **Hypoxia** may result from right main stem bronchus intubations, pneumothorax, venous carbon dioxide embolism, or pulmonary edema.
   c. **Tachycardia and hypertension**: Light anesthesia, hypoxia, and hypercapnia must be ruled out first. These conditions may be treated with increments of esmolol (short acting β blocker) or labetalol (a mixed α and β blockers).
4. Serious intraoperative problems include:
   a. **CO_2 embolism**. This serious complication is diagnosed by a sudden decrease in end-expired CO_2 partial pressure and a rapid decrease in pulse oximetry values. Despite the fact that CO_2 is highly soluble in plasma, this may be a life-threatening complication if the volume of intravascular gas is large. Precordial Doppler monitoring and transesophageal echocardiography are very sensitive monitors of intravascular gas but are not routinely used during laparoscopy. Use might be considered when it is anticipated that during the course of the surgery a large raw area will be exposed to high gas pressures or when the surgical field is vascular in a hypovolemic patient.

Table 3.2. Physiologic changes associated with pneumoperitoneum and their implications for anesthesia management

Change	Physiologic consequence	Implication for management
• Elevation of diaphragm	• Decreased functional residual capacity • Increased ventilation-perfusion mismatch • Increased intrapulmonary shunting • Increased alveolar-arterial gradient of oxygen partial pressures	• Increase mechanical ventilation and FiO_2
• Decreased venous return with increased cardiac filling pressures	• Initial decrease in cardiac index • Cardiac index then increases • Cardiac axis of heart shifts, causing electrocardiographic alterations	• Adequate volume load
• Carbon dioxide load	• CO_2 absorbed by peritoneum must be excreted by lungs • Respiratory acidosis if CO_2 not adequately eliminated	• Increase mechanical ventilation

b. **Pneumothorax.** The diagnosis is made by the finding of sudden increase in airway pressure, desaturation, and increase in end-expiratory values of CO_2 partial pressures.

c. **Main stem bronchus intubations** may occur if the tip of the endotracheal tube is close to the carina. Pneumoperitoneum will move the diaphragm and tracheobronchial tree cephalad.

d. **Other complications** include subcutaneous emphysema, and facial and airway swelling (if the patient was kept in Trendelenburg position for prolonged periods of time).

E. Pain Management

Pain is at its worst during the first 3 to 4 hours postoperatively and contributes a great deal to the occurrence of PONV in laparoscopic cholecystectomy.

1. **Opioids** are the mainstay of postoperative pain control.
2. Because postoperative pain is produced by surgical tissue injury, stimulation of pain receptors, and activation of central pain pathways, a multimodal approach appears logical and is reported to be highly effective. This approach includes:
    a. Intramuscular administration of **ketoralac** and **meperidine** preoperatively. The influence of ketoralac on coagulation mechanisms may limit its use.
    b. **Infiltration** of the wound sites with a long-acting local anesthetic, e.g., 0.25% bupivacaine (about 10 minutes before incision).
    c. **Intraperitoneal instillation** of bupivacaine provides pain relief following laparoscopic gynecologic procedures but not following laparoscopic gallbladder resection.
    d. Finally, **evacuating gas from the peritoneal cavity** at the end of procedure is important since residual pneumoperitonium contributes to the occurrence of postoperative pain.

F. Selected References

Lobato EB, Glen BP, Brown MM, Bennett B, Davis JD. Pneumoperitoneum as a risk factor for endobronchial intubation during laproscopic gynecological surgery. Anesth Analg 1998;86:301–303.

Loughney AD, Sarma V, Ryall EA. Intraperitoneal bupivacaine for the relief of pain following day case laparoscopy. Br J Obstet Gynaecol 1994;101(5):449–51.

Michaloliachou C, Chung F, Sharma S. Preoperative multimodal anesthesia facilitates recovery after ambulatory laparoscopic cholecystectomy. Anesth Analg 1996;82:44–51.

Neuman GG, Sidebotham G, Negoianu E, et al. Laparoscopy explosion hazards with nitrous oxide. Anesthesiology 1993;78(5):875–879.

Nishanian E, Goudsouzian NG. Carbon dioxide embolism during hip arthrography in an infant. Anesth Analg 1998;86:299–300.

Puri GD, Singh H. Ventilatory effects of laparoscopy under general anesthesia. Br J Anaesth 1992;68:21–213.

Tang J, Wang B, White P, Watcha MH, Qi J, Wender RH. The effect of timing of ondansetron on its efficacy, cost-effectiveness, and cost-benefit as a prophylactic antiemetic in the ambulatory setting. Anesth Analg 1998;86:274–282.

Tatlor E, Feinstein R, White PF, Soper N. Anesthesia for laparoscopic choleycstectomy: Is nitrous oxide contraindicated? Anesthesiology 1992;76:541–543.

Wahba RW, Beique F, Kleiman SJ. Cardiopulmonary functions and laparoscopic chole-
    cystectomy [Review]. Can J Anaesth 1995;42(1):51–63.
Wittgen CM, Andrus CH, Fizgerald SD, Baundendistel LJ, Dahms TE, Kaminski DL.
    Analysis of the hemodynamic and ventilatory effects of laparascopic cholecystec-
    tomy. Arch Surg 1991;126:997–1001.

4. Access to Abdomen

Nathaniel J. Soper, M.D.

A. Equipment

Two pieces of equipment are needed to gain access to the abdomen: an insufflator and a Veress needle (or Hasson cannula, see section C).

1. Insufflator

Turn the insufflator on and check the CO_2 cylinder to ascertain that it contains sufficient gas to complete the procedure. If there is any doubt, bring an extra CO_2 container into the OR. In any event, always keep a spare tank of CO_2 immediately available.

Check the insufflator to assure it is functioning properly. Connect the sterile insufflation tubing (with in-line filter) to the insufflator. Turn the insufflator to high flow (>6 L/min); with the insufflator tubing not yet connected to a Veress needle, the intra-abdominal pressure indicator should register 0 (Fig. 4.1).

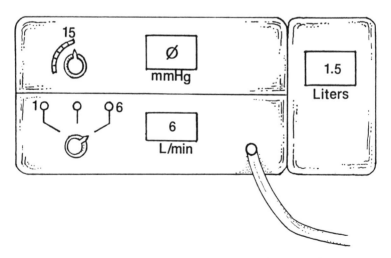

Figure 4.1. **Insufflator testing**. With insufflator tubing open (i.e., not connected to Veress needle) and flow rate set at 6 L/min, the intra-abdominal pressure reading obtained through the open insufflation line should be 0 mm Hg.

Lower the insufflator flow rate to 1 L/min. Kink the tubing to shut off the flow of gas. The pressure indicator should rapidly rise to 30 mm Hg and flow indicator should go to zero (Fig. 4.2). The pressure/flow shutoff mechanism is essential to the performance of safe laparoscopy. These simple checks verify that it is operating properly.

Next, test the flow regulator at low and high inflow. With the insufflator tubing connected to the insufflator and the Veress needle (before abdominal insertion), low flow should register 1 L/min and at high flow should register 2 to 2.5 L/min; measured pressure at both settings should be <3 mm Hg. A pressure reading ≥3 mm Hg indicates a blockage in the insufflator tubing or the hub or shaft of the Veress needle; if this occurs, replace the needle. Maximal flow through a Veress needle is only about 2.5 L/min, regardless of the insufflator setting, because it is only 14 gauge. A Hasson cannula has a much larger internal diameter and can immediately accommodate the maximum flow rate of most insufflators (i.e., >6 L/min).

During most laparoscopic procedures, the pressure limit should be set at 12 to 15 mm Hg; intra-abdominal pressures higher than this limit can diminish visceral perfusion and vena caval return.

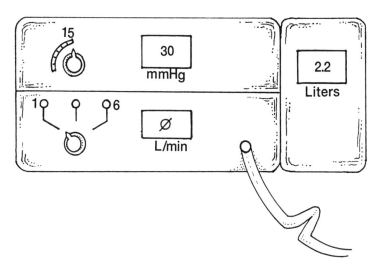

Figure 4.2. **Insufflator testing.**With the insufflation tubing kinked, the intra-abdominal pressure should rapidly rise (e.g., 30 mm Hg), thereby exceeding the preset 15 mm Hg pressure set point. The flow of CO_2 should immediately cease (0 L/min) and an alarm should sound.

2.   Veress needle

Both disposable and reusable (nondisposable) Veress needles are available. The former is a one-piece plastic design (external diameter, 2 mm; 14 gauge;

length, 70 or 120 mm), whereas the latter is made of metal and can be disassembled. Check the Veress needle for patency by flushing saline through it. Then occlude the tip of the needle and push fluid into the needle under moderate pressure to check for leaks. Replace a disposable Veress needle if it leaks; check the screws and connections on a reusable Veress needle.

Next, push the blunt tip of the Veress needle against the handle of a knife or a solid, flat surface to be certain that the blunt tip will retract easily and will spring forward rapidly and smoothly (Fig. 4.3). A red indicator in the hub of the disposable needle can be seen to move upward as the tip retracts.

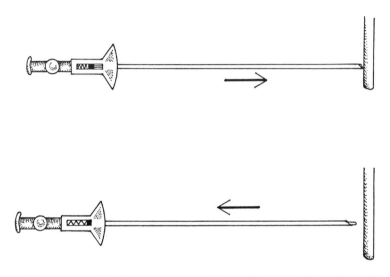

Figure 4.3. **Testing retractable tip of disposable Veress needle**. A. Blunt tip retracts as it contacts resistance (e.g., a knife handle). B. When the needle is pulled away from the point of resistance, the blunt tip springs forward and protrudes in front of the sharp edge of the needle.

B. "Closed" Technique with Veress Needle

1.   **Umbilical puncture**

Place the supine patient in a 10- to 20-degree head-down position. If there are no scars on the abdomen, choose a site of entry at the superior or inferior border of the umbilical ring (Fig. 4.4). There are several ways to immobilize the umbilicus and provide resistance to the needle. The inferior margin of the umbilicus can be immobilized by pinching the superior border of the umbilicus between the thumb and forefinger of the nondominant hand and rolling the superior margin of the umbilicus in a cephalad direction. Alternatively, in the anesthetized patient, a small towel clip can be placed on either side of the upper margin of the umbilicus; this makes it a bit easier to stabilize the umbilicus and lift it upward.

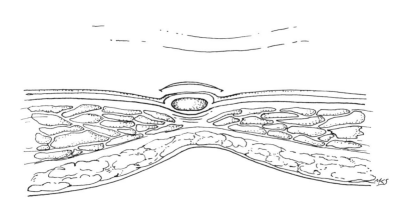

Figure 4.4. Site of Veress needle insertion at superior crease of umbilicus; stab incision has been made. Transverse oblique section at superior crease of umbilicus; the peritoneum is closer to the skin at the umbilicus and is more densely adherent to the umbilicus than at any other site along the abdominal wall.

Next, make a stab incision in the midline of the superior or inferior margin of the umbilicus. With the dominant hand, grasp the shaft (not the hub) of the Veress needle like a dart and gently pass the needle into the incision—either at a 45-degree caudal angle to the abdominal wall (in the asthenic or minimally obese patient) or perpendicular to the abdominal wall in the markedly obese patient. There will be a sensation of initial resistance, followed by a give, at two points. The first point occurs as the needle meets and traverses the fascia and the second as it touches and traverses the peritoneum (Fig. 4.5). As the needle enters the peritoneal cavity, a distinct click can often be heard as the blunt-tip portion of the Veress needle springs forward into the peritoneal cavity.

Connect a 10-ml syringe containing 5 ml of saline to the Veress needle. There are five tests that should be performed in sequence to confirm proper placement of the needle.

a. Aspirate to assess whether any blood, bowel contents, or urine enter the barrel of the syringe.
b. Instill 5 ml of saline, which should flow into the abdominal cavity without resistance.
c. Aspirate again. If the peritoneal cavity has truly been reached, no saline should return.
d. Close the stopcock and disconnect the syringe from the Veress needle, then open the stopcock and observe as any fluid left in the hub of the syringe falls rapidly into the abdominal cavity (especially if the abdominal wall is elevated slightly manually). This is the so-called drop test. If free flow is not present, the needle is either not in the coelomic cavity, or it is adjacent to a structure.

e.   Finally, if the needle truly lies in the peritoneal cavity, it should be possible to advance it 1 to 2 cm deeper into the peritoneal cavity without encountering any resistance. Specifically, the tip indicator or the hub of the needle should show no sign that the blunt tip of the needle is retracting, thereby indicating the absence of fascial or peritoneal resistance.

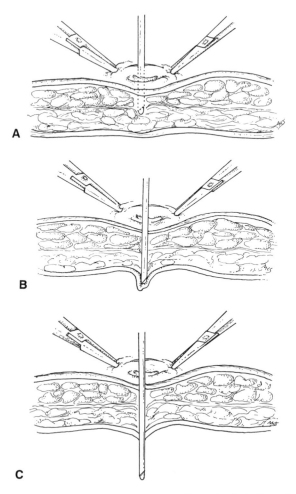

Figure 4.5. A. Veress needle inserted at umbilicus (sagittal view; the blunt tip retracts as it encounters the fascia of the linea alba. B. As the sharp edge of the needle traverses the fascia, the blunt tip springs forward into the preperitoneal space and then retracts a second time as it encounters the peritoneum. C. Blunt tip springs forward as Veress needle passes across the peritoneum to enter the abdominal cavity.

Always be cognizant of anatomic landmarks when placing the needle, and carefully stabilize the needle during insufflation. Minimize side-to-side and back-and-forth movements of the needle to avoid inadvertent injuries.

After ascertaining that the tip of the Veress needle lies in the peritoneal cavity, connect the insufflation line to the Veress needle. Turn the flow of CO_2 to 1 L/min, and reset the indicator on the machine for total CO_2 infused to 0. The pressure in the abdomen during initial insufflation should always register less than 10 mm Hg (after subtracting any pressure noted when the needle was tested by itself and with the insufflator) (Fig. 4.6).

If high pressures are noted or if there is no flow because the 15 mm Hg limit has been reached, gently rotate the needle to assess whether the opening in the shaft of the needle is resting against the abdominal wall, omentum, or the bowel. The opening is on the same side of the needle as the stopcock. If the abdominal pressure remains high (i.e., needle in adhesion, omentum, or pre-peritoneal space), withdraw the needle and make another pass of the Veress needle. If necessary, repeat this process several times until you are certain that the needle resides within the peritoneal cavity. Do not continue insufflation if you are uncertain about the appropriate intraperitoneal location of the tip of the Veress needle. Multiple passes with the Veress needle are not problematic, provided the error is not compounded by insufflating the "wrong" space.

One of the first signs that the Veress needle lies freely in the abdomen is loss of the dullness to percussion over the liver during early insufflation. When the needle is correctly placed, the peritoneum should effectively seal off the needle around the puncture site; if CO_2 bubbles out along the needle's shaft while insufflating, suspect a preperitoneal location of the needle tip. During insufflation, a previously unoperated abdomen should appear to expand symmetrically, and there should be loss of the normal sharp contour of the costal margin.

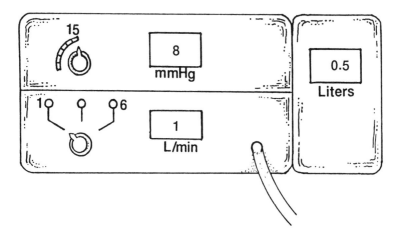

Figure 4.6. Initial insufflation readings: proper inflow at beginning of CO_2–Veress needle insufflation.

Monitor the patient's pulse and blood pressure closely for a vagal reaction during the early phase of insufflation. If the pulse falls precipitously, allow the CO_2 to escape, administer atropine, and reinstitute insufflation slowly after a normal heart rate has returned.

After 1 L of CO_2 has been insufflated uneventfully, increase the flow rate on the insufflator to ≥ 6 L/min (Fig. 4.7). Once the 15 mm Hg limit is reached, the flow of CO_2 will be cut off. At this point approximately 3 to 6 L of CO_2 should have been instilled into the abdomen (Fig. 4.8). When percussed, the abdomen should sound as though you are thumping a ripe watermelon.

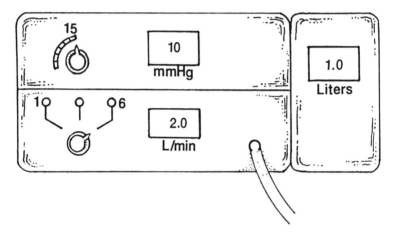

Figure 4.7. After 1 L is insufflated, the set flow is increased to the highest rate.

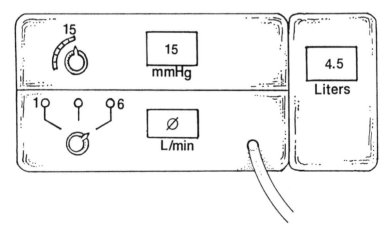

Figure 4.8. At 15 mm Hg intra-abdominal pressure, 3 to 6 L of CO_2 will usually have been insufflated; the registered flow should then fall to 0.

2. **Alternate Puncture Sites**

Prior abdominal surgery mandates care in selection of the initial trocar site, and may prompt consideration of use of the open technique (see section C). If the previous incisions are well away from the umbilicus, the umbilical site may still be used, with either a closed or open technique.

A midline scar in the vicinity of the umbilicus increases the risk that adhesions will be tethering intra-abdominal viscera to the peritoneum at that level. In this situation, the closed technique may still be used, but it is safer to use an alternate insertion site. This site should be well away from the previous scar and lateral to the rectus muscles, to minimize the thickness of abdominal wall traversed and avoid the inferior epigastric vessels.

In general, patients with prior low vertical midline scars should be approached through a trocar placed at the lateral border of the rectus muscle in either the left or right upper quadrant (Fig. 4.9). With previous upper vertical midline incision or multiple incisions near the midline, the right lower quadrant site may be appropriate. Alternatively, it is possible to perform an open technique with the Hasson cannula.

Upper abdomen: In the upper abdomen, the subcostal regions are good choices. Carefully percuss the positions of the liver and spleen to avoid inadvertent injury to these organs, and decompress the stomach with a nasogastric or orogastric tube.

Lower abdomen: The right lower quadrant, near McBurney's point, is preferable to the left because many individuals have congenital adhesions between the sigmoid colon and anterior abdominal wall. Decompress the bladder when using a closed insertion technique at, or caudad to, the umbilicus.

3. **Placement of Trocar**

A wide variety of trocars are available in both disposable and reusable forms. Most have sharp tips of either a tapered conical or pyramidally faceted configuration. Several new disposable trocar designs incorporate unique design features such as direct serial incision of the tissue under visual control, or serial dilatation of the Veress needle tract. This section describes blind entry with the basic sharp trocar, with or without a "safety shield."

Always inspect the trocar to ensure that all valves move smoothly, that the insufflation valve is closed (to avoid losing pneumoperitoneum), and that any safety shields work properly. Make sure you are familiar with the trocar; with the variety of designs available, it is not uncommon to be handed a different device (especially if it is less costly!).

Once you have attained a full pneumoperitoneum, remove the Veress needle. Most surgeons augment the pneumoperitoneum by lifting up on the fascia or abdominal wall to provide additional resistance against which to push the trocar. In a slender individual, the distance to the viscera and retroperitoneal structures is slight, and it is prudent to aim the trocar down into the pelvis. In an obese patient, this is less of a problem and the trocar may be passed in a more direct path. There should be moderate resistance as the trocar is inserted. Excessive resistance may indicate that the trocar is dull or the safety shield (if one is present) has not released, or that the skin incision is too small. The resistance suddenly decreases when the peritoneum is entered. Open the stopcock briefly to confirm intraperitoneal placement by egress of CO_2. Insert the laparoscope and visually confirm entry. Connect the insufflator tubing and open the valve to restore full pneumoperitoneum. Subsequent trocars may be placed under direct vision.

If the trocar has been placed preperitoneally, it is rarely possible to redirect it. Time is often saved in this situation by converting to an open technique for placement of the initial trocar.

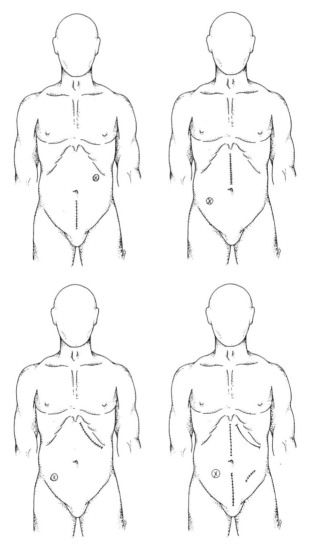

Figure 4.9. Optional trocar sites in previously operated abdomen. Consider the open-cannula technique.

C. "Open" Technique with Hasson Cannula

The open (e.g., Hasson) cannula provides the surgeon with an alternative, extremely safe method to enter the abdomen, especially in a patient who has previously undergone intra-abdominal procedures. In these patients in particular, the blind insertion of a trocar would be fraught with the potential for injury to the abdominal viscera. Some surgeons use the open cannula routinely in all patients for placement of the initial umbilical trocar.

The open cannula consists of three pieces: a cone-shaped sleeve, a metal or plastic sheath with a trumpet or flap valve, and a blunt-tipped obturator (Fig. 4.10). On the sheath or on the cone-shaped sleeve, there are two struts for affixing two fascial sutures. The cone-shaped sleeve can be moved up and down the sheath until it is properly positioned; it can then be tightly affixed to the sheath. The two fascial sutures are then wrapped tightly around the struts, thereby firmly seating the cone-shaped sleeve into the fasciotomy and peritoneotomy. This creates an effective seal so the pneumoperitoneum will be maintained.

Make a 2- to 3-cm transverse incision at the selected entry site (in the quadrant of the abdomen farthest away from any of the preexisting abdominal scars or in the periumbilical skin crease if there has been no prior midline surgery). Dissect the subcutaneous tissue with scissors, and identify and incise the underlying fascia (Fig. 4.11). Gently sweep the preperitoneal fat off the peritoneum in a very limited area. Grasp the peritoneum between hemostats and open sharply. This incision should be just long enough to admit the surgeon's index finger. Confirm entry into the abdominal cavity visually and by digital palpation, to ensure the absence of adhesions in the vicinity of the incision. Place a 0-absorbable suture on either side of the fascial incision. Some surgeons place the fascial sutures first, use these to elevate the fascia, and then make the fascial incision.

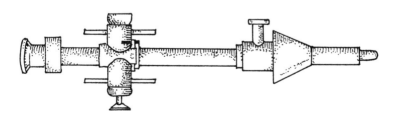

Figure 4.10. Open (Hasson) cannula; reusable type.

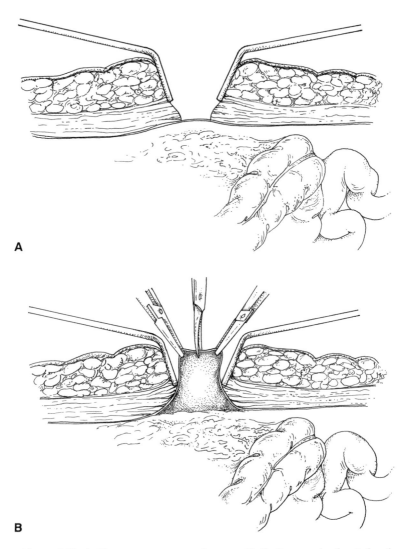

Figure 4.11. A. Retractors expose peritoneum. B. Peritoneum is elevated and sharply incised. Two fascial sutures are secured to the struts on the sheath of the open cannula. The cone-shaped sleeve is then pushed firmly into the incision and the setscrew is tightened, thereby fixing the sleeve to the sheath of the open cannula. The sutures are wound tightly around the struts on the sheath, thereby securing it in place and sealing the incision.

Insert the completely assembled open cannula through the peritoneotomy with the blunt tip of the obturator protruding. Once the obturator is well within the abdominal cavity, advance the conical collar of the open cannula down the sheath until it is firmly seated in the peritoneal cavity. Secure the collar to the sheath with the setscrew. Next, twist or tie the two separate fascial sutures around the struts on the sheath or collar of the open cannula, thereby fixing the cannula in place. Connect the CO_2 line to the sidearm port of the cannula and withdraw the blunt-tipped obturator. Establish pneumoperitoneum with the insufflator set at high flow. Increase intra-abdominal pressure to 12 to 15 mm Hg.

With facility, it is possible to establish pneumoperitoneum just as fast (or faster) with the open technique as can be done with Veress needle and "closed" trocar passage. Indeed, many surgeons consider this to be the safest way to establish pneumoperitoneum.

If a Hasson cannula is not available, a standard cannula from an open trocar can be placed by an open technique. In this case, place two concentric purse-string monofilament sutures in the midline fascia and make an incision into the free peritoneal cavity through the center of the purse strings. Keep both sutures long, and pass the tails of each suture through a 3-cm segment of a red rubber catheter, thereby creating two modified Rummel tourniquets. Place a standard laparoscopic sheath (with the sharp-tipped trocar removed), cinch the purse-string sutures against the sheath, and secure by placing a clamp on the red rubber catheter. At the conclusion of the operation, close the fascia by simply tying the sutures.

D. Avoiding, Recognizing, and Managing Complications

1. **Bleeding from abdominal wall**
    a. **Cause and prevention:** This problem usually manifests itself as a continuous stream of blood dripping from one of the trocars, and/or as blood seen on the surface of the abdominal viscera or omentum. Less commonly, delayed presentation as a hematoma of the abdominal wall or rectus sheath may occur. This source of bleeding is usually the inferior epigastric artery or one of its branches. Abdominal wall hemorrhage may be controlled with a variety of techniques, including application of direct pressure with the operating port, open or laparoscopic suture ligation, or tamponade with a Foley catheter inserted into the peritoneal cavity (Fig. 4.12).
    b. **Recognition and management:** To determine the point at which the vessel is injured, cantilever the trocar into each of four quadrants until the flow of blood is noted to stop. Then place a suture in such a manner that it traverses the entire border of the designated quadrant. Specialized devices have been made that facilitate placement of a suture, but are not always readily avail-

able. The needle should enter the abdomen on one side of the trocar and exit on the other side, thereby encircling the full thickness of the abdominal wall. This suture can either be passed percutaneously using a large curved #1 absorbable suture as monitored endoscopically, or using a straight Keith needle passed into the abdomen and then back out using laparoscopic grasping forceps. The suture, which encircles the abdominal wall, is tied over a gauze bolster to tamponade the bleeding site.

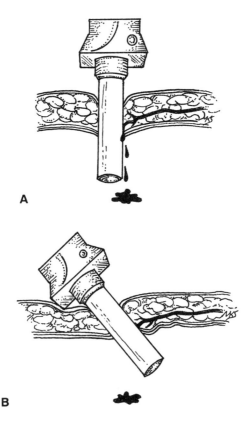

A

B

Figure 4.12. A. **Bleeding from a trocar site**. B. Cantilevering the sheath into each quadrant to find a position that causes the bleeding to stop. When the proper quadrant is found, pressure from the portion of the sheath within the abdomen tamponades the bleeding vessel, thus stopping the bleeding. A stitch can then be passed under laparoscopic guidance.

2. **Visceral injury**
   a. **Cause and prevention:** Careful observation of the steps enumerated above will minimize the chance of visceral injury. However, placement of the Veress needle is a blind maneuver, and even with extreme care puncture of a hollow viscus is still possible.
   b. **Recognition and management:** If aspiration of the Veress needle returns yellowish or cloudy fluid, the needle is likely in the lumen of the bowel. Due to the small caliber of the needle itself, this is usually a harmless situation. Simply remove the needle and repuncture the abdominal wall. After successful insertion of the laparoscope, examine the abdominal viscera closely for significant injury.

If, however, the laparoscopic trocar itself lacerates the bowel, there are four possible courses of action, depending on the surgeon's experience: formal open laparotomy and bowel repair or resection; laparoscopic suture repair of the bowel injury; laparoscopic resection of the injured bowel and reanastomosis; minilaparotomy, using an incision just large enough to exteriorize the injured bowel segment for repair or resection and reanastomosis (similar to the technique of laparoscopic-assisted bowel resection). If possible, leave the trocar in place to assist in identifying the precise site of injury.

3. **Major vascular injury**
   a. **Cause and prevention:** Major vascular injury can occur when the sharp tip of the Veress needle or the trocar nicks or lacerates a mesenteric or retroperitoneal vessel. It is rare when the open (Hasson cannula) technique is used.
   b. **Recognition and management:** If aspiration of the Veress needle reveals bloody fluid, remove the needle and repuncture the abdomen. Once access to the abdominal cavity has been achieved successfully, perform a full examination of the retroperitoneum to look for an expanding retroperitoneal hematoma.

If there is a central or expanding retroperitoneal hematoma, laparotomy with retroperitoneal exploration is mandatory to assess for and repair major vascular injury. Hematomas of the mesentery and those located laterally in the retroperitoneum are generally innocuous and may be observed. If during closed insertion of the initial trocar there is a rush of blood through the trocar with associated hypotension, leave the trocar in place (to provide some tamponade of hemorrhage and assist in identifying the tract) and immediately perform laparotomy to repair what is likely to be an injury to the aorta, vena cava, or iliac vessels.

E. References

Baadsgaard SE, Bille S, Egeblad K. Major vascular injury during gynecologic laparoscopy: report of a case and review of published cases. Acta Obstet Gynecol Scand 1989;68:283–285.

Chapron CM, Pierre F, Lacroix S, Querleu D, Lansac J, Dubuisson J-B. Major vascular injuries during gynecologic laparoscopy. J Am Coll Surg 1997;185:461–465.

Deziel DJ, Millikan KW, Economou SG, Doolas A, Ko ST, Arian MC. Complications of laparoscopic cholecystectomy: a national survey of 4,292 hospitals and an analysis of 77,604 cases. Am J Surg 1993;165:9–14.

Oshinsky GS, Smith AD. Laparoscopic needles and trocars: an overview of designs and complications. J Laparoendosc Surg 1992;2:117–125.

Riza ED, Deshmukh AS. An improved method of securing abdominal wall bleeders during laparoscopy. J Laparoendosc Surg 1995;5:37–40.

Soper NJ. Laparoscopic cholecystectomy. Curr Probl Surg 1991;28:585-655.

Soper NJ, Odem RR, Clayman RV, McDougall EM, eds. Essentials of Laparoscopy, St. Louis: Quality Medical Publishing, 1994.

Wolfe WM, Pasic R. Instruments and methods. Obstet Gynecol 1990;75:456–457.

5.1. Pneumoperitoneum

Claudia L. Corwin, M.D.

A. Choice of Insufflating Gases

Understanding the physiology of pneumoperitoneum is essential for performing laparoscopy in a safe manner. This section first describes the characteristics of the ideal insufflating agent, and the advantages and disadvantages of various gases that have been used for this purpose. The second part of this section describes the physiologic changes observed with carbon dioxide pneumoperitoneum, the most common agent used in the United States.

Air was the first gas used to produce pneumoperitoneum, but has largely been abandoned for this purpose.

1. The **main disadvantage of air** is the risk of air embolism. Air embolism is the introduction of air into the venous or arterial circulatory system.
    a. During laparoscopy, venous embolism is the most likely mechanism for air embolism to occur, as small veins are inevitably transected during the procedure.
    b. Venous air embolism may reduce or stop the flow of blood through the heart, or may cause neurological complications. Death occurs because an airlock forms in the right ventricle, and the heart compresses the air rather than pumping blood. It is estimated that as little as 300 ml of venous air can be fatal.
    c. Arterial air embolism occurs when air enters the left side of the heart, and then enters the aorta. Subsequently the air may flow into the coronary or cerebral circulation. Experiments have shown that as little as 1 ml of air in the coronary circulation can lead to death.

2. **Characteristics of the ideal insufflating agent**
    a. The ideal agent for insufflation during laparoscopic procedures should be colorless, physiologically inert, and nonexplosive in the presence of electrocautery or laser coagulation.
    b. The agent's solubility in tissues should be low, conserving use and simplifying the maintenance of pneumoperitoneum for operation.
    c. Solubility in blood should be high, minimizing the effects of inadvertent injection of the gas into the venous or arterial circulation.
    d. The insufflating gas should be readily available, inexpensive, and nontoxic.

Several gases have been tested for laparoscopic applications (Table 5.1.1). Each gas will be considered individually.

B. Carbon Dioxide

Carbon dioxide (CO_2) is an odorless, colorless gas that results from the oxidation of carbon. It is a readily available stable gas, naturally formed in the tissues and eliminated by the lungs. Carbon dioxide is the most commonly used gas for insufflation during laparoscopic procedures.

1. **Advantages of carbon dioxide**
   a. **Relatively low risk of venous gas embolism.** Venous gas embolism is a life-threatening laparoscopic complication with an incidence of 0.0016% to 0.013%. Carbon dioxide bubbles rapidly dissolve in the bloodstream, due to the high aqueous solubility of this gas. Thus, if a gas embolism should occur, it will rapidly dissolve in the bloodstream, increasing the safety margin of this rare event.
   b. **CO_2 does not support combustion.** It is therefore safe to use electrocautery during laparoscopy.
2. **Disadvantages of carbon dioxide**
   a. **Hypercarbia and acidosis** resulting from carbon dioxide insufflation during laparoscopy has been well documented over the past 30 years and remains a significant limitation to laparoscopic surgery in the 1990s.

Carbon dioxide instilled into the abdominal cavity normally diffuses across the peritoneal surface into the venous circulation. After the carbon dioxide is carried away by the venous system, it may be eliminated by the lungs or stored elsewhere in the body. Total body stores of carbon dioxide approaches 120 L. While blood and alveolar storage sites often come to mind first, bone actually serves as the single largest reservoir for carbon dioxide. Under sustained exposure to carbon dioxide, such as during carbon dioxide pneumoperitoneum, other short-term visceral storage sites, such as skeletal muscle, become important. During pneumoperitoneum, body stores of carbon dioxide continuously increase.

Following a long laparoscopic procedure, it may take several hours for the accumulated carbon dioxide to be eliminated and for the body's acid-base balance to be restored to a steady state. This may affect postoperative respiratory recovery. Several studies have shown that hypercarbia is due to increased absorption of carbon dioxide from the peritoneum, rather than from increased ventilatory dead space after expansion of the peritoneal cavity secondary to impairment of diaphragmatic excursion and alveolar expansion. Bicarbonate levels have also been shown to remain constant, providing further supporting evidence that the hypercarbia and acidosis during pneumoperitoneum is of respiratory origin.

   b. The **circulatory effects of increased carbon dioxide** load are due to both the direct local effects of carbon dioxide and to the centrally mediated effects of carbon dioxide on the autonomic

5.2. Abdominal Wall Lift Devices

Edmund K.M. Tsoi, M.D.
Albert K. Chin, M.D.
Claude H. Organ, Jr., M.D.

A. Types of Abdominal Wall Lifting Devices

Although pneumoperitoneum provides exposure and access for laparoscopic surgery, it is associated with potential complications (see Chapter 5.1) and restricts instrument design due to the constraints of working in a sealed environment. Various investigators have sought alternative ways to obtain exposure by a variety of abdominal wall lifting devices. These devices provide vertical upward forces to lift the anterior abdominal wall, creating a space similar to that produced by pneumoperitoneum. Virtually every open procedure can be performed with minimally invasive techniques using these devices, which thus may serve as a bridge between open and conventional laparoscopic techniques. In this section, three types of abdominal lifting devices are described, and the technique for using one type of device (planar lift) is given in detail. References at the end of the chapter give further information about the other techniques mentioned in the text.

1. **Low-pressure pneumoperitoneum and "sequential" lifting devices**. Before the current standard of 15 mm Hg was adopted, laparoscopists used pressures as high as 30 mm Hg. Recognizing the detrimental cardiopulmonary effects of such elevated pressures, the first abdominal wall lifting devices were developed to allow exposure without elevated intra-abdominal pressure. These devices were placed after exposure was obtained, and were variously employed with low-pressure pneumoperitoneum.

    a. A **T-shaped** instrument was described in 1991 by Gazayerli. This was designed to be inserted into a trocar port to elevate a small portion of the abdominal wall, thus providing an increased ceiling in obese patients, or allowing exposure without cardiopulmonary compromise in patients unable to tolerate more than 8 mm Hg. Low-pressure pneumoperitoneum was generally needed.

    b. A **U-shaped** retractor was described in 1992 by Kitano. Once the retractor is in place, the pneumoperitoneum can be evacuated and the procedure completed without insufflation.

    c. Banting and associates introduced a **falciform lift** device in 1993. Consisting of a long, curved 4-mm trocar to which a flexible polyethylene tube is attached, this was inserted through a stab wound in the left upper quadrant lateral to the falciform ligament. Under direct visual guidance, the trocar, together with the tubing, is passed beneath the falciform ligament to exit in the right upper quadrant. A similar design by Inoue et al., which is inserted from the supraumbilical area to the right upper quadrant, is reported to provide comparable exposure to intra-abdominal pressure of 15 mm Hg. Go and colleagues placed a Kirschner wire at the subcostal region for lifting to reduce the amount of pneumoperitoneum needed for adrenalectomy (Fig. 5.2.1). Recently, Angelini and colleagues report a new abdominal lifter, which is designed to be used with or without pneumoperitoneum. The authors suggested that by combining the use of an optical trocar and subcutaneous abdominal wall retraction, both pneumoperitoneum-related side effects and trocar injuries can be reduced.

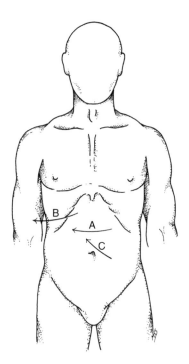

Figure 5.2.1. Diagram demonstrating the placement of flexible tubing or wire in combination with low-pressure pneumoperitoneum: (A) Banting et al., (B) Inoue et al., (C) Go et al. These techniques can be adapted using readily available materials and hence should be part of the laparoscopist's armamentarium.

2. **Gasless devices** are designed to provide the requisite exposure without utilizing pneumoperitoneum, even in the initial stages of exposure.

   a. In 1991, a Japanese team led by Nagai used an abdominal wall wire lifting system to perform laparoscopic cholecystectomy without pneumoperitoneum. In this system, Kirschner wires are placed in the subcutaneous tissue of the abdomen to act as a handle for lifting. Small winching devices connected by an L-shaped bar fixed to the side rail of the operating table are connected to the Kirschner wires to elevate the abdominal wall. An alternate wire lifting method reported by Hashimoto and associates in 1993 used two 30-cm stainless steel wires connected to a Kent retractor (Fig. 5.2.2). Subsequent refinements in the design of these wire lifting systems have simplified and extended their use to a wide variety of advanced laparoscopic procedures.

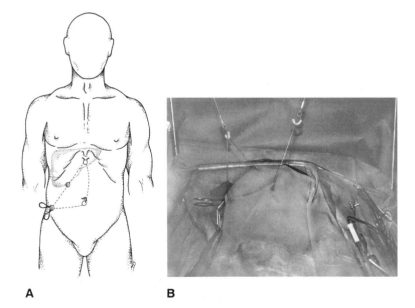

A   **B**

Figure 5.2.2. Hashimoto's subcutaneous lift method. (Reprinted with permission from Tsoi EKM, Organ CH Jr., eds.) Abdominal Access in Open and Laparoscopic Surgery. New York: Wiley-Liss, 1996.

b. **Planar lifting devices.** Chin and Moll developed a planar lifting technique to elevate the abdominal wall. Unlike the wire lifting devices, the planar lifting device is widely available around the world; it can elevate the abdominal wall with minimal trauma and can be used in heavier patients. Because this device has gained wide acceptance, the technique of its use will be described in detail (section B). The advantages and disadvantages of this device are summarized in Table 5.2.1.

Table 5.2.1. Advantages and disadvantages of planar abdominal wall lifting devices

Advantages	Disadvantages
• Minimally invasive	• Exposure is less than ideal in the lateral gutters
• Avoids cardiopulmonary side effects associated with pneumoperitoneum	• Exposure is poor in patients with a muscular abdominal wall, such as highly conditioned athletes, or who are morbidly obese
• Operates in an isobaric environment (a "sealed environment" not needed)	• Abdominal contents can shift with mechanical ventilation
• Conventional as well as laparoscopic instruments can be used by surgeon interchangeably	• The abdominal lifting devices can be an obstacle for the surgeon during the conduct of the operation
• High-volume suction device and a large volume of irrigation solution can be used to maintain a clear operating field	
• Tactile examination of intra-abdominal contents is possible	
• Less contamination risk for the surgical team since the operating field is semi-enclosed in an isobaric environment where abdominal fluids will not be force out of the abdomen by CO_2 insufflation	

c. **Conventional retractors** (Richardson or Army-Navy pattern), used in strategically placed small incisions, can provide the necessary exposure for selected procedures performed under laparoscopic guidance with laparoscopic instruments. Examples of such procedures include laparoscopic cholecystectomy performed through the "minimal stress triangle" described by Tyagi et al. This corresponds to the subxiphoid regions, and is bounded by the medial costal margins of the sixth to eighth ribs (Fig. 5.2.3). Similar approaches have been used for other procedures, including tube gastrostomy construction and closure of Hartmann's procedure.

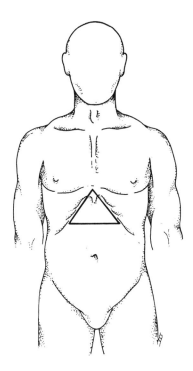

Figure 5.2.3. Boundaries of "minimal stress triangle" described by Tyagai et al. Incisions placed within this triangle are well tolerated.

B. Technique for Planar Lifting Device

The use of the most widely available device, both intra- and extra-peritoneally, is briefly described here. For further information, consult the references at the end of this section.

1. **Intraperitoneal exposure**
   a. Secure the abdominal wall lifter (Laparolift, Origin Medsystoms, Lathrop Engineering Inc., San Jose, CA) to a side rail before draping the patient. Prep the abdomen in the usual sterile fahion. Drape the abdominal wall lifter with a transparent plastic cover before the abdomen is draped.

b. Initial access for the abdominal procedure is made in the peri-umbilical area.

c. Make a small incision in the abdomen to allow the placement of the lifting device.

d. Both fan-shaped and donut-shaped devices are available

e. Open the device within the abdomen (Fig. 5.2.4).

f. Connect the planar lifting device to the Laparolift (Fig. 5.2.5). The Laparolift is then activated to raise the abdominal wall to provide exposure equivalent to 15 mm Hg of pneumoperito-neum.

g. Place the laparoscope into the abdomen through the peri-umbilical incision.

h. Insert additional instruments through trocars or small incisions (generally less than 2 cm in length). Through these incisions, both conventional laparoscopic instruments or extra long tradi-tional instruments for open surgery may be used. A clear oper-ating field can be maintained with traditional high volume suc-tion and copious irrigation without the fear of losing exposure.

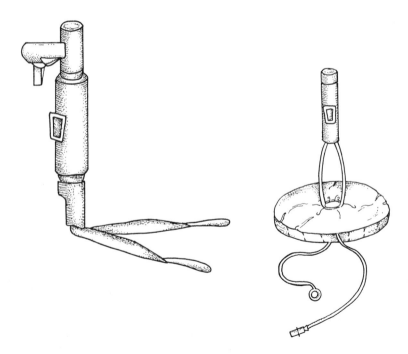

Figure 5.2.4. Both a fan-shaped and an inflatable donut-shaped device are available. Each is inserted into the abdomen in a collapsed configuration, then expanded within the peritoneal cavity.

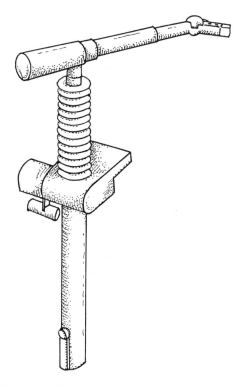

Figure 5.2.5. The Laparolift is a powered articulating arm that attaches to the operating table. The arm lifts up on the lifting device, providing upwards displacement of the anterior abdominal wall and producing retraction.

2. **Extraperitoneal exposure**
    a. Obtain initial access into the extraperitoneal space via a small incision (<2 cm).
    b. Enter the extraperitoneal space by using a muscle-splitting technique.
    c. Place a dissecting balloon into this newly created space to create an operating field.
    d. Place the abdominal wall retractor into the extraperitoneal space through this incision. Connect the abdominal wall retractor to the lifter and elevate the abdominal wall to a maximum pressure equivalent to 15 mm Hg pneumoperitoneum.

     e.   Insert the laparoscope.

     f.   Place inflatable laparoscopic bowel retractors into the extra-peritoneal space to push the peritoneum (together with the abdominal viscera) away from the operating field.

3.   A **wide variety of procedures** have been performed with the planar abdominal wall lift device. (Table 5.2.2)

Table 5.2.2. Intra- and extraperitoneal procedures

Intraperitoneal procedures	Extraperitoneal procedures
• Diagnostic laparoscopy	• Aortic surgery
• Gastrostomy	• Inguinal hernorrphy
• Gastrojejunostomy	• Retroperitoneal lymph node dissection
• Gastric resection	• Retroperitoneoscopic assisted spine surgery
• Nissen fundoplication	• Bladder neck suspension
• Closure of perforated viscus	
• Adrenalectomy	
• Appendectomy	
• Colectomy and colostomy	
• Derotation of volvulus	
• Cholecystectomy	
• Common bile duct exploration	
• Liver biopsy	
• Liver resection	
• Pancreatic pseudocysts	
• Hysterectomy and myomectomy	
• Closure of diaphragmatic hernia	
• Tubal ligation	
• Peritoneal dialysis catheter management	
• Salpingo-oophorectomy	

C. Selected References

Angelini L, Lirici MM, Papaspyropoulos V, et al. Combination of subcutaneous abdominal wall retraction and optical trocar to minimize pneumoperitoneum-related effects and needle and trocar injuries in laparoscopic urgery. Surg Endosc 1997;11:1006–1009.

Banting S, Shimi S, Velpen GV, et al. Abdominal wall lift: low pressure pneumoperitoneum laparoscopic surgery. *Surg Endosc* 1993;7:57–59.

Barr LL. Minimally invasive tube gastrostomy. Surg Laparosc Endosc 1997;7(4):285–287.

Chin AK, Eaton J, Tsoi EKM, et al. Gasless laparoscopy using a planar lifting technique. J Am Coll Surg 1994;178:401–403.

Gazayerli MM. The Gazayerli endoscopic retractor model I. Surg Laparosc Endosc 1991;1:98–100.

Go H, Takeda M, Imai T, et al. Laparoscopic adrenalectomy for Cushing's syndrome: comparison with primary aldosteronism. Surgery 1995;117:11–17.

Hashimoto D, Nayeem AS, Kajiwara S, et al. Laparoscopic cholecystectomy: an approach without pneumoperitoneum. Surg Endosc 1993;7:54–56.

Inoue H, Muraoka Y, Takeshitak K, et al. Low pressure pneumoperitoneum using newly design devised flexible abdominal wall retractor. Surg Endosc 1993;7:133 (abstr).

Kitano S, Tomikawa M, Iso Y, et al. A safe and simple method to maintain a clear field of vision during laparoscopic cholecystectomy. Surg Endosc 1992;6:197–8.

Nagai H. Subcutaneous lift system (SCLS) for laparoscopic surgery. In: Tsoi EKM, Organ CH Jr., eds. Abdominal Access in Open and Laparoscopic Surgery. New York: Wiley-Liss, 1996;99–128.

Nagai H, Inaba T, Kamiya S, et al. An new method of laparoscopic cholecystectomy: an abdominal wall lifting technique without pneumoperitoneum. Surg Laparosc Endosc 1991;1:126 (abstr).

Navarra G, Occhionorelli S, Marcello D, et al. Gasless video-assisted reversal of Hartmann's procedure. Surg Endosc 1995;9:687–689.

Tsoi EKM, Organ CH Jr., eds. Abdominal Access in Open and Laparoscopic Surgery. New York: Wiley-Liss 1996.

Tyagi NS, Meredith MC, Lumb JC, et al. A new minimally invasive technique for cholecystectomy: subxiphoid "minimal stress triangle" microceliotomy. Ann Surg 1994;220(5):617–625.

Vogt DM, Goldstein L, Hirvela ER. Complications of CO_2 pneumoperitoneum. In: Tsoi EKM, Organ CH Jr., eds. Abdominal Access in Open and Laparoscopic Surgery. New York: Wiley-Liss, 1996;75–98.

5.3. Generation of Working Space: Extraperitoneal Approaches

David M. Brams, M.D.

A. Indications

Extraperitoneal endoscopic surgery (EES) was first described by Bartel in 1969. Wickham and Miller described the use of CO_2 and videoscopic control in 1993. Gaur introduced balloons for retroperitoneal dissection in 1993, and Hirsch and coworkers described the use of a trocar mounted balloon for extraperitoneal dissection in 1994. There are both advantages and disadvantages to this approach (Table 5.3.1).

Table 5.3.1. Advantages and disadvantages of extraperitoneal endoscopic surgery

Advantages	Disadvantages
• Decreased risk of bowel injury	• Small working space
• Decreased problems with bowel retraction	• Orientation can be confusing
• Less postoperative ileus	• Inadvertent entry into peritoneum causes loss of working space
• Closure of peritoneum not required when mesh implanted retroperitoneally	• Retractors often needed to displace peritoneal sac
• Less adverse hemodynamic effects from retroperitoneal insufflation	• Prior extraperitoneal dissection is a contraindication to this approach

Procedures in which EES has been utilized include:
1. Totally extraperitoneal (TEP) inguinal herniorrhaphy (see Chapter 34)
2. Retroperitoneal endoscopically assisted spine surgery
3. Renal surgery
4. Adrenalectomy (see Chapter 33)
5. Varicocele ligation
6. Pelvic lymph node dissection (see Chapter 32)
7. Bladder suspension
8. Aortoiliac surgery
9. Lumbar sympathectomy

B. Anatomic Considerations

Knowledge of anatomic landmarks is essential to orientation in the extraperitoneal space. The retroperitoneum can be divided into three spaces:

1. The retropubic space (space of Retzius) is the space between the pubic bone and the bladder. This space is obliterated by prior retroperitoneal urologic surgery such as retropubic prostatectomy.
2. The space of Bogros is lateral and cephalad to the space of Retzius.
3. The lumbar retroperitoneal space is the posterior continuation of the space of Bogros bounded by the vena cava and aorta medially, the psoas dorsally, the colon ventrally, and transversalis fascia laterally. This space contains the kidney, adrenal, ureter, and Gerota's fascia.

C. Access to the Extraperitoneal Space

There are three basic ways to gain access to the extraperitoneal space.

1. The **open approach**
   a. Make a 2-cm incision overlying the space to be developed.
   b. Bluntly dissect down to the preperitoneal space and develop this space.
   c. Place a Hasson cannula or a Structural Balloon (Origin Medsystems, Menlo Park, CA).
   d. Continue dissection with laparoscope or balloon dissector (see dissection, below).
2. Use of a **lens-tipped trocar**
   a. Make a 12-mm skin incision over the desired location.
   b. Place a 0-degree laparoscope into a lens-tipped trocar.
   c. Use this to penetrate the layers of the abdominal wall under direct vision.
   d. Once the correct plane is achieved, place a Hasson cannula or Structural Balloon and continue dissection (see dissection, below).
3. **Dulocq Technique**
   a. Insert a Veress needle suprapubically through the fascial layers into the preperitoneal position. The needle will traverse two palpable points of resistance (the anterior rectus sheath and transversalis fascia).
   b. Insufflate 1 L of CO_2.
   c. Make a skin incision lateral to the midline.
   d. Insert a 10-mm trocar, directed caudad, until the gas-filled space is entered.
   e. Place the laparoscope into the trocar and use it to dissect the space while insufflating CO_2.
   f. The major **disadvantage** is that this procedure is relatively "blind" and risks visceral and vascular injury as well as penetration of the peritoneum. If this technique is used to develop the

lumbar retroperitoneal space, fluoroscopic control with ureteral and nephric imaging is essential.

D. Dissection of Extraperitoneal Space

Just as there are several techniques for obtaining access, there are several methods of dissection of the extraperitoneal space to create working room.

1. **Operating laparoscopes** have a 5-mm instrument channel (in a 10-mm laparoscope). These allow dissection under direct vision while insufflating CO_2.
2. Alternatively, a **30-degree laparoscope** can be used alone to open the space by sweeping tissue away while insufflating CO_2.
3. **Balloon dissection** is the most popular and easiest method of developing the extraperitoneal space.
   a. Insert an air-inflated, trocar-mounted clear plastic dissection balloon into the space to be developed.
   b. Place a 0-degree laparoscope into the balloon and inflate the balloon while identifying landmarks (Fig. 5.3.1). Identify blood vessels, such as the inferior epigastrics, and avoid injury by controlled insufflation.

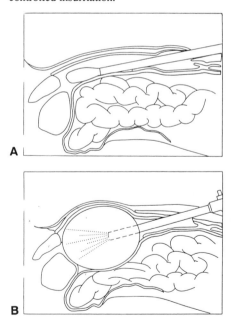

Figure 5.3.1. Balloon used to dissect extraperitoneal space. Reproduced with permission from Tsoi EKM and Organ Jr CH, eds. Abdominal Access in Open and Laparoscopic Surgery (John Wiley & Sons, New York, 1996).

     c.   Spherical balloon dissectors are most useful.

     d.   Kidney-shaped balloon dissectors are available for lateral dissection in bilateral hernia repair.

4.   Insert additional trocars under direct vision after creating the initial space. Develop and enlarge the extraperitoneal space with blunt dissection and atraumatic graspers, "peanut" dissection, and cautery scissors. A 30-degree laparoscope can facilitate exposure.

5.   Avoid subcutaneous emphysema by maintaining a tight seal between skin and fascia.

E. Maintenance of Extraperitoneal Space

There are several ways to maintain an extraperitoneal working space.

1.   Insufflation to 12 to 15 mm Hg CO_2 will maintain a working space.

2.   Planar abdominal wall-lifting devices (laparolift, Origin Medsystems, Menlo Park, CA), allow gasless extraperitoneal endoscopy using conventional instruments (see Chapter 5.2).

3.   In TEP hernia repairs, the Structural Balloon (Origin Medsystems, Menlo Park, CA) replaces a Hassan cannula and displaces peritoneum posteriorly while providing a seal between skin and fascia and providing access for the laparoscope (Fig. 5.3.2).

4.   Peritoneal retraction devices are necessary to displace the peritoneal sac for lumbar and iliac extraperitoneal laparoscopy. Instruments such as the Laparofan (USSC, Norwalk, CT) or the Extrahand Balloon Dissector (Origin Medisystems, Menlo Park, CA) can be used in a gasless or gas extraperitoneal laparoscopic procedure.

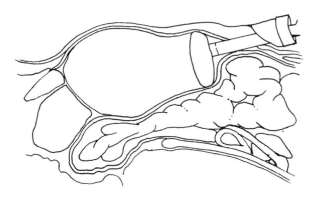

Figure 5.3.2. Structural Balloon provides access for gas insufflation and laparoscope while retracting the peritoneum posteriorly.

F. Potential Problems

1. **Peritoneal holes** allow CO_2 to leak, creating a pneumoperitoneum that decreases the extraperitoneal space. Close peritoneal holes with a pretied suture ligature or by suturing them shut.
2. **Penetration into the peritoneal cavity** during access or dissection may necessitate a transabdominal laparoscopic or open procedure.
3. **Venous bleeding** can be controlled with cautery and will usually stop spontaneously in the limited extraperitoneal space.
4. Cautery, clips, or suture ligation can also be used to control **arterial hemorrhage**. Suction and irrigation should be available.
5. **Prior retroperitoneal dissection** obliterates the potential space and is a contraindication to the extraperitoneal approach.
6. **Prior intra-abdominal surgery** will fuse the peritoneum to the abdominal wall. Begin the dissection away from old scars and leave dissection of these areas for last. This will diminish the risk of peritoneal violation.
7. This procedure is more difficult in **obese patients**, as excess adipose tissue in the extraperitoneal space will obscure planes and landmarks.
8. In retroperitoneal approaches to the kidney and adrenal, **laparoscopic ultrasound** can be used to help identify structures.

G. Selected References

Arregui ME, et al. Laparoscopic mesh repair of inguinal hernia using a pre-peritoneal approach: a preliminary report. Surg Laparosc Endosc 1992;2:53–58.

Bartel M. Die Retroperitoneskopie. Eine endoskopische Methode zur Inspektion und bioptischen Untersuchung des retroperitonealen. Zentralbl Chir 1969;94:377–383.

Coptoat MJ. Overview of extraperitoneal laparoscopy. Endosc Surg 1995;3:1–2.

Eden CG. Alternative endoscopic access techniques to the retroperitoneaum. Endosc Surg 1995;3:27–28.

Gaur DD. Laparoscopic operative retroperitoneoscopy. Use of a new device. J Urol 1993;148:1137–1139.

Himpens J. Techniques, equipment and exposure for endoscopic retroperitoneal surgery. Semain Laparosc Surg 1996;3(2) 109–116.

Hirsch IH, Moreno JG, Lotfi MA, et al. Controlled balloon dilatation of the extraperitoneal space for laparoscopic urologic surgery. J Laparoendosc Surg 1994;4:247–251.

McKernan JG, Laws HL. Laparoscopic repair of inguinal hernias using a totally extraperitoneal prosthetic approach. Surg Endosc 1993;7:26–28.

Tsoi EKM, Organ CH. Abdominal Access in Open and Laparoscopic Surgery. New York: Wiley-Liss, 1996.

Wicham JEA, Milles RA: Percutaneous renal access, in Percutaneous Renal Surgery. New York: Churchill Livingstone, 1983, p. 33–39.

6. Principles of Laparoscopic Hemostasis

Richard M. Newman, M.D.
L. William Traverso, M.D.

Hemostasis has been a key issue from the beginning of laparoscopic general surgery. Precise visualization can only be attained during laparoscopy in a bloodless field. Hemostasis must be attained at the first attempt, because the limitations of access and a small visual field make a second chance much more risky. Prevention of bleeding requires the timely and appropriate use of technology, much of it newly modified for the laparoscopic approach. In this section we present a variety of major hemostatic modalities that can be used during laparoscopic surgery. Monopolar electrosurgery will be emphasized because it is employed during most operations. A practical section on the laparoscopic control of active bleeding is included.

A. Mechanical Methods of Hemostasis

1. Endoscopic clip appliers were developed to facilitate ligation of small (2–5 mm) structures such as ducts and vessels. Metallic (titanium) clips are most often used. The common disposable clip appliers contain up to 20 clips and are available in a 10-mm diameter instrument or more recently a 5-mm instrument. These are expensive, however, and are not necessary for simple procedures such as cholecystectomy, where a limited number of structures must be clipped. High-quality reusable clip appliers are available from several manufacturers that allow the surgeon to considerably decrease costs, but these instruments have to be reloaded after each clip is fired.

Clip application requires visualization of both sides of the clip to ensure adequate tissue purchase and to prevent inadvertent clipping of nontarget tissues. The theoretic risk of clip migration into duct and vascular structures has prompted the advent of absorbable clips usually made of polyglycolic acid polymers (Dexon or Vicryl). These clips have identical ligation properties but may pose less threat to adhesion formation or migration. Our bias has been to use pretied ligatures underneath clips when clip migration could be a problem, as with the cystic duct stump.

Inadvertent mechanical ischemic necrosis can occur from metallic clips placed in close proximity to bile duct or bowel wall, resulting in stricture or perforation. These complications can be prevented by better visualization of the structures prior to placing the clip or not relying on a clip when a loop ligature would be more applicable.

2. Linear stapling devices: Although these instruments are used primarily for anastomotic purposes, they are of vital use to prevent major hemostatic complications. Endoscopic linear cutters that deploy two or three parallel rows of hemostatic staples (height = 2.5 mm vascular or 3.5 mm intestinal applications) on each side of a simultaneously produced linear incision are available to facilitate **hemostatic** division of tissue. The tissue is atraumatically crushed between the stapler and its opposing anvil before firing. With effective cutting lengths from 30 to 60 mm, larger vessels or highly vascularized tissues such as in the lung or bowel mesentery can be controlled and divided in one motion. Inspection of both sides of the device is mandatory prior to firing in order that unintended structures are not damaged and to ensure that the entire target tissue is within the active area as indicated in marks or numbers on the side of the device. Depending on the manufacturer, the shaft diameters of these linear cutters vary from 12 to 18 mm. Appropriately large trocars must be strategically placed to allow opening of the active portion of these instruments within the desired operative field.

3. Pretied suture loops with slip knots have a limited use in *primary* hemostasis because the vessel or vascular pedicle must first be divided, grasped, and then encircled with the loop. This leaves a bleeding structure for a period of time while being encircled by the loop. However, the loops are extremely useful to secure bleeding vessels after transection. The bleeding structure is grasped, and the field irrigated. An atraumatic grasper is passed through another port, and passed through the loop of the suture ligature. The first grasper is then released, and the second grasper grasps the stump of the bleeding structure. The loop is snugged down over the shaft of the instrument, securing the bleeder. More information about specific strategies is given in section D.

4. Simple ligatures need to be nothing more than a long suture (at least 42 inches) that is passed around a clearly dissected vessel. Care must be taken to employ an instrument to act as a fulcrum and prevent "sawing" of the tissue or vessel as the ligature is being passed and redelivered out the entry port (for an extracorporeally tied knot). If an intracorporeal knot is planned, the suture material should be fashioned about 6 inches long (length of a scalpel handle is a convenient reference). Further details on knot tying are given in Chapter 7, Principles of Tissue Approximation).

5. Suturing in laparoscopic surgery has been used primarily for tissue approximation. When tissue approximation will result in hemostasis, suturing is a valuable adjunct. An obvious example is the use of figure-of-eight suture to secure a bleeding vessel.

B. General Principles of Energy Induced Hemostasis

Even before the laparoscopic revolution, surgeons relied on energy sources, rather than mechanical means such as sutures and clips, to aid in hemostasis in the operating room. Electricity, laser energy, and ultrasonic waves have been the energy sources most often employed. These modalities all function by the same mechanism, i.e., an energy source is delivered to tissue, resulting in hemostasis via a predictable pattern of **thermal tissue destruction**. The temperature attained in the tissues may predict the changes observed:

1. **At 45°C**, collagen uncoils and may reanneal, allowing apposed edges to form covalent bonds and fuse.
2. **At 60°C**, irreversible protein denaturation occurs and coagulation necrosis begins. This is characterized by a blanching in color.
3. **At 80°C**, carbonization begins and leads to drying and shrinkage of tissue.
4. **From 90° to 100°C**, cellular vaporization occurs and vacuoles form and coalesce, leading to complete cellular destruction. The surgeon observes a plume of gas and smoke that represents water vapor.
5. **Above 125°C**, complete oxidation of protein and lipids leads to carbon residue or eschar formation.

Variations in the rate of tissue heating and the degree of thermal spread accounts for the differences seen between the various energy sources. A basic understanding of how each energy source functions, as well as their limitations and potential complications, allows the surgeon to make careful choices of operative settings and avoid potential problems.

C. Energy Sources Used in Laparoscopy

1. Electrical Energy

Electrosurgery has evolved into the gold standard of energy sources for achieving laparoscopic hemostasis because of familiarity, cost, and versatility. The **active electrode** is a conductor connected directly to the **electrosurgical unit (ESU)** generator. The **return electrode** is a conductor that accepts current from the active electrode and returns it to the ESU, thus completing the electrical circuit. The configuration of the active and return electrode determines the path of current or "mode" during electrosurgery.

a. **In monopolar electrosurgery**, current from the active electrode (hook, spatula, or any instrument tip such as insulated scissors) is allowed to return through the patient to a large return electrode (grounding plate). The path taken by the current is unpredictable, but generally diffuses over a large-enough volume of tissue outside the immediate surgical field.

b. **In bipolar electrosurgery** the active electrode can be intermittently apposed to the return electrode (usually in a forceps-type arrangement). Electrical current passes between the electrodes to complete the circuit, and flow of current beyond the surgical field is minimal. Safe, slow tissue heating leads to controlled coagulation. The rate of tissue heating is not great enough to achieve cutting. The same properties that make bipolar electrosurgery safe in many coagulation applications limit its versatility in routine laparoscopic general surgery.

The ESU can produce two general types of current, depending on the waveform:

    a.   **Cutting current (continuous wave, high frequency, lower voltage)** produces focal and rapid tissue heating and a cutting effect. Heating occurs so rapidly that there is minimal associated coagulation necrosis and therefore no hemostasis.

    b.   **Coagulating current (pulsed waveform, low frequency, high voltage)** produces a slower heating that causes protein denaturation. Hemostasis occurs via coagulative necrosis in and around the target tissue. In laparoscopic surgery, due to its limited visual field, the control of even the smallest amount of bleeding is desirable; therefore, pure cutting is rarely employed. Often the cutting mode is turned completely off by the surgeon and all laparoscopic electrosurgery is performed with the pulsed coagulation current.

Since laparoscopic surgery requires cutting as well as coagulation, how can monopolar electrosurgery accomplish bloodless division of tissues using pure coagulating current? The answer is through current density. Reducing the surface area of the active electrode increases current density. This produces a cutting effect as is illustrated by a comparison of Figs. 6.1 and 6.2.

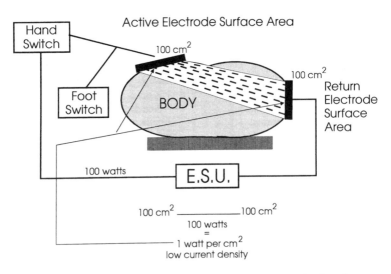

Figure 6.1. Low current density is depicted by this schematic that shows an active electrode with a large surface area (low density of current in the larger surface area). The amount of current going through the patient at this electrode is only 1 watt per cm^2. Heating that may occur here is low and will not result in coagulation or cutting. (Source: Airan MT, Ko ST. Electrosurgery techniques of cutting and coagulation. In: Principles of Laparoscopic Surgery. Arregui ME et al. (eds.). New York: Springer–Verlag, 1995; pp. 30–35.)

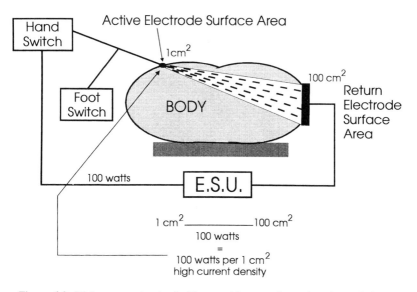

Figure 6.2. High current density is illustrated here as the active electrode has been decreased to 1 cm², raising the current density at this site to 100 watts per cm². Now there will be a rapid rate of temperature rise—quickly with a thin wire electrode (cutting results) and less quickly with a broad electrode (coagulation will result). (Source: Airan MT, Ko ST. Electrosurgery techniques of cutting and coagulation. In: Principles of Laparoscopic Surgery. Arregui ME et al. (eds.). New York: Springer–Verlag, 1995; pp. 30–35.)

Although any instrument can act to deliver a high current density with monopolar electrosurgery the following familiar example of a hook or L-shaped electrode will further illustrate the concept of current density:

A cutting effect is achieved when the tip of the "L," with its small surface area and thus high current density, is applied to Glisson's capsule at the side of the gallbladder to produce a cutting effect utilizing coagulation current (Fig. 6.3). Care must be taken when a pointed electrode is used in this regard because this high current density situation can lead to powerful cutting with little control. Puncture of the gallbladder could result at this point.

Coagulation or desiccation can be achieved by using the outer side of the "L" with its greater surface area and thus lower current density (Fig. 6.4). The use of the active electrode in this manner leads to slower tissue heating, controlled tissue division, and a coagulation effect as the gallbladder is freed from the liver bed. The same effect may be obtained by use of a spatula tip, or the side of a scissors blade connected to electrocautery.

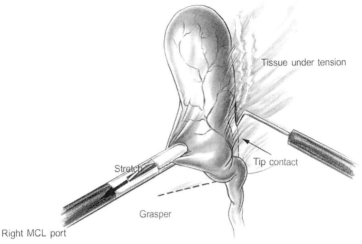

Figure 6.3. Using a coagulation current (low current and high voltage) a cutting effect can be achieved by placing the tissue on tension and using the tip of the thin wire electrode resulting in a high current density. (Source: Airan MT, Ko ST. Electrosurgery techniques of cutting and coagulation. In: Principles of Laparoscopic Surgery. Arregui ME et al. (eds.). New York: Springer–Verlag, 1995; pp. 30–35.)

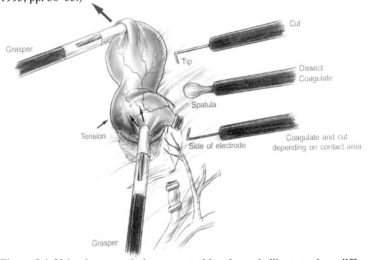

Figure 6.4. Using just coagulation current, this schematic illustrates how different tools can vary the contact area (and the contact density) to achieve cutting or coagulation. The current is constant and only the contact density changes, resulting in the "art" of bloodless electrosurgical dissection with little energy loss for coagulation. (Source: Airan MT, Ko ST. Electrosurgery techniques of cutting and coagulation. In: Principles of Laparoscopic Surgery. Arregui ME et al. (eds.). New York: Springer–Verlag, 1995; pp. 30–35.)

Fulguration is achieved with high power and low current density at the target tissue. This is done by using the outer side of the "L" or other blunt-shaped electrode, but at the same time increasing the distance from a specific bleeding point (liver bed in the example). The increased distance allows further dissipation of the current density, as the current must arc from the active electrode to the liver bed. The result is superficial tissue heating, producing a carbonized eschar and hemostatic coagulum.

These physical principles can be used to predict potential areas of danger as discussed in the next section.

Complications of monopolar electrosurgery. Early attempts to utilize electrosurgery for laparoscopic applications were associated with specific complications. To complete the monopolar circuit, electrical current will take the lowest resistance pathway back to the return electrode. This may result in injuries if current density is sufficiently high. Factors that contribute to this include:

1. Insulation failure. Laparoscopic instruments and electrosurgical electrodes are insulated to prevent electrical current from contacting surrounding structures. Even a break in insulation too small to be noted by the casual observed can allow electrical current to leak or arc to a metal trocar or to an adjacent viscus such as the colon. Current pathway and density are unpredictable in this situation. Often the tissue effects of this current are out of the visual field of the operator. This obvious source of patient injury can be minimized by routine inspection of the insulation covering all electrosurgical instruments. Current leakage detectors can be used to test adequacy of insulation. Modern ESUs have automatic leakage detection that results in system shut off.

2. Direct coupling. This phenomenon occurs when one conductive material touches or arcs to another one. Some surgeons use the direct coupling effect to coagulate tissue grasped in one instrument by touching it with a different active electrode. Caution must be employed as this potentially can lead to current directed toward nontarget structures. The laparoscopic visual field must ensure that no conductive part of any instrument is in contact with nontarget structures prior to ESU activation.

3. Capacitive coupling. This phenomenon will explain many of the inexplicable injuries reported to have occurred during laparoscopic monopolar electrosurgery. It occurs when a conductor has intact insulation but passes through an noninsulated conductor such as a metal trocar, operative laparoscope, or metal suction-irrigation tip. Electromagnetic forces produce a coupled current on the outside conductor, resulting in transfer of energy to unintended structures outside the visual field. The high voltages that are produced when activating the electrode without tissue contact or when the power setting is increased during fulgurization may produce capacitively coupled currents strong enough to produce injury. One way to limit these types of injuries is to use all-metal (conductive) trocar systems. The large conductive surface area dissipates energy via the abdominal wall to the return electrode, preventing a capacitor from forming around the metal instrument. In plastic (nonconductive) trocar systems, the trocar itself does not generate capacitively coupled currents; however, metal suction irrigation tips and operative laparoscopes do, and because the current cannot escape safely through nonconductive trocar to the abdominal wall, it must find its way back to the return electrode through nontarget tissue, potentially injuring it. In hybrid systems, such as metal trocars with plastic abdominal wall stabilizers, capacitively coupled currents on the metal trocar cannot get back to the return electrode safely via the abdominal wall and must go through another unpredictable and potentially dangerous route. Knowledge and attention to the physics behind electrosurgery help the surgeon to prevent potentially dangerous situations.

2. Argon Beam Coagulator

This modality uses electrical circuitry essentially similar to monopolar electrosurgery. The difference is that ionized pressurized argon gas completes the circuit between the active electrode and the target tissue, resulting in denaturation of surface tissue proteins and formation of a shallow eschar. At the same time, argon gas pressure displaces oxygen from the combustion area so that heat is confined to a lower temperature range. This pressurized gas beam also displaces blood and fluid away from the bleeding source and allows for more precise fulguration.

Some studies have shown that this energy source saves time and minimizes blood loss in common laparoscopic applications like cholecystectomy. The significantly limited cutting ability, lack of tactile feedback, and concerns about gas embolism limit routine use. It may have a role in advanced procedures requiring solid organ parenchyma dissection via a minimally invasive approach.

3. Ultrasonic Energy

Ultrasonically activated "scissors" and related instruments use high frequency (>20,000 Hz) to induce mechanical vibration at the cellular level. The result is a localized heat generation from friction and shear, producing a predictable pattern of thermal destruction. The first surgical use of ultrasonic mechanical energy was in the form of the **cavitational ultrasonic aspirator** (CUSA Technologies, Inc, Salt Lake City, UT), Ultrasonic waves from the CUSA (23,000 Hz) cause cavitational fragmentation of parenchyma, which the apparatus then aspirates from the field. The more resistant vessels and ducts remain and are clipped and divided. Though helpful in open solid-organ surgery, CUSA has limited laparoscopic applications.

The modern laparoscopic **ultrasonic scalpel** became available in 1992. It was developed to provide precise, hemostatic cutting and coaptive coagulation, but it also provided a lower risk of lateral thermal injury associated with electrocautery and laser. The ultrasonic scalpel functions by providing electrical energy to a piezoelectric ceramic element that expands and contracts rapidly (55,500 Hz). This mechanical energy is transduced to an imperceptibly moving blade that oscillates to produce heat secondary to friction and shear when coupled to tissue.

In general, lower power causes slower tissue heating and thus more coagulation effect. Higher power setting and rapid cutting is relatively nonhemostatic. In these regards ultrasonic energy is similar to other forms of energy-induced hemostatic modalities. Aside from the power setting, hemostatic tissue effect can be enhanced by blade configuration and tissue traction in a manner analogous to electrode design for electrosurgery (i.e., the broader the blade, the more coagulation effect).

Blade configuration has a significant effect on device performance.

>   a.   **A single blade or hook type of blade** is used in a similar fashion as the familiar monopolar electrosurgical appliances. The activation of the blade creates localized heating and hemostatic

cutting of tissues where tension and countertension (supported tissues) can be created. The cutting effect on tissue not under tension is minimal. Cutting speed is inversely proportional to hemostasis. Coagulation can be achieved with a lower power setting and utilizing the broader side of the activated blade. This allows slower tissue heating that denatures protein to form a hemostatic coagulum.

b. **Ultrasonic coagulating shears** were developed because of the difficulty of applying ultrasonic energy to unsupported tissues. The shears have one ultrasonically activated blade that can be rotated to expose the tissue to a sharp edge, a rounded edge, or a flat edge. A nonactivated pad opposes the active blade and acts as an anvil to hold tissue, enabling the creation of frictional and shearing forces necessary for cutting and coagulating.

In the cutting mode, tissue is compressed against the **sharp blade** edge and cut when the shears are activated. Hemostasis is minimal. In the hemostatic cutting/coagulation mode, moderately to highly vascular tissues are grasped to oppose tissue between one of two blade shapes—the **rounded** or the **flat** blade and the tissue pad. The frictional energy developed between the blade and pad produces coaptive coagulation of vessels in the shears. For vascularized adipose tissue, the **rounded** blade with a medium power setting usually suffices. A larger vessel of around 2 mm would require the **flat edge** of the activated blade on a low power setting to slowly coagulate the vessel. As coagulation occurs, added pressure can be applied opposing the tissue to the anvil, and this will facilitate cutting the coagulated vessel. The opened, activated blade of the co-agulating shears can also be used alone as a single blade.

In the single-blade mode, ultrasonic cutting and coagulation offer little advantage over electrosurgery for routine laparoscopic applications. The real advantage to the coagulation shears is the hemostatic division of unsupported vascular tissues with the coagulating shears. This versatile tool can grasp, bluntly dissect, sharply cut, and coagulate. This technology adds efficiency (with less instrument exchanges) and could reduce costs (by not using expensive disposable clips or staplers). This technology has enjoyed recent application during minimally invasive surgery for division of the short gastric vessels, the mesentery, or the tissues around the adrenal gland.

Because energy (heat production) is localized in ultrasonic wave production, the risk of lateral thermal injury is minimized. There are no electrical grounding devices required and coupling is not a problem. The laparoscopic use of ultrasonic energy appears to be a safe and versatile energy source that has a specialized role to the advanced laparoscopic surgeon. This role may expand as the costs for this technology decrease and the units become more widely available and more familiar to the surgical community.

4. **Laser Energy**

Laser is an acronym for **L**ight **A**mplification by **S**timulated **E**mission of **R**adiation. Laser energy is produced by the electrical stimulation of a medium that causes a change in energy states at the atomic level, leading to the organized emission of photons (parcels of light). This coherent monochromatic light (one wavelength) may be precisely delivered at high intensity. Tissue heating occurs when the cell absorbs laser light energy. This intracellular kinetic energy is stored as heat.

Many types of lasers are used in medicine. They are generally classified with regard to the portion of the electromagnetic spectrum from which the energy is emitted. **Common laser types** are listed in order from the visible spectrum (visible spectrum ends at >700 nm) to the invisible infrared portion of the monochromatic light spectrum—Argon (488 and 514 nm, emits visible blue-green light), KTP (potassium thionyl chloride, 532 nm, emits visible green light), Nd:YAG (composite crystal of neodymium and yttrium aluminum garnet, 1,064 nm, emits invisible light), and carbon dioxide (10,600 nm, invisible light from the far infrared spectrum).

The ability of laser light to heat a particular target tissue depends on the laser type or its wavelength, the amount of light encountering a given area of tissue (power density), and characteristics of the target tissue that determine energy absorption and light energy penetration. These tissue characteristics include water content and concentration of chromophores (macromolecules that absorb light) such as hemoproteins (oxy and methemoglobin) or pigments (melanin, xanthophyll).

These principles can be illustrated by the following clinical examples:

Water is a weak chromophore, and therefore visible or near-infrared laser energy penetrates easily through the cornea and lens (high water content tissues) and maximally heats (or absorbs) on the pigment-bearing retina causing potential damage. Hemoglobin is a strong chromophore for blue and green light, so argon and KTP energy is absorbed quickly in highly vascular or bleeding tissue. Small or very superficial vessels may be successfully coagulated, resulting in hemostasis. Because the energy is absorbed on the surface, larger or deeper vessels will not be coagulated, and the energy is readily absorbed and dissipated by a pool of blood or developing eschar. In the same setting, a Nd:YAG laser with its infrared (invisible) light would be more poorly absorbed by hemoglobin, allowing deeper tissue penetration and effective hemostasis. All laser energy is highly absorbed by black pigments and therefore, when an eschar forms over a bleeding site, heat will penetrate poorly, limiting photocoagulation.

These examples illustrate potential limitations and lack of versatility of the laser as a useful energy source for laparoscopic hemostasis. Laser delivery systems further compound the problem. **Contact-type fibers** transmit energy only when in contact with target tissues, whereas bare laser fibers project light energy from the end of the filament to any structure in the pathway of light. Contact fibers allow versatility by providing tactile feedback while cutting. The contact fiber tip, however, remains hot 5 to 10 seconds after removal from any tissue. A potentially hazardous situation can result if the tip should inadvertently touch nontarget tissue. **Bare fiber systems** are only hemostatic in a line beginning at the end of the fiber. In addition the bare fiber's laser energy can potentially miss the target and be transmitted beyond the target tissue and cause past-pointing injuries. Ocular safety issues are important for all personnel when operating this energy source. Cost and surgeon unfamiliarity are other issues. For all of these reasons, applications of lasers in laparoscopic surgery are limited, and more versatile energy sources like electrosurgical units and ultrasonic dissectors have become more popular. It is important to understand laser technology, however, because this potentially powerful surgical tool may have future application.

D. Laparoscopic Prevention and Management of Active Hemorrhage

Develop an operative plan that includes visualizing and identifying all structures prior to division. Avoid bluntly avulsing adhesions and adipose tissue; contained small vessels tend to retract into the divided tissue and are difficult to control. Safe application of energy to the area of the vascular structure to be divided, prior to its division, helps to prevent uncontrolled hemorrhage. If one is unsure about the vascularity of a structure, it is better to mechanically occlude it with a clip prior to its division or at least to have enough of the structure dissected free to allow manual control if subsequent bleeding is observed after division.

Even with the most careful dissection and hemostatic techniques, laparoscopic surgeons will occasionally encounter active bleeding. Often this leads to panic, culminating in conversion to an open procedure, or, worse, the dangerous and random application of energy and/or clips in the direction of the presumed bleeding point. It is far better to have a plan for bleeding before it occurs. The following are stepwise guidelines for the control of active hemorrhage. An emphasis is placed on visualization. When bleeding is encountered and not easily controlled by electrocautery, the surgeon should:

1. Try to visually identify the bleeding source without moving any instrument that is providing retraction.
2. Avoid Redout that occurs when even small amounts of blood obscure the laparoscope's view.
3. Suction with a large-bore suction cannula (10 mm, if available). Irrigation, while helpful in identifying slow bleeding sites, should be minimized in active bleeding because it adds to blood/liquid pool and potentially can splatter onto the laparoscope and limit visualization.
4. Apply a 5-mm atraumatic grasper to bleeding point when identified. A maneuver specifically for uncontrolled bleeding from the cystic artery may be useful—use the gallbladder infundibulum grasped by the instrument through the right upper quadrant (RUQ) trocar to apply direct pressure over the actively bleeding area. This allows the surgeon to stop the bleeding temporarily by tamponade, aspirate blood from the field, clean the laparoscope, and place new instruments or trocars to control the cystic artery. (This maneuver was first described by S. T. Ko and M. C. Airan, personal communication.)
5. **If the vessel cannot be controlled under direct vision in step 4, the surgeon should convert to an open procedure.**
6. If the bleeding point is controlled with a grasper, the next step is to evaluate the trocar situation. Simply put, there must be enough trocars to control the bleeding and to introduce a clip applier or suture ligature. Most commonly, a clip will be used to control the bleeding. A trocar must be available that can accommodate a clip applier, with-

out removing any instruments that are providing retraction. It is better to add a trocar, rather than to compromise by moving instruments and risk losing control of the bleeder. The added port should be placed at least 15 cm away from the bleeding site in a vector that will allow torque-free clipping and at right angles to the laparoscope (so that the placement of a clip can be easily observed).

7. Place a clip precisely on both sides of the atraumatic grasper with care not to torque or displace the controlling grasper.

8. Irrigate and evaluate. If questions remain as to whether the clips are providing secure hemostasis or whether they have injured surrounding structures, the procedure should be converted to open exploration.

E. Selected References

Airan MC, Ko ST. Electrosurgery techniques of cutting and coagulation. In: Principles of Laparoscopic Surgery. Arregui ME, Fitzgibbons RJ Jr, Katkhouda N, McKernan JB, Reich H (eds.). New York: Springer–Verlag, 1995; pp. 30–35.

Hunter JG. Laser or electrocautery for laparoscopic cholecystectomy. Am J Surg 1991;161:345–349.

Hunter JG, Trus TL. Lasers and argon beam in endoscopic surgery. In: Endosurgery. Toouli J, Gossot D, Hunter JG (eds.) New York: Churchill Livingstone, 1996, pp. 103–109.

Melzer A. Endoscopic instruments—conventional and intelligent. In: Endosurgery. Toouli J, Gossot D, Hunter JG (eds.) New York: Churchill Livingstone, 1996, pp. 69–95.

Tucker RD, Voyles CR. Laparoscopic electrosurgical complications and their prevention. AORN J 1995;62:51–71.

Voyles CR. Education and engineering solutions for potential problems with laparoscopic monopolar electrosurgery. Am J Surg 1992;164:57–62.

7. Principles of Tissue Approximation

Zoltan Szabo, Ph.D., F.A.C.S.

A. Laparoscopic Suturing and Intracorporeal Knot Tying—General Principles

While the benefits to the patient of laparoscopic suturing are considerable, the demands placed on the surgeon are high. For the patient, care is improved by a greater precision of repair, because of better access and minimized access trauma. These results are met by a surgeon who faces the technical challenge to perform intracorporeal maneuvers using optical equipment, illumination, and video that present a less than ideal visual image, and with limited movement because of the use of awkward instrumentation. These challenges can be overcome by following a mental choreography of step-by-step maneuvers and by working slowly, precisely, and patiently to master this new skill.

In laparoscopic tissue approximation, intracorporeal suturing and knot tying is the preferred method because it is highly adaptable, flexible, economical, and utilizes commercially available equipment. In deep crevices and in certain situations, intracorporeal knotting is possible but extracorporeal knotting may be preferred. In either case, learning to suture requires special attention to the setup, visual perception, hand-eye coordination, and motor skill. These factors will be described and illustrated individually in this section.

1. The **position of the surgeon** in relation to the instruments and the intended suture line determines the challenge and the result. The visual path, coaxial alignment, and triangulation of camera and operating ports are crucial aspects of the setup. The positioning of the laparoscopic and instrument ports has the same function as in open surgery. The camera is positioned midway between two instrument ports; this setup mimics the normal relationship between the eyes and two hands. The three ports should be shifted in unison when the surgeon attempts to suture in a different location. The port positioning, relative to the proposed suture line, provides the proper angle of access and a fulcrum for the instruments (Fig. 7.1).

2. **Visual perception** is a significant factor because the operative field is viewed indirectly through a closed-circuit video system. A three-chip camera and high-resolution 19-inch monitor viewed from a distance of no more than 5 to 6 feet are utilized. One of the challenges of this procedure is the magnification of a small operative field, which is inversely proportional to the magnification power and requires a proportionate reduction of the speed and range of instrument movement to maintain control. The visualization is affected by:

    a. The use of optical instrument (the laparoscope),

b. A flat two-dimensional image on the video monitor, and

c. The ability of the surgeon to adjust to the new viewing perspective.

The following factors are found with this visualization setup:

a. Details are magnified and become more appreciable, but the visual field becomes proportionately smaller and the depth of field more shallow.

b. At higher magnification the image becomes better defined with an improved 3-dimensional effect.

c. The surgeon must readjust eye-hand coordination and adapt to the speed of instrument movement.

d. Visual health, 20/20 vision, corrected by regular visits to the optometrist, and well-rested eyes can determine the success of a flawless procedure. Visual memory and a trained eye are the ideal cognitive instruments.

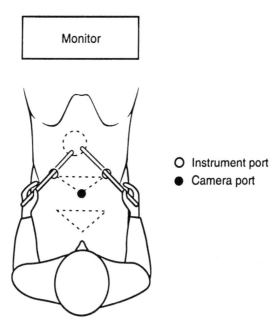

Figure 7.1. Position of the surgeon for visual path coaxial alignment. Note the triangulation of camera and operating ports, which corresponds to the triangulation of the surgeon's eyes and two hands. The surgeon, target tissue, suture line, and monitor are aligned.

3. **Eye-hand coordination:** The movements in laparoscopic surgery should be slower than in open surgery. Seeing one's movements magnified on a screen shows how quickly instruments are perceived to move, even at a normal pace. By slowing the pace of movement, control is restored and sufficient visual information is gathered, but operating time is increased. Eliminating unnecessary movements and tightly choreographing the procedure help to make the most efficient use of time. Choreographed movements increase precision and eliminate unnecessary movements. A proper formal training course and supervised practice kindle the overall success and efficiency of these procedures.

4. **Motor skill** determines the performance of a successful surgical procedure. The balance and coordination of perception, decision making, and motor skill orchestrate the ideal procedure. Because laparoscopic surgery requires adjustment to a magnified field, the motor skills that we have developed over a lifetime in everyday practice are distorted. Magnification and the use of foot-long instrumentation create an imbalance. This is compensated by a special approach that is commonly referred to as principles of microsurgery. Familiarity with open microsurgery eases the transition from open, traditional surgery to laparoscopic surgery.

B. Equipment and Instrumentation

1. **Video equipment.** High standard optical and video components are preferred due to the greater visual acuity necessary to visualize the tissue layers accurately and to track needle and suture movements.

2. **Suturing instruments** have various designs. The handle can have either a pistol grip or an in-line, coaxial handle, with or without a ring for holding it securely (the ringless handle affords greater maneuverability). The **assisting grasper,** used by the nondominant hand, handles the tissue and is more curved and pointed. The **needle driver,** used by the dominant hand, handles the needle and suture material and is short and powerful with a curved and a blunt tip.

3. **Trocars** should be slightly longer than the thickness of the abdominal wall with a preferred diameter of 5 to 10 mm. Trocars that are too long interfere with instrument mobility and function by preventing the opening of the instrument jaws and minimizing movement in the abdomen.

4. The geometry of the **needle tip** controls the characteristics of the tissue penetration and the size and shape of the tunnel cut. To minimize tissue trauma, the ease of penetration is important in laparoscopic surgery. Stronger, sturdier needles are required to penetrate thicker tissue layers; smaller, thinner needles are required to penetrate delicate tissues. A needle tip with a high tapering ratio or a "taper cut" tip will penetrate tissue layers more readily.

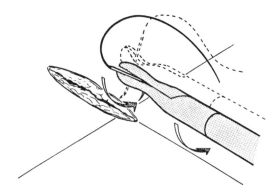

Figure 7.2. Pushing the needle head on against tissue resistance.

5. The selection of **suture material** is based upon favorable tissue response, handling characteristics, and visibility. It is chosen for its particular attributes such as absorbability, strength, and tissue reaction. Because visibility is limited in laparoscopic surgery, pitch black or fluorescent white sutures are preferred over colorless suture. The handling characteristics of the 2-0 and 3-0 silk is optimal for folding and bending memory. Alternatives such as monofilament polypropylene, polydiaxanone, and nylon can be too stiff to readily knot intracorporeally.

6. **Needle handling and passage.** Bicurve geometry affects the handling and scooping characteristics of the needle and can be easily adapted to particular tissues and their access requirements. In difficult situations it is beneficial to take the time necessary to reexamine simple movements to efficiently execute them. Entrance and exit bites and knot tying are the main movements repeated during tissue approximation. In this technique, the needle will follow the tip in passing through tissue layers with the least amount of trauma and effort if the tissue resistance, needle tip, grasping point, and direction of force are assembled on the same axis. If the needle is pushed in any angle other than 90 degrees, head-on against tissue resistance (Fig. 7.2), the driving force will to deflect the needle and turn in the jaws of the needle holder. A high level of concentration is integral to performing even simple needle driving maneuvers when working in a magnified field. Indirect tissue manipulation complicates this matter further. In the main function of needle driving, taking the entrance and exit bites, double indirect manipulation comes into play. The hand holds the instrument handle and the instrument tip grasps the needle. Instrument movement and special needle-driving techniques need to be employed to accommodate the necessary needle control. There are

limitations to the instrument approach because complicated equipment such as single-use needle holders, stiff opening, closing power, and other problems are presented. The strength of the needle holder, in particular the locking and unlocking maneuver, can inadvertently jar the instrument and tear the tissue, as in thin-walled vascular structures. To avoid this situation, it is advised to develop and learn needle-driving techniques that depend more on skill than on gadgetry.

C. Knot-Tying

Both intracorporeal and extracorporeal knot-tying techniques have an important role in laparoscopic surgery. For most purposes, intracorporeal knot-tying is preferred. **Intracorporeal knots** are placed by a process that virtually duplicates the methods used during open surgical procedures. Intracorporeal tying is faster and uses less suture. **Extracorporeal tying** use a special knot that is designed to slip one way but not the other. Both methods are illustrated in Figs. 7.3 and 7.4.

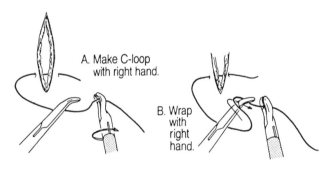

Figure 7.3. **Square and surgeon's knot**. A. **Overhand Flat Knot.** (1) Starting position: Create a C-loop as the right instrument reaches over to the left side of the field, grabs the long tail and brings it back to the right, below the short tail. This loop must be in a horizontal plane, or else it will be difficult to wrap the thread. If a monofilament material is used, the right instrument can rotate the threat counterclockwise until it lies flat against the tissue. The right instrument holds the long tail and the left instrument is placed over the loop. The short tail should be long enough so that it cannot be pulled out accidentally, but not so long that its end is hidden. Use a large loop to allow ample space for both instruments, moving slowly, when retrieving the short tail. Use the right instrument to wrap the long tail around the stationary tip of the left instrument. Rotate the right instrument forward to create an arch in the suture, assisting the wrapping motion. Keep the jaws of the instruments retrieving the short tail closed, until ready to grasp the tail. In the inset, the right instrument is shown wrapping the suture around the left instrument twice, creating a surgeon's knot.

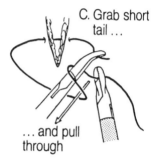

C. Grab short
tail …

… and pull
through

(2) Grasping the short tail: Both instruments should move together toward the short tail. This prevents a tight noose from forming around the instrument, making it difficult to reach the short tail. Grasp the short tail near the end to avoid creating an extra loop when pulling the suture through.

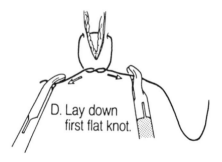

D. Lay down
first flat knot.

(3) Completing the first flat knot: Pull the short tail through the loop and adjust it so that there is an equal length left. The end will be hard to find if the tail is too long. Pull the two instruments in opposite directions, parallel to the stitch. The left instrument then drops the short tail, and the right instrument keeps its grasp on the long tail. The inset illustrates the surgeon's knot that has been created.

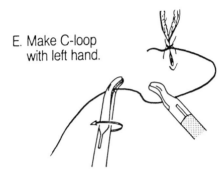

E. Make C-loop
with left hand.

Figure 7.3. B. **Second opposing flat knot.** (1) Creating the reversed C-loop, wrapping the thread, and grasping the short tail: The reversed C loop is created as the right instrument is brought to the left side of the field under the short tail, and rotated clockwise 180 degrees. The right instrument transfers the long tail to the left instrument. The right instrument is placed over the reversed C-loop and the left instrument wraps the thread around the right instrument. The tips of both instruments are moved together in unison toward the short tail, which is grasped with the right instrument.

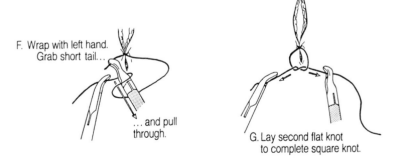

F. Wrap with left hand.
Grab short tail...

... and pull
through.

G. Lay second flat knot
to complete square knot.

(2) Completing the second knot: Pull the short tail through the loop, and then pull both tails in opposite directions, parallel to the stitch, with equal tension. Verify that the knot is configured correctly as the knot cinches up.

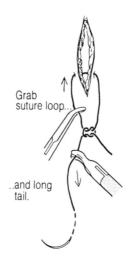

Grab
suture loop...

..and long
tail.

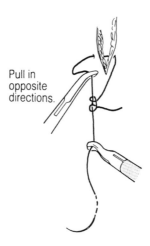

Pull in
opposite
directions.

Figure 7.3. C. **Slip knot for the square knot.** (1) Starting position and pulling: To convert the square knot (locking configuration) to a slip knot (sliding configuration), both instruments must grasp the suture on the same (ipsilateral) side. One instrument grasps the thread outside the knot and the other in the suture loop (between the knot and the tissue). Both instruments pull in opposite directions (perpendicular to the stitch). A snapping or popping sensation can often be felt and the short tail may flip up. The knot looks like a pretzel. If the conversion does not occur after a few attempts, try the maneuver on the other side of the knot. Conversion is easier on monofilament suture.

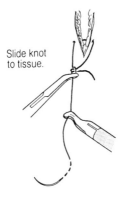

Slide knot
to tissue.

(2) Pushing the slip knot: The right instrument maintains its grasp on the tail
and pulls tightly. The left instrument pushes the knot closer to the tissue by
sliding on this tail.

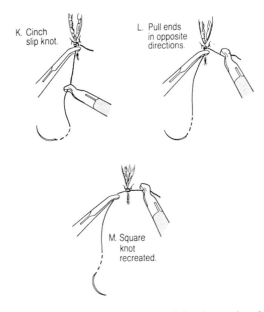

K. Cinch
   slip knot.

L. Pull ends
   in opposite
   directions.

M. Square
   knot
   recreated.

(3) Cinching down. Cinch down the slip knot until the tissue edges have been
approximated to the desired tension. Recenter the knot and recheck the tension.
Reconvert the slip knot to a square knot before making additional overhand
throws. Both instruments regrasp the tails in opposite directions, parallel to the
stitch in the same way as when the square knot was originally tied. An additional overhand knot is necessary on top and is tied in the same manner as the
first throw [Fig. 7.3.A(1)].

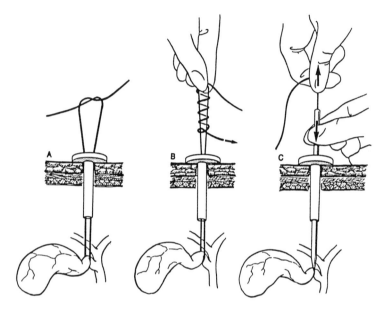

Figure 7.4. **Extracorporeal knot.** Bring a long suture into the laparoscopic field, leaving its tail outside of the port. Place the stitch, then bring the needle end out through the same port. Create a Roeder knot by tying an overhand knot and then wrapping the suture tail back around both arms of the loop three times. Lock the suture by bringing the tail back through the large loop, between the last two twists of the wrap. Slide the knot down with a plastic applicator rod or a knot pusher.

An **extracorporeal knot** is tied externally and slid down to the tissue with the aid of knot pusher. This method requires long threads and while extracorporeal knotting appears to be a simpler approach, it requires a systematic and careful application to avoid traumatizing the tissues and contaminating or damaging the suture.

The Roeder knot is widely used in laparoscopic surgery for extracorporeal tying. It was developed around the turn of the century and introduced to laparoscopic practice before intracorporeal knotting was developed. This is the knot used in commercially available pre-tied suture ligatures. This method is described and illustrated in Fig. 7.4. Another method of extracorporeal knot tying uses a modified square knot, tied extracorporeally.

D. Suturing Techniques

Suturing and intracorporeal knotting is the final challenge following a laparoscopic procedure, testing the surgeon's skill and endurance. A surgeon's skill level can be measured to some degree, e.g., the ability to tie a square knot correctly in 30 seconds or less. These techniques are a challenge that can be achieved after 20 to 40 hours of formal training with confidence and skill (as observed by the author). Intracorporeal knotting can be the starting and finishing point of continuous and interrupted suture lines.

Tissues should be prepared and positioned in anticipation of either interrupted, continuous, or a combination of both types of sutures, so that minimal tension exists.

1. **Interrupted suturing:** When constructing a linear suture line, the factors that are involved in creating entrance and exit bites include length of incision or laceration, type of tissue layers to be approximated and their function, needle and thread combination selection, and length of suture.

   a. Place the instrument port positions so that the laparoscope port is inline with the needle driver, essentially parallel with the suture line, and the assisting grasper port is 45 to 90 degrees apart.

   b. Place the needle perpendicular to the suture line, and the ports should be at least 6 inches apart. The entrance and exit scooping motion should follow a 3 o'clock to 9 o'clock direction relative to the surgeon's frontal plane.

   c. Interrupted stitches can be utilized with a suspension slip-knot technique if there is tension in the tissues or poor visibility. Evenly spaced stitches approximate the tissue precisely without tension.

2. **Continuous suturing:** This type of suture is more rapid, yet it is more difficult to accomplish correctly. This technique begins and ends with an anchoring knot, the last of which can be tied to the loop of the last stitch. The tissue edges must be identified by carefully shifting the tension on the suture loops as the approximation continues.

3. **Suture choice** is a necessary component since monofilament and braided materials behave differently. Monofilament is stiff, springy, and slides smoothly through tissue. Braided material can drag through the tissue, lock unexpectedly, and can be more cumbersome to work with since each stitch must be taut before proceeding to the next.

4. **Anastomosis:** Laparoscopic ductal anastomosis is a challenge that can be met using methods from microvascular anastomoses and from duplicating open surgical techniques. It can be performed end-to-end, end-to-side, or side-to-side.

   a. End-to-end anastomosis is the preferred method for approximating ducts of equal caliber and wall thickness. The number of stitches, their configuration, and the size of the bites are calculated, depending on the function of the structure. Either interrupted or continuous sutures could be used. Interrupted sutures provide better precision and control; continuous sutures are performed more rapidly but are less forgiving.

b. Conduits with different lumina and wall thickness can be joined with end-to-side anastomosis in a less invasive procedure.

c. Side-to-side anastomosis is a practical method for conduits that lie side by side. This method of approximation is similar to the end-to-side anastomosis.

E. Tissue Gluing

Glue can be used in combination with other techniques as an aid that provides a hemostatic or hydrostatic seal. Fibrin and other glues have been used but have never quite gained popularity for tissue approximation as they need anchoring or primary stitches to secure the tissue edges. As the boundaries of laparoscopic surgery expand, there will be more possibilities for and developments in tissue approximation. However, the traditional concept of hand suturing and square/surgeon's knot method of securing two suture ends will undoubtedly remain the most popular as it has already endured centuries of trials.

F. Stapling

As a method of tissue approximation, stapling borrows the same principle as used in open surgery but is technically more demanding and more expensive. Some general principles were discussed in Chapter 6, and details are given in sections II-IX where procedures in which stapling is routinely used are described.

Despite the use of staplers in laparoscopic procedures, the ability for surgeons to place stitches and tie knots should not be compromised. Staplers may lead to complications and the surgeon must be aware of tissue ischemia if any procedure is inadequate. Proper mastery and knowledge of these techniques with many prior successful practice runs is essential for their use.

G. Selected References

Bowyer DW, Moran ME, Szabo Z. Laparoscopic suturing in urology: a model for vesicourethral anastomosis following radical prostatectomy. Min Invas Ther 1993;4(2):165–170.

Buncke HJ, Szabo Z. Introduction to microsurgery. In: Grabb WC, Smith JW, eds. A Concise Guide to Plastic Surgery. Boston: Little, Brown, 1980;653–659.

Cushieri A, Szabo Z. Tissue Approximation in Endoscopic Surgery. Oxford: Isis Medical Media, 1995.

Guthrie CC. Blood vessel surgery and its application: a reprint. Pittsburgh: University of Pittsburgh, 1959;1–69.

Szabo Z. Laparoscopic suturing and tissue approximation. In: Hunter JG, Sackier JM, eds. Minimally Invasive Surgery. 1993;141–155.

Wolfe BM, Szabo Z, Moran ME, Chan P, Hunter JG. Training for minimally invasive surgery: need for surgical skills. Surg Endosc 1993;93–95.

8. Principles of Specimen Removal

Daniel J. Deziel, M.D.

A. General Considerations

A major advantage of laparoscopic surgery, small incisions, must be balanced with the need to remove and preserve specimens that may be larger than the laparoscopic port site. Specimens vary in dimensions, physical characteristics (hollow versus solid), and ease of extraction. Special considerations apply to specimens that may be infected or malignant, where improper removal may lead to wound infection or tumor dissemination. The best method for removal depends on the size, location, and nature of the specimen and whether there is a need to preserve the specimen intact for pathologic evaluation.

B. Routes of Specimen Removal

Ideally the site selected for specimen removal should be along the path of least resistance that produces the least pain, prevents contamination, and provides the best cosmesis. If a specimen cannot be removed from the abdominal cavity immediately after it has been resected, it must be secured in a position that will permit ready identification and retrieval later. Several potential routes for removal of abdominal and pelvic specimens are listed in Table 8.1 and will be considered individually here.

Table 8.1. Routes for removal of abdominal and pelvic specimens

- Port sites
- Separate abdominal wall incisions
- Transanal (if colon resection performed)
- Transvaginal (via culpotomy incision)

1. **Small specimens** can be removed directly through an appropriate cannula (usually 10 mm or larger) with or without a reducing sleeve. Use a toothed grasper to secure the specimen as it is retrieved under direct laparoscopic visualization and control. Open the valve mechanism of the cannula to allow the specimen to pass through unimpeded, if a reducing sleeve is not used.

2. Specimens originally **larger than the size of the cannula** can be retrieved **at the port site** by several methods:

    a. Reduce the size of the specimen while it is still within the peritoneal cavity; that is, remove contents of hollow structures (fluid, stones) or cut up solid structures. This technique permits removal without enlarging the incision. The major disadvantages include the risk of losing portions of the specimen and contamination of the peritoneal cavity. This method may be appropriate for the removal of specimens such as lymph node packets and benign solid tumors of moderate size.

b. Exchange the existing cannula for a **larger cannula** at the port site (20–40 mm), by placing it over a blunt probe with a tapered introducer. This method protects the wound from direct contact with the specimen. A major disadvantage is that the specialized cannulae are not always available. This method is sometimes used for removal of specimens such as an inflamed appendix, gallbladder, fallopian tube, and ovary.

c. **Exteriorize portions of the specimen** and then remove the contents so that the specimen can be pulled through the port site. This is most commonly used for removal of the gallbladder following laparoscopic cholecystectomy. Hold the specimen firmly against the end of the cannula as both are pulled out together under laparoscopic visualization. Grasp a portion of the gallbladder outside of the abdomen with clamps and open the gallbladder. Aspirate fluid, and remove stones (fragmenting them if necessary) with stone forceps or ring forceps. This technique avoids enlarging the incision and requires no special equipment. However, it risks wound contamination and is tedious if the stones are multiple or large.

d. **Enlarge the incision at a port site**. This is perhaps the simplest, most efficient, and most commonly used method in many circumstances. It works particularly well at umbilical or other midline port sites since only a single fascial layer requires division. Either stretch the fascia or elevate it with a right-angled clamp and divide it with scissors or a scalpel. Perform this maneuver under direct laparoscopic visual control, with the specimen held in a relaxed manner (**not** taut against the abdominal wall) to avoid puncturing the specimen. This is frequently the best method of removing a large, stone-filled gallbladder. This is also the typical method for removing larger organs such as the colon and spleen.

The length of incision necessary in these cases varies but is usually only several centimeters. When the port site incision is not midline, use a muscle spreading technique to avoid dividing abdominal wall musculature. During colectomy the colon is often exteriorized through an extended port site incision prior to complete resection. After resection the anastomosis can be constructed extracorporally. These are considered "laparoscopically assisted" operations.

A disadvantage of this technique is the loss of pneumoperitoneum that occurs during specimen extraction. To reestablish the pneumoperitoneum, completely close the incision if that port site is no longer needed. Alternatively, close or tighten the fascia around a cannula. Another disadvantage of incision enlargement for specimen retrieval is the increased discomfort that patients may have at that site. Regardless, this is often the most practical method.

3. **Separate abdominal wall incision.** In some situations it may be most practical to remove the specimen through a separate abdominal wall incision that does not incorporate any of the existing port sites. These incisions can generally be limited to a few centimeters in length, and a muscle-splitting technique can be used for nonmidline sites. Examples of this technique include removal of the right or left colon through transverse incisions lateral to the rectus in the right or left abdomen, respectively, removal of the sigmoid colon through a suprapubic or left lower abdominal incision, and removal of an intact spleen through a low midline or Pfannenstiel incision. During colon resection the site of incision can be gauged by holding the mobilized specimen up to the abdominal wall; this location may or may not correspond to an existing cannula site.

4. **Transanal route.** Transanal extraction has been used for some laparoscopic low anterior colon resections. This route can be considered when the lower limit of transection is near or below the pelvic brim and the specimen is not too bulky. Place the specimen in a bag. Slowly dilate the anus and pass a ring forceps or similar instrument transanally. Grasp the bag and gently pull it through the rectal stump and anus. During laparoscopic abdominoperineal resection the specimen is readily delivered through the perineal incision in a similar manner.

5. **Transvaginal route.** Another alternative to abdominal incision for intact removal of larger specimens is an incision in the posterior vaginal fornix (cul de sac), which is termed culdotomy or posterior colpotomy. This has most frequently been used for removal of ovarian masses or the uterus during laparoscopic-assisted vaginal hysterectomy and occasionally for other solid organs.

C. Retrieval Bags

Use of a specimen retrieval bag minimizes the risk of contamination and specimen loss. This is particularly important when the specimen may be malignant, infected, leaking or friable. Commercially manufactured bags and retrieval devices are available for this purpose but sterile gloves, glove fingers, condoms, or other containers may suffice. The important features to consider in selecting a retrieval bag are its strength, size, aperture, maneuverability, ease of deployment and retrieval, and porosity. Bags are typically made of polyurethane or of nylon with a polyurethane coating. Nylon bags are more resistant to tearing and are preferred for removing larger specimens that must be fragmented in the bag, such as the spleen or kidney.

The precise technique of specimen retrieval in a bag varies according to the specific specimen and bag employed but there are several common principles.

1. **Bag insertion:** Tightly roll the bag and insert it through an appropriately located cannula. Depending upon the size of the bag, either insert it directly through the cannula, through a reducing sleeve, or through the port incision with the cannula removed. A special two-pronged introducer facilitates insertion of larger bags. Coat the outside of the bag with water-soluble lubricant to make it slide easily

2. **Bag deployment:** Pull the bag gently out of the cannula or sleeve. Use two graspers, placed through other cannula sites, to unroll it. Grasp the edges of the bag and open the mouth by pulling in opposite directions. Use a third instrument, if necessary, to help open the bag by moving along the front edge in a circular direction. A commonly used commercial device consists of a bag with a flexible metal ring at its mouth, contained in a plastic sheath. The sheath is introduced through a cannula and the device deployed by advancing a plunger. A flexible ring automatically holds the bag open. Once the specimen is contained, a ring is pulled to close the bag.

3. **Specimen entrapment:** This is generally the most difficult step, particularly for large organs. Hold the mouth of the bag open with two, or preferably three (to allow triangulation of the opening), graspers. Manipulate the open bag so it lies behind the specimen, with the mouth facing the surgeon. Allow sufficient working distance for comfortable manipulation. For example, when retrieving the spleen, the closed end of the bag is positioned toward the diaphragm. Advance the grasper holding the specimen all the way to the depth of the bag. The specimen should enter the bag, and the entire specimen must fit within the bag prior to closure. Manipulating large organs can be difficult and care must be taken not to rupture the specimen. Wherever possible, grasp connective tissue around the organ rather than the organ itself. In some instances it may be useful to leave a portion of the organ attached (for example, ligaments attaching the spleen to the diaphragm) and to divide this attachment only when the rest of the specimen has been maneuvered into the bag. Proper positioning of the patient may also facilitate entrapment (i.e., Trendelenburg, reverse Trendelenburg, rotation).

4. **Bag closure:** Commercial bags are usually equipped with a drawstring that must be tightened. Close small plastic bags, glove fingers, or condoms with a preformed endoscopic ligature.

5. **Bag extraction:** Keep the bag under constant laparoscopic visual control as it is pulled to the cannula site. Withdraw the bag and cannula (if still in place) through the abdominal wall as a unit. Small bags may be directly removed through a 10- to 12-mm port site. Usually the bag is partially pulled through the abdominal wall and secured externally. The bag and contained specimen are removed by either enlarging the port site, as described above, or by reducing the specimen in size by fragmentation (for example, spleen or kidney) or removing portions (for example, gallstones). Resist the temptation to pull hard, and use care to avoid puncturing or tearing the bag.

D. Specimen Fragmentation/Morcellation

Morcellation or fragmentation is an appropriate method for removing large solid specimens when it is not necessary to preserve the gross architecture of the organ for pathology. Classic examples include the spleen removed for immune thrombocytopenic purpura or the kidney removed for benign parenchymal disease. Fragmentation is contraindicated for the removal of known or potentially malignant tumors.

Place the specimen in a sturdy, nonporous retrieval bag. Partially externalize the bag and open it. Break up the specimen and remove it piecemeal using ring forceps, clamps, suction catheters, or a commercial tissue morcellator. Maintain direct laparoscopic visualization of the sac and take care to avoid rupture of the sac and peritoneal spillage.

E. Complications of Specimen Retrieval

Attention to the technical details of specimen retrieval is critical to avoidance of some potentially vexing and devastating problems. The principal complications related to removal of laparoscopic specimens are self evident and include:

1. **Internal specimen loss.** This is less likely to happen if adequate time and care are taken during removal. Confining manipulations to a region of the abdomen where the specimen can be easily retrieved if dropped, or tagging it with a long suture, are two precautions that can safeguard against loss if the specimen is dropped.

2. **Specimen rupture** (consequences of which can include infection, splenosis, tumor dissemination, and inadequate pathologic assessment). This can be avoided by individualizing the technique of specimen removal, considering the size of the specimen and its physical characteristics, and handling it gently.

3. **Wound infection.** Grossly infected specimens (for example, a perforated appendix) should be placed in specimen bags rather than pulled through the abdominal wall.

4. **Tumor implantation at port site.** The mechanism of this complication is not fully understood. Common sense suggests that malignant or potentially malignant specimens (for example, thick-walled gallbladders) should be placed in specimen bags rather than pulled directly through the abdominal wall.

5. **Visceral injury** (due to entrapment during extraction). This can be avoided by maintaining constant visual laparoscopic control. Large specimen bags may obscure visualization of the area behind the bag and extra care must be taken during bag extraction. Awareness of the potential for this complication, and a bit of extra vigilance, should prevent its occurrence.

6. **Incisional hernia.** All trocar sites must be closed in an appropriate fashion to avoid this complication.

F. Selected References

MacFadyen Jr BV, Ponsky JL, eds. Operative Laparoscopy and Thoracoscopy. Philadelphia: Lippincott-Raven, , 1996.

Petelin JB. Technologies and techniques for telescopic surgery. In: Hunter JG, Sackier JM, eds. Minimally Invasive Surgery. New York: McGraw-Hill, 1993.

Way LW, Bhoyrul S, Mori T, eds. Fundamentals of Laparoscopic Surgery. New York: Churchill Livingstone, 1996.

9. Documentation

Daniel J. Deziel, M.D.

A. General Considerations

Modern video technology converts the optical image from a laparoscopic lens to an electronic signal that can be displayed, transmitted, and recorded. Electronic images can be recorded in a variety of formats either as videos or as still images. The value of these recorded images lies in the ability to subsequently communicate information for clinical, scientific, educational, and medicolegal purposes. New formats for video imaging and laparoscopic documentation will continue to become available as technology develops. Cost, equipment, storage requirements, and general availability of a particular format are important practical considerations.

B. Components of Video Imaging

Important components of a video image include luminance (brightness), resolution, color, light sensitivity, signal to noise ratio, and image size.

The development of the Hopkins rod lens system used in modern laparoscopes was key to allowing photographic and video documentation. Light is transmitted through a series of glass rods with lenses at the ends rather than through air as in previous lens systems. This provides improved light transmission with higher resolution, a wider viewing angle, and a larger image. The problem of insufficient illumination for laparoscopic documentation was overcome by the development of the high intensity (300 W) xenon lamp, which is now the standard light source. Newer light sources have been developed for use with cameras that are more light sensitive. Light is transmitted from the lamp to the laparoscope through cables. There are two types of cables: fiberoptic and fluid. Fiberoptic cables are flexible but do not transmit a precise light spectrum. Fluid cables transmit more light and a complete spectrum but are more rigid. Fluid cables require soaking for sterilization and cannot be gas sterilized.

The basis of laparoscopic cameras is the solid-state silicon computer chip or CCD (charge-coupled device). This consists of an array of light-sensitive silicon elements. Silicon emits an electrical charge when exposed to light. These charges can be amplified, transmitted, displayed, and recorded. Each silicon element contributes one unit (referred to as a pixel) to the total image. The resolution or clarity of the image depends upon the number of pixels or light receptors on the chip. Standard cameras in laparoscopic use contain 250,000 to 380,000 pixels. Of course the clarity of the image eventually displayed or recorded will also depend on the resolution capability of the monitor and the recording medium. Standard consumer-grade video monitors have 350 lines of horizontal resolution; monitors with about 700 lines are preferred for laparoscopic surgery.

The importance of the operator and of maintenance personnel for obtaining a quality video image cannot be underestimated. Besides assuring proper electronics, the operator must attend to mechanical details such as lens cleaning, focusing, and framing. No improvements in electronic signal processing can overcome the limitation of a scope that is damaged or a lens that is fogged, smeared, or out of focus. The ocular (proximal) and objective (distal) lenses of the laparoscope as well as the camera lens must be checked. The objective lens can be cleaned internally with irrigation and externally by wiping with cotton gauze soaked in warm water (not saline) and then wiping with dry gauze before applying anti-fogging solution. It is imperative that the cannulas are clean and that no tissue is in the way during introduction of the scope.

C. Types of Video Signals

The video systems used in laparoscopic surgery and elsewhere grew out of television broadcast technology. Television analog systems read and transmit an image using scanning lines. In digital systems, a row of silicon elements on the CCD chip replaces the scanning line. The number of scanning lines represents the number of lines of information that can be transmitted and displayed on a monitor. The standard NTSC (National Television Systems Committee) format used in North America and Japan consists of 525 lines scanning at a rate of 30 frames per second. Systems used in other parts of the world (PAL or Phase Alternating Line and SECAM or Sèquentiel Couleur et Mèmoire) use 625 lines at 25 frames per second. Computer-enhanced high-definition television (HDTV) systems that are under development may have more than 1,000 scanning lines and can incorporate 5 or 6 times more information than standard television and video formats. By comparison, the human eye can distinguish the equivalent of some 1600 scan lines and the resolution of 35mm photographic film is about 2300 scan lines.

Standard television and simple video signals are **composite** signals, meaning that all of the image information is carried over a single channel. These signals are subject to a certain amount of degradation during transmission and processing. Dividing the signal into **components** that are transmitted over separate channels provides a higher quality image. Super VHS (S-VHS or S-Video) splits the signal into separate components for brightness (luminance=Y) and color (chrominance=C). An RGB signal divides the color into red, green, and blue components that are transmitted over separate channels. A fourth channel carries brightness information. Modern laparoscopic cameras have multiple output slots on the camera box that permit the operator to select the type of signal output. Obviously the monitor or recording equipment receiving the signal must be compatible in order to reconstruct the information (Fig. 9.1).

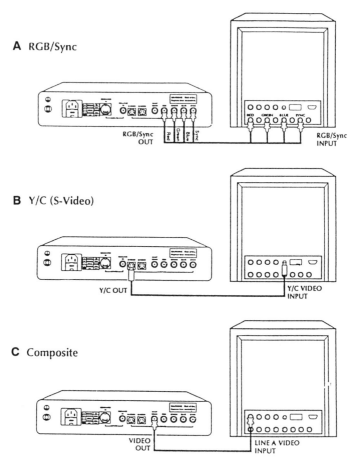

Figure 9.1. Signal output from the camera box and signal input to the monitor or recording equipment must be compatible. (From SAGES Video Production Guidelines.)

Image quality can also be improved by digital processing of the CCD signal. The original image is captured as an analog signal. This signal is transmitted as a continuous electronic waveform that is subject to interference and distortion. Digital systems convert the analog signal into binary code, which better preserves the original information and lessens distortion during reconstruction. Unlike analog images, digital recordings retain the quality of the original when duplicated or copied. Digital recordings can also be enhanced and modified for other applications in ways that analog images cannot.

D. Recording Media

There are multiple options for documenting laparoscopic procedures as either continuous recordings or still pictures. In this era of electronic data management the present state of the art would be to digitalize images for storage on magnetic or optical disks. For practical purposes most documentation is done using videotapes or still video printers.

Videotapes obtained by attaching a videocassette recorder to the imaging system have become the standard for continuous documentation. A variety of videotape formats are available; $\frac{1}{2}''$ VHS and 8mm are acceptable but inferior in quality to $\frac{1}{2}''$ S-VHS, $\frac{3}{4}''$ U-Matic, Betacam, and high 8 mm. Digital video recorders provide higher quality than analog recordings but are more expensive and to date not as widely used. Although there are many choices of videotape format, realistic considerations such as cost, equipment, widespread availability and anticipation of changing technology generally limit selection. $\frac{1}{2}''$ S-VHS or VHS are standard for most applications. The Y/C component signal of the S-VHS format provides better resolution than the single-channel composite signal of VHS systems. S-VHS machines can also record and play either S-VHS or conventional VHS tapes.

The best quality still images are photographs taken through a 35mm camera attached directly to the eyepiece of the laparoscope. Unfortunately, this method can be inconvenient. Still images are usually obtained from commercially available video printers or slide makers that receive the electronic image from the camera. Laparoscopic images can also be put on a disk recorder and stored on optical (laser) or floppy disk for later retrieval.

The way in which the video recording equipment is connected to the imaging system is important. If the camera box has multiple outlets for component signals (Y/C or S-Video, RGB), then both the recorder and the primary monitor can be hooked up to the camera directly (Fig. 9.2). For example, one Y/C port can be connected to the recorder and the second Y/C outlet or the RGB outlet (depending upon the camera control unit) can be connected to the monitor. This is a parallel arrangement and neither the recorded image or the image displayed on the monitor will be degraded. In a serial hookup the camera, recorder, and monitor are connected in a line. If the signal goes to the recorder first and to the monitor second, the image on the monitor may be somewhat degraded. If the signal goes to the monitor first, the quality of the recorded image will not be as high. As the complexity of the system increases, problems due to loose or incorrect connections become more likely. Chapter 1, Equipment Setup and Troubleshooting, and the SAGES Laparoscopy Troubleshooting Guide provide helpful information for problem solving.

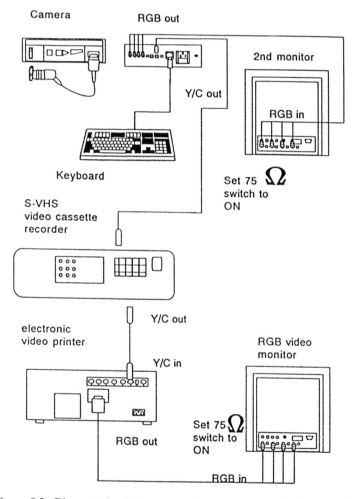

Figure 9.2. Diagram showing one way to connect several documentation sources and monitors. (From Berci G, Paz-Partlow M. Video imaging. In: MacFayden BV, Ponsky JL, eds. Operative Laparoscopy and Thoracoscopy. Philadelphia: Lippincott-Raven, 1996. Used with permission.)

E. Selected References

Berci G, Paz-Partlow M. Video imaging. In: MacFayden BV, Ponsky JL, eds. Operative Laparoscopy and Thoracoscopy. Philadelphia: Lippincott-Raven, 1996.

Cartmill J, Aamodt D. Video systems in laparoscopy. In: Graber JN, Schultz LS, Pietrafitta JJ, Hickok DF, eds. Laparoscopic Abdominal Surgery. New York: McGraw-Hill, 1993.

Szabo Z, SAGES Educational Resources Committee. Video Production Guidelines. Society of American Gastrointestinal Endoscopic Surgeons, 1996.

10.1. Special Problems: Massive Obesity

Cornelius Doherty, M.D., F.A.C.S.

A. Physiologic Alterations Associated with Massive Obesity

Massively obese patients should increasingly be considered acceptable candidates for basic and advanced minimal access laparoscopic procedures as technology and surgical skills improve. Massive obesity denotes a body mass index of 40 or greater, where body mass index is calculated as weight in kilograms divided by the square of the height in meters (kg/m^2).

As the body mass index increases, pathophysiological alterations add complexity and risk to laparoscopic surgery. Central or android fat distribution magnifies these alterations, which include thick anterior abdominal wall, large fatty liver, massive omentum, prominence of the colon, and increased intra-abdominal pressure. Massively obese patients have a fat mass that is 60% or more of their ideal body mass. The cardiovascular and respiratory demands necessary to support such a fat mass must not be jeopardized by anesthesia and pneumoperitoneum. Intensive monitoring and important perioperative care enhancements are required for a safe and effective outcome. Physiologic changes that accompany morbid obesity are summarized in Table 10.1.1.

Table 10.1.1. Pathophysiologic alterations of morbid obesity that correlate with excess body weight

• Significantly increased total blood volume
• Increased cardiac output
• Increased oxygen cost of breathing compared to the increased mechanical work of breathing
• Decreased pulmonary compliance

Simply placing a morbidly obese patient supine significantly impairs a number of cardiopulmonary parameters. The changes that occur when a morbidly obese patient moves from the sitting to the supine position are detailed in Table 10.1.2.

In addition to the changes summarized in Table 10.1.2, the pulmonary closing volume (CV) becomes a greater proportion of the pulmonary functional residual capacity (FRC). Changes in pulmonary closing volume result in small-airway closure in the supine position. Mechanical ventilation using appropriate ventilatory patterns can minimize the work of breathing, improve oxygenation through improving the closing volume–to–functional residual capacity ratio, and reduce the tendency toward pulmonary congestion found in massively obese patients when supine.

Table 10.1.2. Hemodynamic changes associated with the change from sitting to supine position, morbid obesity

• 11% ↑ in oxygen consumption (Vo_2)
• 35.5% ↑ in cardiac output (CO)
• 35.8% ↑ in cardiac index (CI)
• 17.85% ↓ in arteriovenous oxygen difference
• 31% ↑ in mean pulmonary artery pressure (PAP)
• 44% ↑ in pulmonary wedge pressure (PAWP)
• 21.5% ↓ in peripheral resistance (PR)
• 6% ↓ in heart rate {HR)
• 17.7% ↑ in venous admixture (Q_s/Q_t)

B. Measures to Decrease Risk of Complications in Morbidly Obese Patients Undergoing Laparoscopy

When a massively obese patient is in the supine position, the heart responds to the increased preload and increased work of breathing by increasing output. This response minimizes the rise in filling pressure and resulting pulmonary congestion and simultaneously masks the effects of increased intrapulmonary shunting on arterial oxygenation.

Morbidly obese patients are at higher risk of thromboembolic complications in the perioperative period. Several measures can be taken to minimize these risk. These are summarized in Table 10.1.3.

Table 10.1.3. Measures to decrease risk of thromboembolic phenomena in the severely obese patient

• Preoperative hydration with dextrose and water to overcome the hypercoagulation associated with mobilized free fatty acids that occurs in the massively obese during fasting
• Low-dose heparin
• No venipunctures of the lower extremities
• External venous compression stockings that overcome stasis and venous return problems that accompany pneumoperitoneum and reversed Trendelenburg positioning (Venodyne, Division of Advanced Instruments, Inc., Norwood, MA, manufactures a comfort lined compression sleeve designed especially for the morbidly obese; the extra-large size accommodates a calf circumference of 20 to 24 inches or 50 to 61 centimeters)

Table 10.1.3. continued

• Ambulation soon after operation and frequently throughout the postoperative period

C. Technical Considerations for Laparoscopic Surgery in the Morbidly Obese

1. **Production of pneumoperitoneum and general considerations:** The open Hasson technique of trocar placement has disadvantages in the massively obese. The depth of the wound requires retraction that interferes with direct vision and frequently widens the wound, making it very difficult to maintain a tight seal. The trauma associated with the retraction of the wound plus the avascular adipose tissue predispose to infection. A Veress needle technique in the left upper quadrant has the advantages of less trauma, better seal, and equal safety. Maintain intra-abdominal pressure at 14 to 16 mm Hg. This pressure represents a compromise between the poor exposure of intra-abdominal structures afforded by lower intra-abdominal pressures and the adverse hemodynamic consequences of higher pressures. At operating pressures of 15 mm Hg, venous return through the inferior vena cava is reduced by approximately 50%.

Intermittent compression stockings overcome or diminish the hemodynamic consequences of pneumoperitoneum. Complete relaxation of the abdominal muscular wall increases the intra-abdominal operative space. The tensile strength of the relaxed abdominal wall rests in its fascial-aponeurotic layers. The dosage of muscle relaxants used must be individualized. Clinical observations have repeatedly confirmed that obliteration of the neuromuscular junction between the ulnar nerve and the hypothenar muscles does not reliably indicate complete relaxation of the abdominal musculature in the massively obese.

Placement of dilators and tubes into the stomach through the mouth should be a cooperative activity between the anesthesiologist and the surgeon to avoid inadvertent perforation of the esophagus.

2. **Enhancements that facilitate upper abdominal exposure**: The majority of experience with laparoscopic procedures in these patients has been upper abdominal. Laparoscopic cholecystectomy, hiatal hernia repair, and even bariatric surgery have all been reported. The usually available operating room table for general surgery procedures has limitations that fail to meet the needs of the morbidly obese patient. A recently developed accessory attachment for the Midmark 7100 General Surgery table with the extreme reverse trendelenburg attachment (ERTA) has expanded the range of the head-up, feet-down tilt position to 62 degrees. Such positioning uses the force of gravity to open the upper abdominal operative field. The Midmark 7100 general surgery table is engineered for use for patients whose body weight is up to 500 pounds or 226 kg.

In the head-up, feet-down tilt position, the transverse colon, omentum, and small bowel drop down from the upper abdomen toward the pelvis. Visualization of the diaphragm, esophagogastric junction, spleen, stomach, and lesser sac is improved. The phrenoesophageal epiphrenic fat pad can be removed or used as a handle to manipulate the stomach and esophagus. Good exposure means less trauma to tissues and shorter operation time. It eliminates time-consuming, repeated steps to maintain unobstructed operative access (e.g., the annoying problem of the omentum obscuring the operative field). Retraction of the transverse colon and omentum risks bleeding from avulsion of the splenic capsule.

Patients tolerate extreme head-up, feet-down tilt positioning remarkably well, when a cautious and orderly protocol is followed. The routine used is summarized in Table 10.1.4.

Table 10.1.4. Routine for extreme reverse trendelenberg positioning in morbidly obese patients

1. Patients are well hydrated.
2. Two large-bore intravenous catheters are in place.
3. Continuous monitoring of systemic arterial blood pressure is done.
4. Activate external intermittent venous compression devices on the lower extremities prior to the induction of general anesthesia.
5. Suspend the upper extremities with skin traction and poles attached to the operating room table.
6. Pad all pressure point sites including the foot plate **while the patient is awake** and can identify points of discomfort. Careful application of padding and securement straps on the lower extremities prevents flexion of the knees in the head-up, feet-down tilt position.
7. Gradually initiate the head-up, feet-down tilt positioning. Some patients require several boluses of 250 to 500 ml of balanced salt solution before they can tolerate the extreme head-up, feet-down tilt position.

D. Selected References

Lord MD, Gourevitch A. The peritoneal anatomy of the spleen with special reference to the operation of partial gastrectomy. Br J Surg 1965;52:202–204.

Mason EE, Gordy DD, Chernigoy FA, Printen KJ. Fatty acid toxicity. Surg Gynecol Obstet 1971;133:992–998.

Millard JA, Hill BB, Cook PS, et al. Intermittent sequential pneumatic compression in prevention of venous stasis associated with pneumoperitoneum during laparoscopic cholecystectomy. Arch Surg 1993;128:914–919.

Paul DR, Hoyt JL, Boutros AR. Cardiovascular and respiratory changes in response to change of posture in the very obese. Anesthesiology 1976;45:73–78.

Safran DB, Orlando R III. Physiologic effects of pneumoperitoneum. Am J Surg 1994;167:281–286.

Stellato TA. History of laparoscopic surgery. Surg Clin North Am 1992;72:997–1002.

Wilson YG, Allen PE, Skidmore R., Baker AR. Influence of compression stockings on lower-limb venous hemodynamics during laparoscopic cholecystectomy. Br J Surg 1994;81:841–844.

10.2. Laparoscopy During Pregnancy

Myriam J. Curet, M.D., F.A.C.S.

A. Indications for Laparoscopic Surgery During Pregnancy

The field of laparoscopic general surgery has exploded since the first laparoscopic cholecystectomy was performed in the late 1980's. Initially, pregnancy was considered an absolute contraindication to laparoscopic surgery. Recent clinical reports have demonstrated the feasibility, advantages and potential safety of laparoscopic cholecystectomy in the pregnant patient. However, concerns about the effects of a carbon dioxide pneumoperitoneum on mother and fetus persist, resulting in controversy and concern.

Nongynecologic surgery is required in 0.2% of all pregnancies.

1. The safest time to operate on the pregnant patient is during the second trimester when the risks of teratogenesis, miscarriage and preterm delivery are lowest. The incidence of spontaneous abortion is highest in the first trimester (12%), decreasing to 0% by the third. During the second trimester there is a 5-8% incidence of preterm labor and premature delivery which increases to 30% in the third trimester. In addition, the risk of teratogenesis seen in the first trimester is no longer present during the second trimester. Finally, the gravid uterus is not yet large enough to obscure the operative field as is the case during the third trimester.

2. The most common indications for operation on the pregnant patient are acute appendicitis and biliary tract disease.

    a. **Acute appendicitis** occurs in 1 out of 1500 pregnancies. Accurate diagnosis becomes more difficult as the pregnancy progresses resulting in a correct preoperative diagnosis in 85% of patients evaluated in the first trimester of pregnancy, which decreases to only 30-50% in the third. The usual hallmarks of acute appendicitis such as abdominal pain, accompanying gastrointestinal symptoms, and leukocytosis may already be present in a normal third trimester pregnancy, obscuring the correct diagnosis. In addition, the description and location of the pain may change significantly as the uterus enlarges. The morbidity and mortality seen in the pregnant patient with acute appendicitis results from a delay in diagnosis and treatment. This delay leads to a 10-15% perforation rate. Fetal mortality has been shown to increase with perforation from 5% to 28% while premature delivery can be as high as 40% in this situation. Therefore, the pregnant patient suspected of having acute appendicitis should be treated as if she were not pregnant. Immediate exploration after appropriate resuscitation is mandated regardless of gestational age.

b. **Biliary tract disease**: Gallstones are present in 12% of all pregnancies and a cholecystectomy is performed in 3-8 out of 10,000 pregnancies.

  i.   An uncomplicated **open cholecystectomy** in a pregnant patient should be accompanied by a 0% maternal mortality, 5% fetal loss and 7% preterm labor.

  ii. Complications such as **gallstone pancreatitis** or **acute cholecystitis** will increase maternal mortality to 15% and fetal demise to 60%.

  iii. Patients with **uncomplicated biliary colic** should be treated medically with nonfat diets and pain medications until after delivery. Patients who present in the **first trimester** of pregnancy with crescendo biliary colic or persistent vomiting should be medically managed if possible until they are in the second trimester. Pregnant patients in the **second trimester** of pregnancy who present with the above complications of biliary tract disease will need operative treatment during the second trimester after appropriate resuscitation. Patients with these complications who present in the third trimester of pregnancy should be treated conservatively until after delivery if possible or at least until a gestational age of 28-30 weeks in order to maximize fetal viability.

B. Advantages and Feasibility of Laparoscopic Surgery During Pregnancy

Potentially, laparoscopic surgery in the pregnant patient should result in the proven advantages of laparoscopy seen in the nonpregnant patient: decreased pain, earlier return of gastrointestinal function, earlier ambulation, decreased hospital stay and faster return to routine activity. In addition, a decreased rate of premature delivery due to decreased uterine manipulation, decreased fetal depression secondary to decreased narcotic usage and a lower rate of incisional hernias may be seen in the pregnant patient.

To date, approximately 150 laparoscopic cholecystectomies in pregnant patients have been reported in the literature. Average operative time was 55 minutes and average length of stay was 1.3 days. There were no reports of maternal complications or deaths. Of 99 babies delivered at time of publication, 3 were premature and one was born with hyaline membrane disease at 37 weeks gestation. The remaining 95 were fullterm and healthy. There were no intraoperative fetal deaths or complications.

One study has retrospectively compared pregnant patients undergoing open laparotomy to pregnant patients undergoing laparoscopic surgery and found the latter resumed regular diet earlier, required less pain medication and were hospitalized for a shorter time. These differences were statistically significant.

C. Disadvantages and Concerns about Laparoscopic Surgery During Pregnancy

Concerns about laparoscopic surgery in the pregnant patient center on three areas:

1. Increased intraabdominal pressure can lead to decreased inferior vena caval return resulting in **decreased cardiac output**. The fetus is dependent on maternal hemodynamic stability. The primary cause of fetal demise is maternal hypotension or hypoxia, so a fall in maternal cardiac output could result in fetal distress.
2. The increased intraabdominal pressure seen with a pneumoperitoneum could lead to **decreased uterine blood flow** and **increased intra-uterine pressure**, both of which could result in fetal hypoxia.
3. Carbon dioxide is absorbed across the peritoneum and can lead to **respiratory acidosis** in both mother and fetus. Fetal acidosis could be potentiated by the decreased vena caval return.

One clinical study has reported 4 fetal deaths following laparoscopic surgery. Three occurred during the first postoperative week and the last 4 weeks postoperatively. The causes of death are unknown but might be related to prolonged operative time. The operative times in these 4 patients was 106 minutes compared to the average of 55 minutes seen in the other studies. The laparoscopic procedure was performed for pancreatitis in 3 of these women and a perforated appendix in the fourth. It is possible that fetal loss was the result of the inflammatory process itself rather than the laparoscopy per se. There is a 4% fetal mortality rate for all reported laparoscopic cholecystectomies. It compares favorably with a 5% fetal mortality rate seen with open procedures.

Animal studies raise several concerns about the effects of a carbon dioxide pneumoperitoneum on the mother and fetus. Because of the complexity of the maternal-fetal unit, it is useful to summarize these individually:

1. In pregnant baboons, a CO_2 pneumoperitoneum held at 20 mm Hg pressure for 20 minutes resulted in increased pulmonary capillary wedge pressure, pulmonary artery pressure and central venous pressure. The mothers developed a respiratory acidosis despite controlled ventilation and an increase in respiratory rate. One fetus developed severe bradycardia which responded to desufflation.
2. In pregnant ewes, no change in maternal placental blood flow was seen after 2 hours of 13 mm Hg pressure. However, maternal and fetal respiratory acidosis developed. Fetal tachycardia, fetal hypertension, an increase in intra-uterine pressure and a decrease in uterine blood flow were also seen in pregnant ewes undergoing a carbon dioxide pneumoperitoneum at 15 mm Hg.
3. Maternal respiratory acidosis and severe fetal respiratory acidosis are common findings in all studies utilizing a CO_2 pneumoperitoneum in

pregnant animals. Changes in respiratory rate did not completely correct the problems. Despite these problems, one study demonstrated that the ewes delivered fullterm healthy lambs following intraabdominal insufflation to 15 mm Hg pressure with carbon dioxide for one hour.

4. The physiologic changes exhibited by the pregnant ewe and fetus during insufflation with CO_2 are not present with nitrous oxide. Fetal tachycardia, hypertension, and acidosis as well as maternal acidosis are not present when utilizing a nitrous oxide pneumoperitoneum in animal studies. Use of nitrous oxide as an insufflating gas in the pregnant woman has yet to be evaluated, but may prove to be safer than carbon dioxide. (see Chapter 5.1, Pneumoperitoneum, for a discussion of various insufflating agents).

D. Guidelines

The following practices should be followed when performing laparoscopic surgery in the pregnant patient to minimize adverse effects on the fetus or mother. More information is given in the SAGES Guidelines for Laparoscopic Surgery During Pregnancy (see Appendix).

1. Place the patient in the **left lateral decubitus position** as with open surgery to prevent uterine compression of the inferior vena cava. Minimizing the degree of reverse Trendelenburg position may also further reduce possible uterine compression of the vena cava.

2. **Use antiembolic devices** to prevent deep venous thrombosis. Stasis of blood in the lower extremities is common in pregnancy. Levels of febrinogen and factors VII and XII are increased during pregnancy leading to an increased risk of thromboembolic events. These changes, coupled with the decreased venous return seen with increased intraabdominal pressure and the reverse Trendelenburg position used during laparoscopic surgery, significantly increase the risk of deep venous thrombosis.

3. An **open Hasson technique** for gaining access to the abdominal cavity is safer than a closed percutaneous puncture. Several authors have inserted a Verres needle in the right upper quadrant without complications, but the potential for puncture of the uterus or intestine still exists, especially with increasing gestational age.

4. **Maintain the intraabdominal pressure as low as possible** while still achieving adequate visualization. A pressure of less than 12-15 mm Hg should be used until concerns about the effects of high intraabdominal pressure on the fetus are answered.

5. Continuously **monitor maternal endtidal CO_2** and maintain it between 25-30 mm by changing the minute ventilation. Promptly correcting any evidence of maternal respiratory acidosis is critical as the fetus is typically slightly more acidotic than the mother.

6. Use **continuous intraoperative fetal monitoring**. If fetal distress is noted, release the pneumoperitoneum immediately. Monitoring

should be used even if the fetus is not viable, as the desufflation may reverse fetal distress, preventing serious problems. Transabdominal ultrasound fetal monitoring may not be effective because the establishment of the pneumoperitoneum may decrease fetal heart tones, so intravaginal ultrasound may be necessary for intraoperative monitoring.

7. If intraoperative cholangiography is to be performed, **protect the fetus**.

8. **Minimize operative time**. Several studies have demonstrated a correlation between the duration of a CO_2 pneumoperitoneum and an increase in $PaCO_2$.

9. **Tocolytic agents** should not be administered prophylactically but are appropriate if there is any evidence of uterine irritability or contractions.

10. **Trocar placement**
    a. **Biliary tract disease:** Place a Hasson trocar above the umbilicus. Place the remaining ports under direct visualization in the usual locations.
    b. **Appendicitis/diagnostic laparoscopy:** Place a Hasson trocar in the subxiphoid region. Insert the camera and locate the appendix or other inflammatory process. Insert the remaining trocars in locations appropriate to the pathology. For appendicitis, this will usually be the right upper quadrant at the costal margin and in the right lower quadrant. Ocasionally an additional port might need to be placed just above the uterus. If the uterus is too large and appendectomy cannot be performed laparoscopically, then laparoscopic visualization of the appendix may help determine the best location for the open incision.

In conclusion, animal studies indicate that a CO_2 pneumoperitoneum causes fetal acidosis which may not be corrected by changes in maternal respiratory status. These intraoperative findings do not appear to have any longterm adverse effects on the fetus. The pregnant patient clearly benefits from laparoscopic surgery and should be offered this option as long as the above guidelines are followed.

E. Selected References

Abuabara SF, Gross GW, Sirinek KR. Laparoscopic cholecystectomy during pregnancy is safe for both mother and fetus. J Gastrointest Surg 1997;1:48-52.

Amos JD, Schorr SJ, Norman PF, Poole GV, Thomae KR, Mancino AT, Hall TJ, Scott-Conner CEH. Laparoscopic surgery during pregnancy. Am J Surg 1996;171:435-437.

Barnard JM, Chaffin D, Drose S, Tierney A, Phernetton T. Fetal response to carbon dioxide pneumoperitoneum in the pregnant ewe. Obstet Gynecol 1995;85:669-674.

Curet MJ, Vogt DM, Schob O, Qualls C, Izquerdo LA, Zucker KA. Effects of CO2 pneumoperitoneum in pregnant ewes. J Surg Research 1996;63:339-344.

Curet MJ, Allen D, Josloff RK, Pitcher DE, Curet LB, Miscall BG, Zucker KA. Laproscopy during pregnancy. Arch Surg 1996;131:546-551.

Hunter JG, Swanstrom L, Thornburg K. Carbon dioxide pneumoperitoneum induces fetal acidosis in a pregnant ewe model. Surg Endosc 1994;4:268-271.

Kammerer WS. Nonobstetric surgery during pregnancy. Med Clin North Am 1979;63:1157-1163.

McKellar DP, Anderson CT, Boynton CJ, Peoples JB. Cholecystectomy during pregnancy without fetal loss. Surg Gynecol Obstet 1992;174:465-468.

Motew M, Ivankovich AD, Bieniarz J, Albrecht RF, Zahed B, Scomegna A. Cardiovascular effects and acid-base and blood gas changes during laparoscopy. Am J Obstet Gyncol 1973;113:1002-1012.

Reedy MB, Galan HL, Bean JD, Carnes A, Knight AB, Kuehl TJ. Laparoscopic insufflation in the gravid baboon:maternal and fetal effects. J Am Assoc Gynecol Laproscopist 1995;2:399-406.

Soper NJ, Hunter JG, Petri RH. Laparoscopic cholecystectomy in the pregnant patient. Surg Laparosc Endosc 1994;4:268-271.

10.3. Previous Abdominal Surgery

Norman B. Halpern, M.D., F.A.C.S.

A. General Considerations

Previous intra-abdominal operation may have only trivial impact on the performance of a subsequent laparoscopic procedure or may render laparoscopy not only unwise, but impossible. This wide spectrum of influence is related to the substantial variation in patients' tendencies to form postoperative adhesions. The laparoscopic surgeon should not be intimidated by the potential difficulties posed by such adhesions, but should approach the circumstances with an awareness of the strategies and tactics that have been utilized routinely and successfully during decades of traditional (open) operations. The influence of previous abdominal incision on choice of access for induction of pneumoperitoneum was discussed briefly in Chapter 4, and is considered more fully here.

B. Preoperative Analysis and Planning

During preoperative planning, first consider the **geographical relationships of the previous and the intended operations.** For example, the most commonly performed general surgical laparoscopic procedure is cholecystectomy, usually upon women. Since many women have previously undergone transabdominal hysterectomy, infraumbilical body wall adhesions may interfere with periumbilical cannula placement, although the remainder of the cholecystectomy may be entirely uneventful. Unfortunately, however, adhesions are not always limited to the precise area of the incision, but may occupy a much greater expanse of the peritoneal membrane than the cutaneous scar would suggest.

Next, determine **whether the old scar has healed properly or has developed a herniation.** If weakness is detected, the operative plan should include hernia repair. Since laparoscopic techniques for incisional hernia repair have not been widely applied, a suitable approach would be a combined operation. If the hernia is located remotely from the laparoscopic field, then a conventional herniorrhaphy could precede the laparoscopy. If the hernia is in the general area of the anticipated laparoscopy (e.g., an upper midline hernia in a patient being considered for laparoscopic cholecystectomy), it may be preferable to utilize that weakened incision for an open procedure with repair at the time of closure.

Finally, consider **patient positioning, operating table tilt and roll capabilities, and accessories** (ankle straps, footboard) and assure that the benefits of gravity and shifting tissue/organ relationships may be exploited if necessary.

C. Access to the Peritoneal Cavity

Carefully plan the steps to achieve intra-abdominal access. Make the initial entry at a reasonable distance from any obvious scars. Possible access sites relative to common scars are illustrated in Chapter 4.

1. Some surgeons utilize an alternate-site Veress needle puncture technique (for example, the left subcostal region). For most, the Hasson cannula is a straightforward and possibly safer means, and some surgeons use this technique routinely. With practice, this will be found to be an expeditious means for entering any quadrant by making a miniature muscle-splitting incision in the subcostal, hypogastric, flank, or other region. Just as with open operations, however, bowel that happens to be adherent immediately under the chosen site of entry will be damaged by any blind cutting, spreading, or cauterization. If there is any question as to adherent underlying tissue, the initially chosen site may need to be abandoned and another one selected.

2. **Achieving appropriate working distance** is another reason for judicious selection of the entry site. Avoid ending up too close to any tissue of interest. There must be a comfortable working distance available to the surgeon to properly manipulate instruments, either for lysing the interfering adhesions, or for performing the primary procedure. Secondary cannulas must then be placed with these considerations in mind, also.

D. Managing Adhesions

Once the peritoneal cavity has been reached safely, the **presence and extent of any adhesions** will become apparent. The surgeon must resist the common tendency to excessively eliminate adhesions. Only those adhesions that truly interfere with visualization of the area of interest or would prevent the placement of subsequent cannulas under vision should be dealt with. At times, the end of the telescope can be very easily manipulated around the edge of a sheet of omentum, suspended from the elevated body wall like a curtain, or fenestrated areas can be used as windows through which the scope can be advanced toward the operative area. If these maneuvers are not applicable, then adhesion lysis must be begun.

Safe lysis of adhesions requires a **combination of skillful technique and attention to visual cues**. If the line of tissue adherence can be recognized, it will provide the most expeditious path to follow, with the least chance of causing significant bleeding or visceral injury. Principles of traction/countertraction are essential components of this phase of the operation, and the surgeon may occasionally need to experiment with varying directions of pull on the tissues to clearly display the boundary lines. For body wall adhesions, the combination of gravity pulling the tissues down while the distended abdominal wall moves in the opposite direction sometimes provides adequate stretch to allow the dissection to be done with only one working instrument. Frequently, however (and especially with viscera-to-viscera adherence), an assisting grasper is required, with its cannula being carefully positioned according to principles mentioned previously.

E. Instrument Considerations

The best tool to be used for adhesion lysis is determined by the circumstances and the characteristics of the adhesions and surrounding tissues. Naturally weak areas of areolar tissues appear "foamy" and can be swept away using techniques resembling finger dissection. Rounded graspers, the blunt edges of the scissors blades, and even the suction-irrigator all accomplish the same result with these types of adhesions. For more firmly adherent structures, however, scissors may be the next choice. If the fusion of the tissues has not resulted in very much neovascularity, then adding cautery current to the scissors' action is not helpful, as long as the proper plane of dissection is followed.

Use of **the cautery tool** requires diligence and respect for the potential tissue damage that may result from uncontrolled electrical energy. In addition, the surgeon's expectations for hemostasis must be realistic, using coaptive coagulation (pinching while applying current) for some vessels, but clips or ligatures for larger ones. Techniques for utilizing J- or L-shaped cautery devices commonly involve a hook-pull-burn sequence, but if the surgeon places sturdy traction on the tissues, and then gently sweeps or caresses with the elbow of the wire, a more precise and delicate separation of tissues will follow, as if the traction is actually performing the dissection, and the current is merely weakening the adherence. Although bipolar electrocautery instruments and Harmonic scalpel (Ultracision, Ethicon Endo-Surgery, Cinncinati, OH) devices are commercially available, their actual usage and availability is probably somewhat limited compared to conventional monopolar instrumentation.

The loss of natural proprioceptive processes cannot be eliminated but can be minimized by careful attention to instrument design and function. The acceptability of the "feel" of a dissecting or grasping instrument is determined partly by personal preference. For example, some surgeons find rotatable instrument shafts to be very useful; however, others dislike the added bulk and the change in balance produced by the rotating mechanism. Other design features such as length, shaft flexibility, overall weight, and handle configurations must each be considered as a surgeon is determining whether adequate dexterity exists and whether careful tissue handling will be accomplished. It is particularly important for the closing and spreading movements of the jaws to be smooth and effortless, otherwise it will be impossible to sense how much force is being applied to the tissues.

The use of an angled lens laparoscope (for example, a 30-degree laparoscope) is sometimes extremely helpful. Observing adhesions and abnormal tissue relationships from more than a single vantage point renders new, safer, or more productive dissection pathways apparent. Remember that although such lenses are conventionally thought of as "looking down," there may be great advantages to looking "up" or from a "sideways" perspective.

F. Complications

No operative procedure is risk free. If an operation requires more than the usual efforts for tissue dissection or organ manipulation, there likely will be **an increased opportunity for mishaps,** so the surgeon must develop a keen sense of vigilance for any potentially dangerous situations.

1. **Bleeding**
    a. **Cause and prevention:** Although not life-threatening, any additional blood loss during a laparoscopic procedure not only can be time-consuming to control, but can add to the frustration and mental fatigue associated with an already difficult operation. In addition, if tissues become blood stained, ability to recognize structures may be impaired, and illumination is less effective. Careful, painstaking dissection is the best preventive measure.
    b. **Recognition and management:** Minimization of blood loss will be favorably influenced by rigorous attention to tissue planes, by careful observation of tissue characteristics, and by appropriate precautionary use of electrocautery or other hemostatic maneuvers. Such maneuvers, however, may cause injuries to adjacent structures if hurriedly applied, especially during efforts to control active bleeding. Remember that simple pressure—even with the scissors blades that created the problem—is an immediately available solution to consider when confronted with a spurting vessel. (See Chapter 6, Principles of Laparoscopic Hemostasis, for a discussion of management strategies.)

2. **Visceral injury**
    a. **Cause and prevention:** This can result from excessive traction, as well as cutting, burning, or ligating misidentified structures. As previously described, careful controlled dissection in a bloodless field, with identification of all structures as the dissection progresses, is crucial to prevent these injuries.
    b. **Recognition and management:** With solid organ injury (liver, spleen), bleeding is the immediate, as well as the obvious, consequence. Management of these injuries is primarily directed at obtaining hemostasis. Injuries to hollow viscera may be subtle and apparent only because of the appearance of luminal contents. The decision to perform a laparoscopic repair, as contrasted to open conversion, should be influenced by the characteristics of the tissues and associated injury, as well as the surgeon's experience and capabilities. A "delayed" intestinal perforation, manifesting itself as postoperative peritonitis, may very well be an intraoperative injury that was undetected. For that reason, prior to removing the laparoscope, the mandatory final step of the operation should be a methodical inspection of all intra-abdominal areas that had been subjected to adhesion lysis, tissue manipulation, or actions to control bleeding.

G. Selected References

Caprini JA, Arcelus JA, Swanson J, et al. The ultrasonic localization of abdominal wall adhesions. Surg Endosc 1995:9:283–285.

Halpern NB. The difficult laparoscopy. Surg Clin North Am 1996;76:603–613.

Halpern NB. Access problems in laparoscopic cholecystectomy: postoperative adhesions, obesity, and liver disorders. Seminars in Laparoscopic Surgery 1998; 5:92–106.

Patel M, Smart D. Laparoscopic cholecystectomy and previous abdominal surgery: a safe technique. Aust NZ J Surg 1996;66:309–311.

Schirmer BD, Dix J, Schmieg RE, et al. The impact of previous abdominal surgery on outcome following laparoscopic cholecystectomy. Surg Endosc 1995;9:1085–1089.

Sigmar HH, Fried GM, Gazzon J, et al. Risks of blind versus open approach to celiotomy for laparoscopic surgery. Surg Laparosc Endosc 1993;3:296–299.

Weibel MA, Majno G. Peritoneal adhesions and their relation to abdominal surgery: a post mortem study. Am J Surg 1973;126:345–353.

Wongworowat MD, Aitken DR, Robles AE, Garberoglio C. The impact of prior intraabdominal surgery on laparoscopic cholecystectomy. Am Surg 1994;60:763–766.

11. Emergency Laparoscopy

Jonathan M. Sackier, M.D., F.R.C.S., F.A.C.S.

A. General Considerations

Diagnostic laparoscopy can provide important information in the emergency setting. It provides a minimally traumatic way to confirm or exclude a diagnosis. Clinical judgment must be used to exclude problems best served by formal laparotomy. The indications for emergency laparoscopy can be conveniently grouped into those related to abdominal pain and those related to trauma (Table 11.1). Other indications are continually emerging, and it is important to individualize patient management in this area.

Table 11.1. Indications for emergency laparoscopy

Abdominal pain	<ul><li>Right lower quadrant pain (r/o gynecologic pathology)</li><li>Right upper quadrant pain (r/o Fitz-Hugh-Curtis syndrome)</li><li>Peritonitis</li><li>Mesenteric ischemia</li><li>Intra-abdominal abscess, not amenable to image-guided drainage</li><li>Acalculous cholecystitis</li><li>Small bowel obstruction</li><li>Fever of unknown origin</li><li>Gastrointestinal hemorrhage of unexplained etiology</li></ul>
Trauma	<ul><li>Blunt abdominal trauma</li><li>Penetrating trauma<ul><li>Exclude peritoneal penetration</li><li>Evaluate diaphragm</li></ul></li></ul>

The indications for each type of diagnostic laparoscopic examination will be briefly discussed, and specific technical details will be explained.

B. Abdominal Pain

Laparoscopy should be used in a well-reasoned fashion in the algorithm for evaluation of abdominal pain, and should not sidestep other accepted treatment plans such as observation and sequential abdominal examinations. A young woman presenting with **right lower quadrant pain** in whom the differential diagnosis includes acute appendicitis may be well served by diagnostic laparoscopy. This should be performed in the operating room with appropriate consent through laparoscopic appendectomy (see Chapter 25). The gynecologist should be informed of the plans to take the patient to the operating room after he or she has seen the patient, if considered appropriate. In women of reproductive age with right upper quadrant pain and negative studies, the diagnosis of **Fitz-Hughes-Curtis syndrome** should be entertained. Laparoscopy provides the opportunity to confirm this entity and divide the perihepatic adhesions.

In certain individuals with signs and symptoms of **peritonitis**, diagnostic laparoscopy can precede laparotomy and assist in making the appropriate incision. For instance, a stoic individual may have a perforated duodenal ulcer mimicking appendicitis. Laparoscopy provides the correct diagnosis and avoids a misplaced right lower quadrant incision. Good surgical judgment should be exercised, and in the moribund patient it may be wiser to proceed directly to laparotomy.

Laparoscopy may be of use in evaluating the individual with abdominal pain or sepsis of unknown etiology in the emergency setting, **when the clinical picture is confused** by alcohol or drug abuse, senility, or advanced age.

In the **critically ill patient** in the intensive care unit, diagnostic laparoscopy may be performed at the bedside, and yield important information or even be therapeutic in these circumstances:

1. **Mesenteric ischemia**: These patients are often elderly and fragile and if seen to have widespread gangrenous bowel, appropriate clinical decisions can be made. If the patient does go on to have an embolectomy or resection, a cannula can be left in situ for second-look laparoscopy.
2. **Intra-abdominal abscess**: When computed tomography (CT) guided drainage is not feasible, laparoscopic guided drainage may be a useful alternative to formal laparotomy.
3. **Acalculous cholecystitis**: The difficult diagnosis of acalculous cholecystitis may be made at laparoscopy. If percutaneous drainage is not possible for technical reasons, laparoscopically guided cholecystostomy is a useful option.

Small bowel obstruction due to adhesions may be diagnosed and treated laparoscopically (see Chapter 10.3, Special Problems: Previous Abdominal Surgery). This should be reserved for the skilled laparoscopist, and great care must be taken in handling the bowel.

Unexplained shock: In certain very specific circumstances laparoscopy may be of value. For instance, in the young patient with no history of trauma who is admitted in profound shock with an abdomen containing free blood, laparoscopy can be used to confirm spontaneous splenic rupture.

Fever of unknown origin: In the emergency patient presenting with abdominal signs and fever, especially if there is a history of foreign travel or recent immigration, the diagnosis of tuberculosis or brucellosis should be considered. Laparoscopy can assist in confirming these entities.

In a limited number of cases a full range of diagnostic studies will not elucidate the cause of **GI bleeding**. Usually this will be in a young patient with no history of prior surgery, in which case a Meckel's diverticulum may be responsible. The minimally invasive approach can be used to run the bowel, find the cause, and resect the offending lesion.

C. Conduct of Diagnostic Laparoscopy for Abdominal Pain

Diagnostic laparoscopy is **best performed in the operating room**, for it may be necessary to continue and add a therapeutic laparoscopy or convert to laparotomy. It is feasible to perform diagnostic laparoscopy in the ICU, if the staff is familiar with these techniques. Several points of technique simplify the management of these patients.

1. **Stand on the side of the patient** opposite the anticipated pathology. Plan to move to whichever side of the patient is necessary and be prepared to move around to gain access to all four quadrants of the abdomen.
2. The **video monitors** should be mobile, for in most circumstances it is necessary to be able to move them, depending on the source of the pathology in peritonitis. Obviously, for right lower quadrant pain the monitor should be toward the right side of the foot of the bed.
3. Unless prior abdominal surgery suggests otherwise, **insert the laparoscope at the umbilicus.** Five-millimeter laparoscopes are available and may be placed through a 5-mm cannula. Generally a 10-mm laparoscope provides better light and view, and therefore a larger trocar is placed.
4. It will normally be necessary to place **at least one additional trocar** to manipulate, palpate, and move viscera for a thorough exploration. Where this is placed depends on the pathology. If it is necessary to run the bowel, two 5-mm trocars should be placed, equidistant from the umbilical site, in the midline.
5. Both **a 30-degree laparoscope and a 0-degree laparoscope should be available**. If on inserting the telescope it is immediately apparent there is a major abdominal catastrophe requiring laparotomy, the scope should be withdrawn and the abdomen entered in conventional fashion.
6. If a **defined laparoscopic procedure** (for example, appendectomy or plication of a perforated ulcer) is necessary, refer to the appropriate chapter.
7. In the case of **mesenteric ischemia** requiring laparotomy, the procedure should be completed by placing a 10-mm cannula lateral to the

rectus sheath, a purse-string suture placed around the fascial entrance site, and the tip of the cannula buried in a pocket of peritoneum. In this manner the cannula can be moved to free up the tip; pneumoperitoneum is induced at the bedside in the intensive care unit 24 hours later, and after laparoscopy the cannula is withdrawn and the purse-string tightened. This has been used in lieu of second-look formal laparotomy.

D. Laparoscopy for Trauma

Laparoscopy is indicated in **blunt trauma** when there is a suggestion of multisystem injury and it is important to triage the patient. Alternatives include diagnostic peritoneal lavage, CT scan, and ultrasound, all of which by interpretation of data may lead to false negatives and false positives. Again, laparoscopy is not a panacea and should be used appropriately.

Although it is probably not necessary to state the obvious, always remember the priorities of trauma management—airway, breathing, circulation. The patient who clearly has an expanding abdominal girth and hypotension or a mechanism of injury highly suggestive for a major abdominal catastrophe is best served by prompt laparotomy. In patients with a low probability of injury, diagnostic laparoscopy can be performed under local anesthesia in the emergency room, thus enabling efficient triage.

Laparoscopy has also been used as part of selective management technique for **penetrating trauma.** For stab wounds below the nipples, laparoscopy is an alternative technique. If the patient is cooperative, this can be performed in the emergency room under local anesthesia. Similarly, small-caliber tangential gunshot wounds (with one apparent entrance and one apparent exit wound), particularly in obese patients with no abdominal signs, may be managed by a selective policy that includes diagnostic laparoscopy rather than laparotomy.

E. Conduct of Laparoscopy for Trauma

Diagnostic laparoscopy for trauma may be performed in the emergency room or in the operating room. The purpose is to exclude or confirm intraabdominal injury. Attention to a few points will maximize the chance of success.

1. Place the patient supine on the operating table or emergency room gurney.
2. Stand opposite the entrance wound (for penetrating trauma) and position the main video monitor directly opposite.
3. Unless prior surgery or other circumstances dictate, the laparoscope should be inserted through the umbilicus.
4. Triage is the purpose of the laparoscopy and the 5-mm minilaparoscope can be used. It may not be necessary to place further trocars.

5. If further trocars are needed, one should position these in the mid-abdomen on the side opposite to the entrance wound. If the surgeon wishes to run the bowel or manipulate the liver and stomach to examine the diaphragm, 5-mm trocars on either side of the abdomen to accommodate bowel graspers will be necessary. Additionally, the table should be of the variety that can be tilted up, down, right, and left.

6. If the patient has a stab wound between the nipples and costal margin **always check the chest x-ray** to ensure that there is no pneumothorax, for otherwise the possibility of creating a tension pneumothorax exists. An unrecognized diaphragmatic injury will allow the insufflating gas to enter the chest, producing a pneumothorax.

7. For stab wounds **the entrance site must first be closed**, the pneumoperitoneum created, and the laparoscope inserted. The stab wound is indented and if no penetration of the underlying peritoneum is seen, one can assume there has been no intraabdominal damage.

8. In **gunshot wounds** the laparoscope must be positioned in such a way that it is in between the entrance and exit wounds so that both can be evaluated in similar fashion to stab wounds. Obviously if no peritoneal penetration is seen and no expanding hematoma is noted within the abdominal wall, the patient can receive appropriate wound care without formal laparotomy.

9. In the case of **blunt abdominal trauma**, characterize the nature of bleeding using a **standard grading system** such as the one in Table 11.2. Generally grade 2 or grade 3 hemoperitoneum requires formal laparotomy. Depending upon the mechanism of injury, the surgeon may choose to observe patients with grade 1 hemoperitoneum (for example, a minor splenic laceration that has stopped bleeding), and grade 0 is a normal examination.

Table 11.2. Grading system for hemoperitoneum observed at diagnostic laparoscopy

- Grade 0: No blood is seen within the peritoneal cavity.
- Grade 1: Small flecks of blood on the bowel or small amounts of blood in the paracolic gutters. Blood does not recur when aspirated. No bleeding sight is seen.
- Grade 2: Blood is seen between loops of bowel and in the paracolic gutter. Blood recurs after aspiration.
- Grade 3: Frank blood is aspirated from the Veress needle or the intestines are noted to be floating on a pool of blood.

It is difficult to evaluate the spleen for bleeding, for it is usually covered by the omentum. Bulging of the omentum or a large quantity of intra-abdominal blood in the presence of no obvious liver laceration is a clue that the spleen may have been damaged.

Besides hemoperitoneum, bowel content in the paracolic gutter is a clear indication of intestinal injury.

Appropriate use of this algorithm might save 25% of nontherapeutic laparotomies that may occur with diagnostic peritoneal lavage (DPL) or CT scan evaluation.

The **complications of laparoscopy for trauma** include not only the usual complications of anesthesia and laparoscopy, but also some that are unique to the trauma patient.

1. In blunt trauma the patient may have sustained a closed head injury in addition to a suspected abdominal injury. It has been demonstrated that pneumoperitoneum and reverse Trendelenburg position both lead to **increased intracranial pressure** with potentially serious consequences.

2. **Hypothermia**: Insufflation of cold carbon dioxide exacerbates cooling of an already compromised patient with resultant acidosis.

3. In a high abdominal stab wound, **pneumothorax** is a potential danger.

4. **Physiologic changes** such as acidosis, cardiac suppression, arrhythmias, and gas absorption causing subcutaneous emphysema, may have more profound consequences in the trauma patient.

F. Selected References

Bender JS, Talamini MA. Diagnostic laparoscopy in critically ill intensive care patients. Surg Endosc 1992;6:302–304.

Berci G, Sackier JM, Paz-Partlow M. Emergency laparoscopy. Am J Surg 1991;161:355–360.

Carnevale N, Baron N, Delany HM. Peritoneoscopy, as an aid in the diagnosis of abdominal trauma: a preliminary report. J Trauma 1977;17:634–641.

Forde KA, Treat MR. The role of peritoneoscopy (laparoscopy) in the evaluation of the acute abdomen in critically ill patients. Surg Endosc 1992;6:219–221.

Gazzaniga AB, Slanton WW, Bartlett RH. Laparoscopy in the diagnosis of blunt and penetrating injuries to abdomen. Am J Surg 1996;131:315–318.

Halverson A, Buchanan R, Jacobs LK, Shayani V, Hunt T, Reidel C, Sackier JM. Evaluation of mechanism of increased intracranial pressure with insufflation. Surg Endosc (in press).

Ivatury RR, Simon RJ, Wekler B, et al. Laparoscopy in the evaluation of the inthoracic abdomen after penetrating injury. J Trauma 1992;33:101–109.

Paterson-Brown S, Eckersley JRT, Sim AJW, et al. Laparoscopy as an adjunct to decision making in the acute abdomen. Br J Surg 1986;73:1022–1024.

Paw P, Sackier JM. Complications of laparoscopy and thoracoscopy. J Intensive Care Med 1994;9:290–304.

Sackier JM. Second-look laparoscopy in the management of acute mesentery ischemia. Br J Surg 1994;81:1546.

Sosa JL, Sims D, Martin L, Zeppa R. Laparoscopic evaluation of tangential abdominal gunshot wounds. Arch Surg 1992;127:109–110.

Wood D, Berci G, Morgenstern, Paz-Partlow M. Mini laparoscopy in blunt abdominal trauma. Surg Endosc 1988;2:184–189.

12. Elective Diagnostic Laparoscopy and Cancer Staging

Frederick L. Greene, M.D., F.A.C.S.

A. Diagnostic Laparoscopy

The laparoscope has become an important tool in the diagnosis of benign and malignant conditions in the abdominal cavity. This modality should be utilized in conjunction with conventional imaging techniques such as computed tomography (CT), percutaneous ultrasound, magnetic resonance imaging (MRI), and other radiologic and nuclear medicine studies to differentiate between benign and malignant processes as well as to assess the degree of potential metastatic disease in the abdominal cavity. The laparoscope may also be used to identify the underlying cause of unexplained ascites.

1. **Indications for elective diagnostic laparoscopy**: Patients with underlying malignancy may have either primary or metastatic malignant disease within the abdomen. Common lesions such as carcinoma of the pancreas, stomach, and colorectum are reasons to consider diagnostic laparoscopy for full preoperative assessment (Table 12.1). Frequently, melanoma of the trunk or extremities may metastasize to the small bowel, causing unexplained bleeding or chronic intermittent small bowel obstruction. A patient with these findings may benefit from a laparoscopic examination. Other indications for laparoscopic staging include the full assessment of patients with Hodgkin's lymphoma to plan appropriate chemotherapy and/or radiation therapy.

Table 12.1. Indications for laparoscopic staging of abdominal tumors

• Preoperative assessment prior to major extirpation
• Documentation of hepatic or nodal involvement
• Confirmation of imaging studies
• Therapeutic decision making for Hodgkin's disease
• Full assessment of ascitic fluid

The laparoscope may be utilized for general inspection of the abdominal cavity and as a method of obtaining tissue from solid organs such as liver or lymph nodes (Table 12.2). Imaging studies give only indirect evidence of underlying disease and, therefore, the laparoscope may be used for directed biopsy, obtaining of cytolologic specimens by peritoneal lavage, or fine-needle aspiration techniques. In some part of the world, infectious diseases (such as tuberculosis or parasitic infestation) causing abdominal problems may be more prevalent than cancer, and laparoscopic examination assists in the differential diagnosis of these entities. Diagnostic laparoscopy is also beneficial for patients with chronic abdominal pain who have had limited abdominal procedures in the past. This is especially true in women who have undergone hysterectomy and who have chronic pelvic pain. The identification and lysis of adhesions may be beneficial in this group.

Table 12.2. Techniques utilized during diagnostic or staging laparoscopy

• Full abdominal and pelvic evaluation
• Division of gastrohepatic omentum
• Biopsy using cupped forceps or core needle
• Abdominal lavage for cytological study
• Retrieval of ascitic fluid for cytology and culture
• Identification and removal of enlarged lymph nodes
• Laparoscopic ultrasound

2. **Technique of elective diagnostic laparoscopy**: After appropriate pre-operative evaluation, diagnostic laparoscopy may be performed under either general or local anesthesia. General anesthesia is preferred for most cases, especially if cancer staging is to be performed. Diagnostic laparoscopy may be performed in the operating room (most common) or in a treatment area equipped for administration of anesthesia and with full resuscitative support. A proper table that allows the patient to be placed in both full Trendelenburg and reverse Trendelenburg positions during examination is essential. Appropriate time should be taken for a full examination of the upper and lower abdomen. This generally requires creating a pneumoperitoneum using carbon dioxide at 10 to 12 mm Hg.

A 10 mm laparoscope is preferred utilizing both 0-degree and 30-degree laparoscopes for full visualization. Place the laparoscope through a mid-line subumbilical trocar site using a 10/11-mm trocar sleeve. Depending on the area to be examined, place one or two additional 5-mm trocars in each upper quadrant. These will be used for grasping forceps, palpating probes, and biopsy forceps.

Biopsy may be performed with cupped forceps passed through either a 5- or 10-mm trocar sleeve. Alternatively, cutting biopsy needles may be used to obtain liver or nodal tissue (Fig. 12.1). The needle biopsy may be performed percutaneously under laparoscopic guidance, or the biopsy needle may be passed through one of the 5-mm trocar sheaths. It is important to **perform biopsy cleanly** without crushing tissue which might reduce the opportunity for pathological review.

Specific areas of biopsy depend on the nature of the lesion and the tumor undergoing staging, and several malignancies will be discussed individually in the sections that follow. For example, in patients with lower esophageal and gastric cancer, the liver must be closely inspected and any lesions on the surface of the liver should be biopsied. In addition, the gastrohepatic and gastrocolic omental areas may be divided to allow for evaluation of nodal tissue in these areas. Lymph nodes should be removed intact, if possible, to achieve better histologic identification. In assessing the patient with pancreatic cancer, the duodenum may be mobilized using a Kocher maneuver.

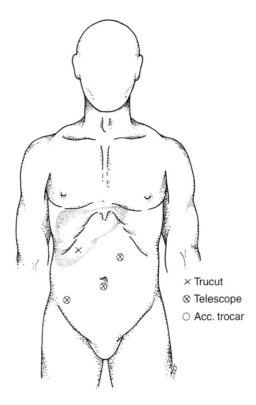

× Trucut
⊗ Telescope
○ Acc. trocar

Figure 12.1. Trocar and needle placement for liver biopsy. The biopsy needle may be passed through a trocar or percutaneously through the abdominal wall.

Retroduodenal tissue may be biopsied and lymph nodes may be assessed using this technique. The gastrocolic omentum should be divided and the superior pancreatic area should be to observe for evidence of local or regional pancreatic cancer. In addition, lavage with 500 ml. of saline should routinely be performed to obtain fluid for cytologic investigation. The fluid should be totally removed and sent to the cytology laboratory to be spun and evaluated for malignant cells. Staging for pancreatic cancer prior to the planning of a Whipple procedure should be a separate event to allow for the assessment of cytology results and any biopsy specimens taken during the procedure. The laparoscope may not completely aid in the examination of the retropancreatic region especially in the region of the superior mesenteric artery and vein. Additional techniques specifically utilizing intraoperative laparoscopic ultrasound may aid in this assessment.

B. Esophageal Carcinoma (Squamous and Adenocarcinoma)

The majority of esophageal cancers occur in the middle and distal third and are predominantly squamous cell. Recently there has been an increase in the incidence of adenocarcinoma of the distal esophagus, seen in association with Barrett's changes, and believed to be related to reflux esophagitis. The classic approach to esophageal cancer management has been esophagectomy with reconstruction using either the stomach or the colon as an interposed organ. Because of the recent advances in esophageal cancer management using chemotherapy and radiation, postoperative or neoadjuvant therapy may be important in many of these patients. In addition, nodal involvement in carcinoma of the esophagus occurs in both the mediastinal area as well as the celiac region and may be advanced even when imaging studies fail to show nodal disease. Patients with advanced esophageal cancer, although amenable to palliation, may not benefit from major extirpative surgery. In these cases radiation with placement of new expandable stents may give appropriate treatment and support quality of life.

Laparoscopic assessment of esophageal cancer is important to identify the group of patients that will not benefit by esophagectomy. Careful assessment of the liver as well as the celiac axis can identify occult nodes in these regions or small metastases that have not been apparent on preoperative imaging studies.

The technique of laparoscopy for the assessment of esophageal cancer utilizes three ports; an umbilical port for the laparoscope and two accessory ports, one in each subcostal region.

1. Begin the assessment of the abdomen by placing the patient in steep Trendelenburg position and inspecting the pelvic peritoneum, looking for small peritoneal metastases.
2. Next, place the operating table in a neutral position. Rotate it sequentially to the right and left decubitus positions (commonly termed "airplaning" the table) and look for ascites. Aspirate any fluid and send it for cytology.
3. Next, inspect the liver. The reverse Trendelenburg position, with the left side down, assists by allowing the liver to drop down out of the subdiaphragmatic space. Look at all visible surfaces of the liver, using an angled laparoscope to facilitate inspection. Carefully assess the liver for any unusual adhesions or plaques, which may initially appear benign yet harbor small metastases. Biopsy any suspicious areas with cup forceps or cutting needle.
4. Biopsy any lesions seen on the peritoneum or omentum with cupped forceps also. Electrocautery is extremely useful, as bleeding may occur; diagnostic laparoscopic examination should not be undertaken without this capability.
5. Next, examine the anterior wall of the stomach and the region of the esophageal hiatus (Fig. 12.2). Place the table in reverse Trendelenburg position and use a 30-degree laparoscope.

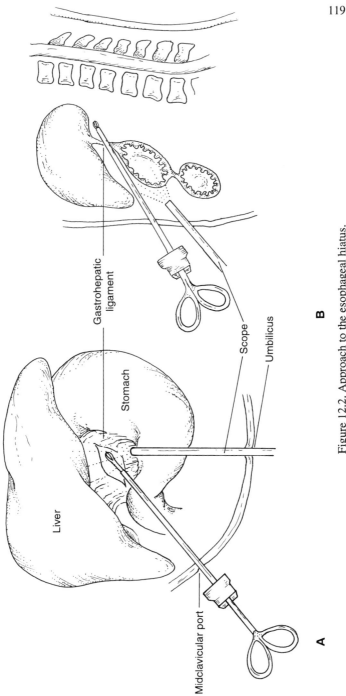

Figure 12.2. Approach to the esophageal hiatus.

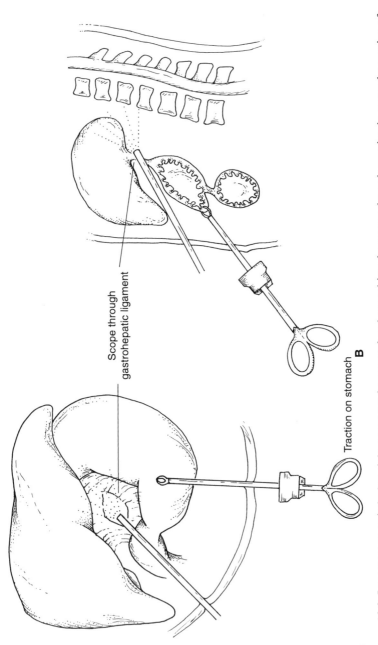

Figure 12.3. Laparoscope switched to right upper quadrant portal and passed into lesser sac through opening in avascular portion of gastrohepatic omentum. Traction on the stomach facilitates this maneuver.

Scope through gastrohepatic ligament

Traction on stomach

A

B

6. Divide the gastrohepatic omentum to search for lymph nodes in the region of the subhepatic space and the lesser curvature extending up to the esophageal hiatus. Lymph nodes in the region of the left gastric and celiac vessels may be inspected by this technique. Pass the laparoscope into the lesser sac for full identification (Fig. 12.3). If large frozen-section–positive nodes are found, place metal clips to facilitate planning of radiation therapy, if appropriate.

C. Gastric Cancer

Although the approach to cancer of the stomach is generally resection whether it be for cure or palliation, laparoscopic evaluation may be important in patients who present with advanced disease and who are unresectable. Recently, there has been a trend of more patients with carcinoma of the cardia and proximal stomach than with the antral carcinomas previously seen. The assessment of the patient with gastric cancer is similar to that noted in esophageal cancer, and many of the same maneuvers are involved. Because of the generally poor results with radiation and chemotherapy in the management of gastric cancer, these patients may be candidates for palliative resection.

D. Tumors of the Liver (Primary and Metastatic)

Laparoscopic assessment of primary hepatic tumors is ideal since many of these tumors involve the surface of the liver. The recent application of laparoscopic ultrasound has aided in the identification of tumors deep to Glisson's capsule. Although metastatic disease of the liver is the most common indication for laparoscopic assessment, given the worldwide incidence of hepatocellular cancer and the increase in hepatic tumors associated with chronic hepatitis, evaluation of hepatocellular cancer is becoming increasingly more important. Traditional imaging studies may underestimate involvement of the liver, and this becomes critically important when hepatic resection is being considered.

1. **A three-trocar technique** is used for hepatic assessment, with an umbilical trocar for the laparoscope, and accessory ports in the left and right upper quadrants. Peritoneal attachments to the liver may need division based on the anatomical findings in the specific patient (Fig. 12.4).
2. Hepatic lesions may have a variety of colors including white, gray, or yellow, and may be nodular or have a depressed center forming a "moon crater" or a "volcano" appearance. These lesions may also have increased vascularity giving a hyperemic appearance.
3. Biopsy techniques using cutting needles or cup forceps are indicated. Electrocautery should be immediately available to achieve hemostasis. If a bleeding vessel is noted it is generally just below the liver capsule and can be handled easily by combining pressure with the cautery tip at the time cauterization is applied.

4.   In patients with hepatocellular cancer, diffuse lesions in both lobes of the liver as well as extrahepatic disease are obvious contraindications to primary resection. These patients may also have associated cirrhosis as a manifestation of chronic alcohol ingestion or hepatitis. Laparoscopy is important in the identification of the cirrhotic liver, which may also be a major contraindication to further resection.

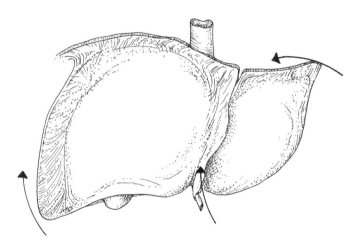

Figure 12.4. Schematic of peritoneal attachments of liver, which may need to be divided for full assessment of the hepatic surface. Generally this is not required, but the laparoscopist should be aware of the regional anatomy.

E. Pancreatic Carcinoma

Currently the most beneficial use of preoperative laparoscopic evaluation is in the management of patients with pancreatic cancer, which may aid in identifying patients in whom cancer cells are already disseminated throughout the abdomen, precluding curative resection. The identification of advanced nodal, peritoneal, or hepatic disease is important prior to undertaking celiotomy. This is especially true in patients with carcinoma of the body and tail since these tumors generally are identified later in the course when compared to patients who have carcinomas of the head of the pancreas and present with early jaundice.

1.   The goals of laparoscopic evaluation in pancreatic cancer are to **assess peripancreatic nodes** as well as **remote sites** that may harbor metastases.
2.   Perform direct inspection of the pancreas by dividing the gastrocolic and gastrohepatic omental areas and inserting the laparoscope into

the **lesser sac**. Needle aspiration or biopsy of peripancreatic masses may be accomplished in this manner, if a tissue diagnosis has not previously been obtained.

3. Pancreatitis and the development of adhesions in this area may render inspection of the lesser sac difficult. Gentle dissection of these adhesions along with electrocautery support may allow for excellent inspection of the pancreatic body and tail with opportunity for laparoscopically guided biopsy in a large number of patients.

4. The major purpose of laparoscopy is to look for superficial peritoneal and hepatic masses that have not been identified by conventional imaging studies. Using a combination of laparoscopy and CT or MRI of the abdomen, at least 90% of unresectible tumors can be identified, which benefits a large group of patients without the need for exploratory celiotomy.

5. Cytologic investigation of peritoneal washings should be performed if other examinations are negative. Carcinoma cells may be obtained from the free peritoneal cavity even when the peritoneum itself is grossly free of metastatic implants.

F. Staging of Other Malignancies, Including Hodgkin Disease

Laparoscopic staging may also be utilized in patients with primary genitourinary malignancies including testicular tumors and prostate cancer. These are discussed in more detail in Chapter 32, Lymph Node Biopsy, Dissection, and Staging Laparotomy. Levels of serum tumor markers are used to delineate a subgroup of these patients that may benefit from preoperative laparoscopic assessment.

Patients with Hodgkin's disease may undergo limited staging laparoscopic procedures or complete laparoscopic staging (equivalent to staging laparotomy) including splenectomy. Hodgkin's disease may present as local, regional, or systemic disease. The traditional open-staging laparotomy includes wedge and needle biopsy of the liver, retroperitoneal and para-aortic nodal dissection, iliac nodal dissection, and splenectomy. Staging laparotomy has largely been supplanted by modern imaging techniques, but still has a role in selected cases where therapeutic decisions require precise assessment of intra-abdominal disease. Staging laparoscopy for Hodgkin's disease combines several procedures that are described in detail in other sections (e.g., laparoscopic splenectomy). A few remarks about the conduct of a staging laparoscopic examination for Hodgkin's disease may be helpful, however.

1. The **Hasson cannula** approach is preferred because tissue must be removed during the procedure (see Chapter 8, Principles of Specimen Removal).

2. Perform **a full abdominal evaluation**, and biopsy any nodules on the surface of the **liver**. If, as is usually the case, the liver appears grossly normal, take a wedge biopsy of the liver (using either suture control

or a laparoscopic stapler for hemostasis). Generally it will be most convenient to take this wedge from the left lobe of the liver. Perform a deep cutting needle biopsy of the other lobe of the liver, generally the right lobe.

3. A **splenectomy** is still considered traditional in full staging for Hodgkin's disease and can be accomplished laparoscopically (see Chapter 31, Laparoscopic Splenectomy). Some protocols utilize a selective approach to splenectomy, based upon imaging studies and intraoperative findings, and this trend may continue.

4. Perform a careful inspection of the spleen in all patients. Identify the region of the tail of the pancreas and hilum of the spleen, and search for **splenic hilar lymph nodes**. Intraoperative ultrasound, discussed later in this section, is extremely helpful. The hilum of the spleen and region of the tail of the pancreas should be identified to assess nodes in this region.

5. Approach the **para-aortic lymph nodes** directly through the base of the transverse mesocolon. Prior study using lymphangiography may identify abnormal nodal regions that could be approached laparoscopically.

6. The nodes in the region of the **common iliac vessels** may be more easily approached and either sampled or totally removed for identification. See Chapter 32 for more information on the technique of node dissection in this region and in the pelvis.

7. Perform a careful assessment of the pelvis in young women and consider oophoropexy if pelvic irradiation is contemplated. Prior consultation with the radiation therapy department will determine whether or not this maneuver is needed. In addition, small clips could be placed in the region of the ovaries to guide the radiation oncologist in treatment planning. Traditionally, oophoropexy may preserve ovarian function in 50% of patients receiving pelvic irradiation, but is less commonly needed with newer treatment protocols.

G. Laparoscopic Ultrasound in Cancer Staging

Laparoscopic cancer staging should include routine adjunctive laparoscopic ultrasound (LUS), which assists in identifying small lesions and directing biopsies. LUS examination uses either linear array or sector scan probes with rigid or flexible tips in frequencies ranging from 5 to 10 MHz. Color Doppler may be available to discern venous or arterial blood flow. These probes allow high-resolution imaging of the liver, bile ducts, pancreas, abdominal vessels, and lymph nodes. Overall, the application of LUS in cancer staging increases the accuracy by approximately 5% to 25% in patients evaluated.

This section gives specific techniques for various anatomic regions, and should be considered complementary to sections B through F (which deal with specific malignancies).

1. **Liver.** Generally three trocars are used, including a 10/11 trocar in the right upper quadrant, an umbilical port for the laparoscope, and a

left upper quadrant port (Fig. 12.5). Pass a flexible or rigid ultrasound probe over the right lobe, medial segment of the left lobe, and lateral segment of the left lobe to identify lesions in the hepatic parenchyma. The anterior and posterior surfaces may be scanned easily without mobilization of the liver.

a. Contact between the ultrasound probe and the liver surface may be improved by lowering the pressure setting on the insufflator and allowing the pneumoperitoneum to partially collapse.

b. Identify hemangiomas and differentiate these from metastatic lesions by their compressibility, elicited either by contact with the ultrasound probe directly or by palpation with an instrument. Small hemangiomas are usually hyperechoic.

c. Small liver metastases are usually hypoechoic compared to normal liver parenchyma or isoechoic with a hypoechoic halo. Biopsy suspicious lesions with a cutting needle or biopsy forceps. Lesions as small as 3 mm may be identified by LUS.

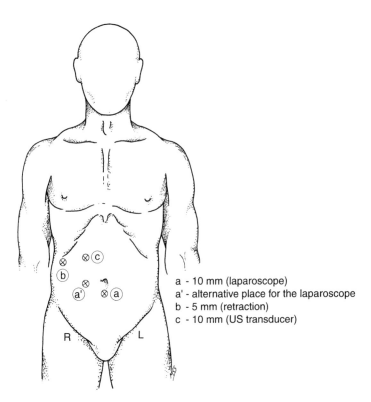

a - 10 mm (laparoscope)
a' - alternative place for the laparoscope
b - 5 mm (retraction)
c - 10 mm (US transducer)

Figure 12.5. Trocar sites for laparoscopic ultrasound examination.

2. **Biliary tract** (See also Chapter 13.3, Laparoscopic Cholecystectomy: Ultrasound and Doppler)

   a. Image the intrahepatic bile ducts, the bifurcation and proximal common bile duct by placing the probe on the anterior surface of segment IV of the liver. Use the umbilical and subcostal trocars alternately to obtain longitudinal and transverse scans. Bile duct dilatation, inflammatory bile duct thickening, and localized bile duct tumors of 1 cm or less may be seen.

   b. Image the **gallbladder** either through the liver or by placing the probe on the gallbladder itself.

   c. Tumors of the bifurcation or the proximal **common bile duct** are usually isoechoic when compared to liver parenchyma. In some patients the falciform ligament prevents the appropriate application of the laparoscopic ultrasound probe during the evaluation of tumors of the left hepatic duct and surrounding area. This may be resolved by scanning segment IV as well as segments II and III to the left of the falciform ligament.

3. **Pancreas and periampullary region**

   a. Visualize the pancreas, pancreatic duct and common bile duct by placing the LUS probe on the stomach and duodenum. Tumors in this region are best imaged through the left and right subcostal trocars, which produce transverse or oblique sections of the pancreas.

   b. The portal venous system may also be imaged with LUS. The superior mesenteric vein is best evaluated from the left subcostal trocar, while the more obliquely oriented portal vein is best imaged from the right subcostal trocar. Vessels of the low-pressure portal system are easily compressed by the ultrasound probe, falsely implying stenosis when in fact the vessel is normal. Tumor infiltration into the portal vein is characterized by loss of the hyperechoic interface between the vessel lumen and the tumor.

   c. Adenocarcinomas of the pancreas as well as small cholangiocarcinomas and carcinomas of the papilla of Vater (approximately 1 cm) may be seen as a hypoechoic mass when compared to normal pancreas. In contrast, neuroendocrine tumors of the pancreas and duodenal wall show higher echogenicity than adenocarcinomas.

   d. Differentiation between pancreatic inflammation and tumor may be quite important. Generally inflamed pancreatic tissue is hypoechoic compared to normal pancreatic parenchyma.

4. **Lymph Nodes**: LUS is an ideal technique for evaluating nodes without performing a formal node dissection. Ultrasound features suggesting benign nodes include a hyperechoic center, which represents hilar fat within the lymph node. If the image is more rounded and more hypoechoic with a loss of the hyperechoic center, metastasis must be assumed. There is overlap on occasion between benign and malignant features of nodes on ultrasound exam. Enlargement of

lymph nodes by itself is not a characteristic of either benign or malignant lesions.

a. Nodes in the **hepatoduodenal ligament** and **celiac axis** are best seen through the left lobe of the liver or by direct approximation of the LUS probe directly on the hepatoduodenal ligament or celiac axis. Localization of these nodes will then allow for laparoscopic biopsy. This is especially helpful in the preoperative staging of gastric carcinoma, or during staging laparoscopy for Hodgkin's disease.

b. Tumors of the gastric cardia or distal esophagus have an isoechoic appearance on LUS. Nodal involvement especially in the **celiac and lesser curve areas** is apparent on LUS.

H. Selected References

Conlon KC, Dougherty E, Klimstra DS, Coit DG, Turnbull AD, Brennan MF. The value of minimal access surgery in the staging of patients with potentially resectable peripancreatic malignancy. Ann Surg 1996;223:134–140.

Feld RI, Liu J-B, Nazarian L. Laparoscopic liver sonography: preliminary experience in liver metastases compared with CT portographpy. J Ultrasound Med 1996;15:289–295.

Fleming ID, Cooper JS, Henson DE, eds. AJCC Cancer Staging Manual, 5th ed. Philadelphia: Lippincott-Raven, 1997.

Greene FL. Laparoscopy in malignant disease. Surg Clin North Am 1992;72:1125–1137.

Greene FL, Rosin RD. Minimal Access Surgical Oncology. Oxford: Radcliffe Medical Press, 1995.

Hunerbein M, Rau B, Schlag PM. Laparoscopy and laparoscopic ultrasound for staging of upper gastrointestinal tumours. Eur J Surg Oncol 1995;21:50–54.

John TG, Greig JD, Carter DC, Garden OJ. Carcinoma of the pancreatic head and periampullary region: tumor staging with laparoscopy and laparoscopic ultrasonography. Ann Surg 1995; 221:156–164.

John TG, Greig JD, Crosbie JL, Miles WF, Garden OJ. Superior staging of liver tumors with laparoscopy and laparoscopic ultrasound. Ann Surg 1994; 220:711–719.

Johnstone P, Rohde DC, Swartz SE, Fetter J, Wexner S. Port site recurrences after laparoscopic and thoracoscopic procedures in malignancy. J Clin Oncol 1996;14:1950–1956.

Ramshaw BJ. Laparoscopic surgery for cancer patients. CA 1997;47:327–350.

Ravikumar TS. Laparoscopic staging and intraoperative ultrasonography for liver tumor management. Surg Oncol Clin North Am 1996;5:271–282.

Warshaw AL, Tepper J, Shipley W. Laparoscopy in the staging and planning of therapy for pancreatic cancer. Am J Surg 1986;151:76–80.

Watt I, Stewart I, Anderson D, Bell G, Anderson JR. Laparoscopy, ultrasound, and computed tomography in cancer of the esophagus and gastric cardia: a prospective comparison for detecting intra-abdominal metastases. Br J Surg 1989;76:1036–1039.

13.1. Laparoscopic Cholecystectomy

Karen Deveney, M.D.

A. Indications

The indications for cholecystectomy remain the same and should not be liberalized because the laparoscopic procedure is viewed as lower in morbidity than its open counterpart. Conditions for which the procedure is used include:

1. **Symptomatic cholelithiasis.** Ultrasound confirmation of gallstones in conjunction with a classic history is sufficient to make the diagnosis.

    a. The most common symptom pattern consists of episodic epigastric or right upper quadrant pain occurring several hours after meals.

    b. Patients with nonspecific symptoms, such as nausea, bloating, indigestion, and flatulence, are sometimes benefited by cholecystectomy; however, the more the symptoms differ from the classic pattern of biliary pain, the less likely the patient is to experience relief after cholecystectomy.

2. **Acute cholecystitis,** typically causing constant right upper quadrant discomfort accompanied by objective signs of right upper quadrant tenderness, with or without a Murphy's sign or a palpable mass: Fever and leukocytosis are common but not necessary for cholecystitis to be present. Despite inflammation, laparoscopic cholecystectomy may be accomplished in most patients without conversion to an open procedure.

    a. **Calculous biliary tract disease** causes most acute cholecystitis, and stones are seen on ultrasound examination.

    b. **Acute acalculous cholecystitis** occurs in critically ill patients, those on prolonged total parenteral nutrition, and some immunosuppressed patients. Thickening of the gallbladder wall on ultrasound, pericholecystic fluid, or delayed emptying all suggest the diagnosis. Although laparoscopic cholecystectomy may be performed, percutaneous cholecystostomy or laparoscopic cholecystostomy are attractive alternative management options for critically ill patients.

3. Individuals with **asymptomatic cholelithiasis** may be appropriate candidates for laparoscopic cholecystectomy under **specific circumstances** such as candidacy for renal transplant.

4. Patients with episodes of right upper quadrant pain, which are "classic" for **biliary pain without evidence of cholelithiasis** on objective tests such as ultrasound or endoscopic retrograde cholangiopancrea-

tography (ERCP) may also be referred for laparoscopic cholecystectomy, but sustained resolution of symptoms is less likely in these patients. Biliary dyskinesia, determined by objective measurement of gallbladder emptying after fatty meal or cholecystokinin infusion, may be present in some of these patients.

5. **Gallstone pancreatitis** occurs when small stones pass through the cystic duct. To prevent recurrence, cholecystectomy should be performed after the pancreatitis has resolved. Cholangiography is prudent to exclude small stones in the common duct.

Contraindications to laparoscopic cholecystectomy include the inability to tolerate general anesthesia, significant portal hypertension, and uncorrectable coagulopathy. The patient must be a suitable candidate for the equivalent open surgical procedure, since conversion to an open procedure may be necessary. Multiple prior operations (causing adhesions, see Chapter 10.3), inflammation from acute cholecystitis or pancreatitis, or unclear anatomy may preclude safe laparoscopic dissection and may require conversion to an open procedure. Conversion to an open procedure represents good judgment under these circumstances.

B. Patient Preparation, Position and Room Setup

Preoperative evaluation should include verification of gallstones and assessment of common duct size by ultrasound, as well as liver function tests. An electrocardiogram (or even specialized cardiac tests) may be prudent to exclude the rare patient in whom cardiac ischemia masquerades as biliary colic. Serum amylase and lipase to exclude acute pancreatitis are ordered selectively.

1. The operating table should be compatible with any radiographic equipment used for cholangiography (see Chapter 13.3, Cholangiography), even if the routine use of this modality is not planned.
2. Position the patient supine on the operating table. The arms are usually extended, but may be tucked at the side if the patient is slender.
3. The surgeon stands at the left side of the patient.
   a. Some surgeons place the patient in the low lithotomy position and operate from between the patient's legs.
   b. Place a single monitor at the head of the operating table if this position is used.
4. Two monitors are used, placed on the right and left of the patient near the head. The typical room setup is shown in Fig. 13.1.1.
5. An orogastric tube is placed after induction of anesthesia. Most surgeons place sequential compression stockings to avoid venous stasis (it is important to note that there are insufficient data in the literature to support this). Some surgeons place a Foley catheter in the bladder.

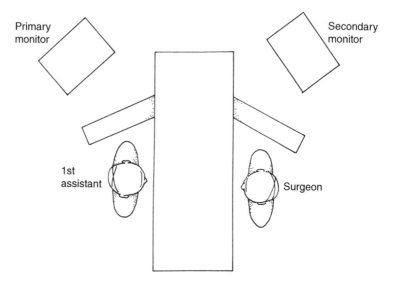

Figure 13.1.1. The most common patient and equipment positions are shown here. The cabinet containing the laparoscopic equipment should be placed on the side of the operating table opposite the main door, so that a C-arm or other radiographic equipment can be brought in if needed. Suction, cautery, and other ancillary equipment are similarly placed behind the monitor on the side away from the door.

C. Trocar Position and Choice of Laparoscope

1. Laparoscopic cholecystectomy usually is performed with four trocars: two 10-mm trocars (in the mid-epigastrium and umbilicus) and two 5-mm trocars along the right costal margin (Fig. 13.1.2).
   a. Place the first 10-mm trocar at the umbilicus, insert the laparoscope, and perform a general exploration of the abdomen.
   b. Although a 0-degree laparoscope can be used, a 30-degree laparoscope allows more flexibility in obtaining a complete view of all structures in the portal area.
2. Place the patient in reverse Trendelenburg position and turn the operating table to the left.

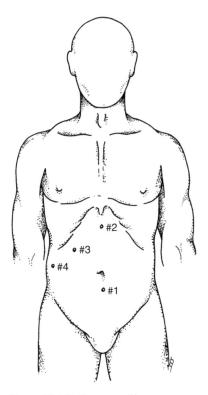

Figure 13.1.2. Trocar positions

a. Under laparoscopic visual control, place two 5 mm trocars along the right costal margin. The usual location is two fingerbreadths below the costal margin at the mid-clavicular and anterior axillary lines. These trocars should be approximately 8 to 10 cm apart. Exact position may need to be modified depending upon patient habitus and the location of the liver relative to the costal margin.

b. The fourth trocar will be the main operating trocar, so good placement is crucial. Some surgeons place graspers into the two lateral ports and manipulate the liver to estimate where Calot's triangle will be during dissection. The most usual location for the fourth trocar is epigastric, at least 10 cm from the laparoscope. The trocar is placed under laparoscopic visual control and should be directed to the right of the falciform ligament as it enters the abdominal cavity.

c.   It is often possible to place the epigastric and two subcostal incisions along the line of an incision suitable for conversion to open procedure.

d.   Modify these trocar positions slightly if the lithotomy position is used. Move the 10/11-mm epigastric trocar to the left upper quadrant, and place one of the 5-mm trocars to the right of the umbilicus. This facilitates two-handed operation from the lithotomy position.

D. Performing the Cholecystectomy

1.   Pass two **atraumatic graspers** through the right subcostal trocars. Gently elevate the liver by passing these graspers beneath the visible liver edge. The gallbladder may be immediate apparent, or may be surrounded by omental adhesions.

2.   Adhesions to the underside of the liver and gallbladder may contain omentum, colon, stomach, or duodenum, and hence must be dissected with care. It is prudent to use cautery as little as possible to avoid transmission of energy to the attached structures (which might result in delayed perforation of a viscus).

3.   If the gallbladder is acutely inflamed and tense, decompress it before attempting to grasp it.

   a.   Pass a Veress needle through the abdominal wall under laparoscopic visual control.

   b.   Use the graspers, closed, to lift the liver and elevate the gallbladder.

   c.   Stab the gallbladder with the Veress needle and connect the needle to suction.

   d.   Remove the Veress needle and place the fundic grasper on stab wound to hold it closed during retraction. Alternatively, use a pretied suture ligature to close this small stab wound.

4.   After the fundus of the gallbladder is exposed, the first assistant grasps the fundus with an atraumatic locking grasper passed through the most lateral of the right subcostal ports. The assistant pushes the gallbladder over the liver toward the right shoulder, opening the subhepatic space and exposing the infundibulum of the gallbladder.

5.   The surgeon or assistant then places a second atraumatic grasper on the gallbladder at its base. This grasper is generally also a locking grasper, although some surgeons will prefer a nonlocking grasper (particularly if a two-handed dissection technique is used).

   a.   Throughout dissection, the direction of traction by this infundibular grasper is critical to prevent errors in identification of the ductal structures in this area.

   b.   Retract the infundibular grasper laterally to expose Calot's triangle (Fig. 13.1.3).

6. Begin dissection directly adjacent to the gallbladder. Take down any additional adhesions to the base of the gallbladder sharply.

7. Identify the cystic duct where it enters the gallbladder. The gallbladder should be seen to funnel down and terminate in the cystic duct. Move the infundibular grasper backward and forward, from side to side, so that the gallbladder–cystic duct junction may be carefully delineated.

8. Some surgeons incise the peritoneum for a centimeter or two upward along the edge of the gallbladder and elevate the gallbladder to create a large space behind the gallbladder, making it easy to identify structures.

9. Dissect the cystic duct free over an adequate length for cholangiography, if desired (see Chapter 13.3). Generally at least 1 cm of length is necessary.

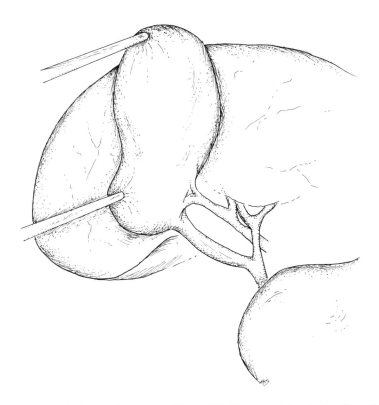

Figure 13.1.3. Retract the fundus of the gallbladder toward the right axilla and the infundibulum laterally to expose Calot's triangle. Retracting the infundibulum anteriorly or even upward tends to collapse Calot's triangle and increase the risk of ductal injury.

10. Place two clips side by side as close to the gallbladder as possible and two similar clips on the cystic duct. Leave enough space between the sets of clips to divide the duct with a scissors. Take care not to retract the cystic duct so forcefully that the clips impinge on the cystic duct–common duct junction (Fig. 13.1.4).

11. Reposition the infundibular grasper to grasp the gallbladder adjacent to the cystic duct. Use this grasper to retract the gallbladder anteriorly and laterally so that the surgeon can expose the cystic artery by gentle spreading and dissecting with a Maryland dissector or laparoscopic right angle clamp. The cystic artery will be noted to terminate by running onto the gallbladder, and visible pulsations may be observed. Generally 1 cm of length is necessary for safe division.

12. Divide the cystic artery with clips, leaving a minimum of two clips on the cystic artery stump. Division of the cystic artery will generally permit the gallbladder to be pulled farther away from the porta hepatis by traction on the infundibular grasper.

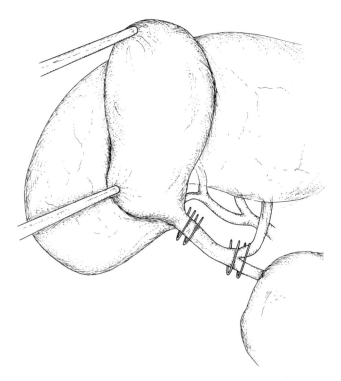

Figure 13.1.4. Excessive traction on the gallbladder infundibulum may "tent up" the common duct, increasing the likelihood that a clip will impinge on the duct and obstruct it.

13. The remainder of the operation consists of dissection of the gallbladder from its bed, taking care to stay away from the porta hepatis and liver bed and to avoid perforating the gallbladder. The infundibular grasper is used to elevate the gallbladder and at a certain point it will become possible to use this grasper to push the gallbladder over the liver edge. Generally better exposure will be obtained if this is postponed until late in the dissection.

   a. Most surgeons use a hook cautery for this phase of the operation. The blunt edge of the hook can be used "cold," without cautery, as a dissector. Bands of connective tissue are hooked, placed on traction, and divided with cautery. Traction and countertraction facilitate the dissection.

   b. Some surgeons prefer cautery scissors or a spatula.

   c. Other energy sources such as laser or Harmonic scalpel (Ultracision, Ethicon Endo-Surgery, Cinncinati, OH) may be used, but are generally unnecessary, less versatile, and more expensive than simple electrocautery (see Chapter 6, Principles of Laparoscopic Hemostasis).

14. When the gallbladder is dissected virtually free from the liver bed but a few strands remain, inspect the gallbladder bed and ducts for evidence of bleeding. Once the gallbladder is removed, exposure of this region is more difficult.

15. Irrigate with saline, but take care not to suction directly on the cystic duct or artery stumps to prevent clip dislodgment.

16. After achieving hemostasis, divide the remaining attachment of the gallbladder to the liver.

17. Place a gallbladder grasper through one of the 10-mm trocars and grasp the gallbladder at or near the cystic duct.

18. Remove the gallbladder from the abdomen.

   a. Consider using a specimen bag if the gallbladder is thick-walled (consider gallbladder carcinoma) or infected.

   b. Frequently bile or stones must first be aspirated from the gallbladder before it can be withdrawn through the trocar site. Open the gallbladder outside the abdominal wall and suction bile from it.

   c. Crush and remove stones with stone forceps, ring forceps, or Kelly clamp. More details of specific extraction techniques are given in Chapter 8, Principles of Specimen Removal.

19. After the gallbladder has been removed, replace the epigastric trocar and inspect the surgical site for bleeding. Irrigate the surgical field, and aspirate the irrigant from the subphrenic space and other areas.

20. If a drain is needed, it can be placed through one of the lateral trocar sites.

   a. Pass an atraumatic grasper into the abdomen through the lateral trocar site.

   b. Align the grasper with the epigastric trocar and pass it out of the abdomen via the epigastric trocar (release the valve in the trocar to accomplish this).

    c.   Grasp the "outside" end of a closed suction drain and pull it into the abdomen.

    d.   Pull the grasper and trocar together out of the abdominal wall, thus pulling the "outside" end of the closed suction drain out. Clamp the closed suction to avoid loss of pneumoperitoneum.

    e.   Position the tip of the drain in the subhepatic space.

21.   Remove the trocars and close the wounds in the usual fashion. Many surgeons inject the trocar sites with a long-acting local anesthetic to minimize pain and facilitate early discharge from hospital.

E. Selected References

Hunter JG. Avoidance of bile duct injury during laparoscopic cholecystectomy. Am J Surg 1991;162:71–76.

Lillemoe KD, Yeo CJ, Talamini MA, Wang BH, Pint HA, Gadacz TR. Selective cholangiography: current role in laparoscopic cholecystectomy. Ann Surg 1992;215:669–676.

Orlando R III. Laparoscopic cholecystectomy: a statewide experience. Arch Surg 1993;128:494–499.

Schirmer BD, Edge SB, Dix J, Hyser MJ, Hanks JB, Jones RS. Laparoscopic cholecystectomy: treatment of choice for symptomatic cholelithiasis. Ann Surg 1991;213:665–677.

Soper NJ, Stockmann PT, Dunnegan DL, Ashley SW. Laparoscopic cholecystectomy: the new "gold standard"? Arch Surg 1992;127:917–923.

Southern Surgeons Club. A prospective analysis of 1,518 laparoscopic cholecystectomies. N Engl J Med 1991;324:1073–1078.

Troidl H, Spangenberger W, Langen R, et al. Laparoscopic cholecystectomy: technical performance, safety and patient's benefit. 1992;24:252–261.

Voyles CR, Petro AB, Meena AL, Haick AJ, Koury AM. A practical approach to laparoscopic cholecystectomy. Am J Surg 1991;161:365–370.

13.2. Laparoscopic Cholecystectomy: Avoiding Complications

Joseph Cullen, M.D., F.A.C.S.

A. Hemorrhage

1. **Cause and prevention:** Bleeding during laparoscopic cholecystectomy can vary from inconsequential oozing to major hemorrhage.
   a. Bleeding can occur at a **trocar insertion** site and drip into the operative field. Obtain hemostasis in the skin before placing a trocar, and avoid any obvious vessels during insertion.
   b. Blunt dissection of adhesions from the gallbladder and liver can result in bleeding from **vessels in the omentum**. Cautious use of electrocautery when dividing omental adhesions prior to applying traction on the gallbladder, can be helpful in preventing this type of bleeding.
   c. Dissection in the **triangle of Calot** can result in sudden and often pulsatile bleeding. Careful and meticulous dissection in this area with accurate identification of the cystic artery and subsequent application of clips can often avoid this complication.
   d. One of the more difficult sources of bleeding is from the **gallbladder fossa**. If bleeding occurs in the area between the posterior wall of the inflamed gallbladder and liver bed, it should be controlled immediately rather than waiting until the entire operative field is obscured.
2. **Recognition and management**
   a. **Trocar site bleeding** may drip into the abdominal wall, or run down instruments to drip into the operative site. There are several strategies for dealing with this kind of bleeding. Identify and gain temporary control by angling the trocar against the abdominal wall; when the trocar is pressed against the region of the bleeding, it will slow or stop. Injection of epinephrine solution (1:10,000) in the vicinity of the bleeding site may stop the bleeding. If disposable trocars are being used, screwing in the anchoring device may compress and stop the bleeding. Finally, a suture ligature may be advanced through the abdominal wall, into the peritoneal cavity, and back out again, thus encompassing the bleeding site. Remember to double-check the area for hemostasis at the conclusion of the case. Remove the trocar under laparoscopic visual control and watch for recurrence of bleeding.

b. When significant, unexpected bleeding occurs in the **triangle of Calot**, do not apply clips blindly. Indiscriminate application of clips in this area may injure the right hepatic artery, right hepatic duct, or common bile duct. If bleeding obscures the laparoscope, remove it and clean the lens. Do not hesitate to insert an additional trocar in the midline between the epigastric and umbilical ports, to provide an extra port for manipulation. Gently pushing the gallbladder against Calot's triangle by manipulating the fundic and infundibular graspers may provide temporary hemostasis while the situation is assessed and additional trocars inserted. Irrigate and aspirate the bleeding area to determine the exact area of bleeding. Grasp and elevate the bleeding vessel and perform any needed additional dissection around the area. Apply clips after precise isolation of the bleeding vessel. If bleeding continues or worsens, laparotomy should be performed.

c. Bleeding from the **gallbladder fossa** can usually be controlled by judicious use of electrocautery. If the cautery tip tends to dig into the liver, apply the metal tip of a suction irrigator to the liver and cauterize on the suction tip instead. Multiple, small areas of bleeding in this area can be controlled by application of oxidized cellulose or topical collagen hemostatic agents. If a bleeder retracts into the liver, a figure-of-eight suture ligature may be necessary. (See Chapter 6, Principles of Laparoscopic Hemostasis, for additional information)

B. Gallbladder Problems

1. **Cause and prevention**

a. The tensely **inflamed gallbladder** often proves difficult to grasp and hold. Preliminary needle decompression (see Chapter 13.1) is sometimes helpful. Stabilize the fundus of the gallbladder and pass a large gauge needle percutaneously into the part of the gallbladder closest to the anterior abdominal wall. A Veress needle works well for this purpose. Connect the needle to suction and aspirate the contents. Close the hole with a grasping forceps or a pretied suture ligature. A large selection of laparoscopic forceps has been designed specifically for retraction of an inflamed and edematous gallbladder. Sometimes an endoscopic Babcock clamp is the best instrument.

b. Despite care, **perforation of the gallbladder** still occurs frequently in the setting of acute cholecystitis. Perforation of during dissection can lead to contamination of the peritoneal cavity with potentially infected bile and gallstones. Tears in the gallbladder wall can also lead to further disruption of the wall, making subsequent dissection difficult. Preliminary decompression, as mentioned before, helps minimize contamination if it occurs.

    c.   Gallbladders containing **large stones** or those with a thickened wall may also be difficult to remove from the abdominal cavity.

    d.   Occult **carcinoma of the gallbladder**, although rare, is occasionally found in the setting of long-standing chronic cholecystitis. Trocar site recurrence has been reported when laparoscopic cholecystectomy was performed in this setting. Some surgeons routinely request pathologic examination of the gallbladder mucosa with frozen section examination of any suspicious areas. The incidence of gallbladder carcinoma is increased in elderly patients with chronic cholecystitis and those with calcifications within the wall of the gallbladder. If preoperative ultrasound is suspicious, or the patient has a calcified gallbladder, consider open (rather than laparoscopic) cholecystectomy.

2. **Recognition and management**

    a.   When **acute cholecystitis** is encountered, partially decompress the tense, distended gallbladder by aspirating its contents through the fundus. Occlude the aspiration site by applying a grasping forceps over the opening or a pretied laparoscopic suture.

    b.   If disruption of the wall has occurred with **spillage**, copious irrigation and suctioning can remove the majority of stones and bile, while larger stones may be placed in a laparoscopic tissue pouch and removed. Placement of closed suction catheters may be indicated for extensive bile spillage. These drainage catheters can be introduced through a lateral cannula. The tip of the catheter is then held in place in the subhepatic space while the cannula is removed.

    c.   Gallbladders containing **large stones** may be placed in a retrieval bag to avoid spillage of stones if the gallbladder tears during attempted removal. Alternatively, the neck of the gallbladder may be pulled partially out of the abdomen and the stones within the gallbladder crushed and removed piecemeal. Gallbladders with thickened walls should be placed in a retrieval bag prior to removal; on rare occasion an occult carcinoma of the gallbladder will be found, and this method minimizes contamination of the trocar site. Finally, enlarging the skin and fascial incisions at the extraction site will usually suffice in completing the removal of the gallbladder from the abdomen. If the adjacent rectus muscles are not incised, enlarging the incision will add minimal additional postoperative pain or cosmetic defects. (See Chapter 8, Principles of Specimen Removal, for additional information.)

    d.   **Carcinoma of the gallbladder** is best recognized and dealt with at the time of the original operation. Maintain a high index of suspicion and request frozen section examination in doubtful cases. If carcinoma of the gallbladder is identified, consider conversion to open with excision of the gallbladder bed, regional lymphadenectomy (depending upon depth of penetration), and excision of trocar sites. Implantation of carcinoma of the gallbladder has been reported to occur as rapidly as one week after laparoscopic cholecystectomy, and is not limited to the trocar used for specimen removal.

C. Postoperative Bile Leakage

1. **Cause and prevention:** Postoperative bile leaks or collections may be the result of common duct or right hepatic duct injury (discussed below), cystic duct stump leakage, or injury to an accessory bile duct. Severely edematous tissues from acute cholecystitis will result in failure of standard clips to completely occlude the cystic duct, resulting in postoperative bile leak. When dissection of the gallbladder is difficult in the setting of acute cholecystitis or when there is significant bile spillage, place a closed suction drain. This may prevent bile collections from minor leaks from the liver bed or aid in controlling cystic duct stump leaks.

2. **Recognition and management:** During operation, a number of conditions that predispose to bile leaks can be recognized, and if managed correctly, the complication can be avoided. If the cystic duct appears edematous and inflamed, both surgical clips and pretied laparoscopic sutures can be used to securely occlude the cystic duct. Bile leakage from small accessory ducts in the gallbladder may not be recognized at the time of laparoscopic cholecystectomy but may be the source of later bile leak. These accessory ducts should be suspected if the gallbladder fills with contrast during intraoperative cholangiography despite occlusion of the junction of the gallbladder and cystic duct. When this filling is noted at operation, these ducts should be recognized and clipped, ligated, or coagulated. Placement of closed suction drains are also recommended. When a collection is suspected, an ulrasound or computed tomography scan of the abdomen will establish the diagnosis and any collections may be aspirated and drainage established.

   If a bile collection occurs, the biliary tree should be investigated by radionuclide scan and endoscopic cholangiography (ERCP). ERCP is useful in both the diagnosis and treatment. Cholangiography often demonstrates extravasation from the cystic duct stump. When a leak is noted, treatment consists of decreasing the pressure at the distal end of the common bile duct and may include passage of a nasobiliary drain, endoscopic sphincterotomy, or placement of a transpapillary stent. All of these methods decrease the pressure in the duct and allow rapid closure in cases of both cystic duct stump leaks and accessory bile duct leaks. Early investigation of bile leaks with ERCP also allows prompt diagnosis of bile duct injury, facilitating early repair and increasing the chance of long-term success.

D. Bile Duct Injury

1. **Cause and prevention:** Injury to the ductal system usually occurs during the dissection at the triangle of Calot, exposing the cystic duct. Cephalad traction will often cause the cystic duct to lie in a straight line with the common bile duct, allowing the common duct to be mistaken for the cystic duct. To prevent this from happening, retract the infundibulum of the gallbladder laterally to fully expose the cystic duct and gallbladder from the common duct.

   Excessive retraction of the gallbladder when the clips are applied to the proximal cystic duct may result in trapping a portion of the common duct in the clips. To prevent this, leave a longer cystic duct remnant. Dissect the cystic duct from the infundibulum of the gallbladder downward, incising the medial and lateral peritoneal attachments of the infundibulum to the liver. Remove all connective tissue and fat to clearly expose the junction of the cystic duct with the gallbladder. Avoid excessive use of electrocautery in the triangle of Calot, which may lead to late injury and strictures to the ductal system. Intraoperative cholangiography will outline the biliary anatomy and may avoid major ductal injuries (see Chapter 13.3, Cholangiography).

2. **Recognition and management:** Major injuries to the ductal system may be noted with continued dissection as bile leaks into the operative field, or later, when the patient presents with jaundice or an intraabdominal bile collection.

   When recognized at operation, conversion to laparotomy is advised. If a significant portion of the ductal system has been excised, reconstruction with a hepaticojejunostomy is indicated. When only a small choledochotomy has been made, reconstruction over a T-tube may be attempted. A clean transection without tissue loss may require a ductal anastomosis over a T-tube. Patients with injury to the biliary system recognized several days later need cholangiography to adequately define the injury. If cholangiography reveals total occlusion or transection of the ductal system, immediate operative repair, usually by hepaticojejunostomy, is indicated. Injuries to the lateral wall of the common duct may be treated with external drainage of any intra-abdominal collections and biliary stenting.

E. Selected References

Airan M, Appel M, Berci G, et al. Retrospective and prospective multi-institutional laparoscopic cholecystectomy study organized by the Society of American Gastrointestinal Endoscopic Surgeons. Surg Endosc 1992;6:169–176.

Gadacz TR, Talamini MA. Traditional versus laparoscopic cholecystectomy. Am J Surg 1991;161:336–338.

McSherry CK. Laparoscopic cholecystectomy: time for critical analysis. Surg Endosc 1992;6:177–178.

Moosa AR, Easter DW, Van Sonnenberg E, et al. Laparoscopic injuries to the bile duct. Ann Surg 1992;215:203–208.

Ponsky JL. Complications of laparoscopic cholecystectomy. Am J Surg 1991;161:393–395.

Ponsky JL. Incidence and management of complications of laparoscopic cholecystectomy. Adv Surg 1994;27:21–40.

Ponsky JL. Management of the complications of laparoscopic cholecystectomy. Endoscopy 1992;24:724–729.

Rossi RL, Schirmer WJ, Baasch JW, et al. Laparoscopic bile duct injuries. Arch Surg 1992;127:596–602.

13.3. Laparoscopic Cholecystectomy: Cholangiography

George Berci, M.D., F.A.C.S.

A. Introduction

Routine intraoperative cholangiography (RIOC) (preferably utilizing fluoroscopy) is practiced by many surgeons and advocated by the author of this chapter for the following reasons:

1. RIOC allows immediate recognition of anatomy and anomalies or stones.
2. Discovery of partial or total transection of ducts or clip placement across the CBD, facilitating immediate repair, can be performed.
3. It allows removing a common duct stone during laparoscopic cholecystectomy, by either the transcystic duct or laparoscopic choledochotomy method (see Chapter 14).
4. It precleuds unnecessary preoperative endoscopic retrograde cholangiopancreatography (ERCP) or endoscopic sphincterotomy.

The variety of anomalies and intraoperative hazards that may be detected by RIOC are shown in Figs. 13.3.1 to 13.3.5.

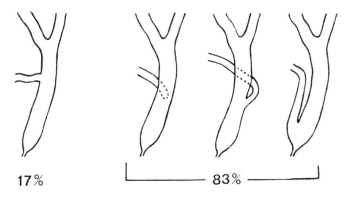

17% 83%

Figure 13.3.1. The textbooks state that the cystic duct enters the common duct along a relatively straight line in 75% of cases. The author has noted that this occurs in only 17% of operative cholangiograms; in the majority of cases, the cystic duct enters posterior, spiral, or parallel to the common duct.

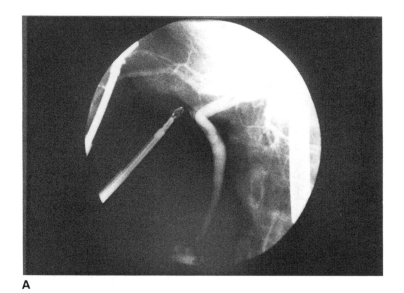

A

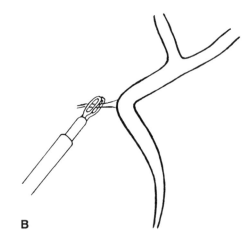

B

Figure 13.3.2. A. Slight traction on the cholangiograsper can tent the common duct, especially if the cystic duct is very short. In the two-dimensional view seen on the monitor, the common duct may be misinterpreted as the cystic duct and transected. The length of the cholangiograsper jaws is 10 mm. B. Schematic diagram of cholangiogram seen in A. It is very important to recognize the short cystic duct.

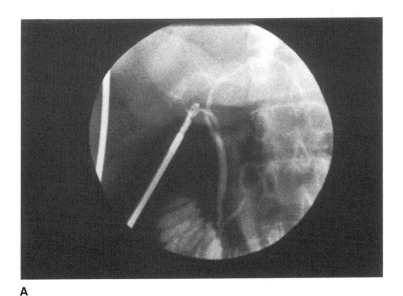

Figure 13.3.3. A. A very close spiral drainage of the cystic duct into the common duct. B. Schematic of cholangiogram.

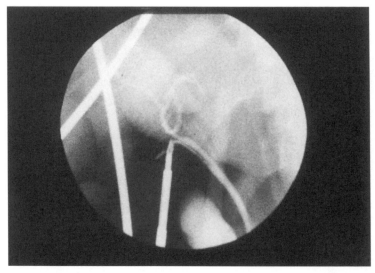

A

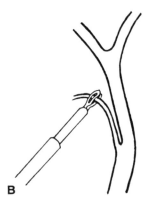

B

Figure 13.3.4. A. Close parallel run of cystic duct and common duct. Note how close the cholangiograsper jaw is to the common hepatic duct. B. Schematic diagram of cholangiogram. The cholangiograsper jaw is only 10 mm long; this gives some hint of distances and proximities.

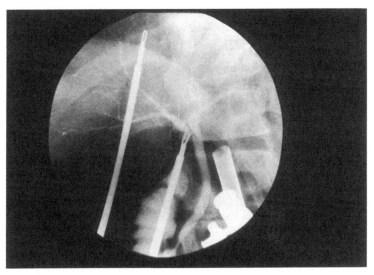

A

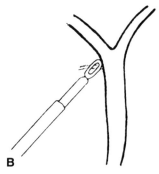

B

Figure 13.3.5. A. Dangerously short cystic duct draining directly into right hepatic duct. B. Schematic drawing of cholangiogram.

B. Radiographic Equipment

Fluoroscopy is preferred for the following reasons:
1. It allows immediate observation of adequacy of filling using small increments of contrast to avoid obscuring small calculi and overlapping structures (e.g. the cystic duct drainage into the CBD).
2. It confers a tremendous savings in time; the anatomy or anomalies are immediately discovered but images are recorded and processed later, and the surgeon does not need to wait for films to be developed (and, all too often, find the film quality suboptimal necessitating repeat studies).
3. Tiny calculi may be flushed from the common duct without duct exploration.

The surgeon should be thoroughly familiar with the equipment and its operation, because after hours and on weekends, a fully trained technician may not available. In some states one must pass a simple fluoroscopy-operator test. This is worthwhile, as the surgeon then has a license to operate the unit. Close collaboration with the Department of Radiology is advised; in some hospitals, it may be possible to transmit images via a simple coaxial cable to a radiologist, who can then watch as the cholangiogram is performed. An audio link allows communication between radiologist and surgeon. Such links are becoming more and more commonplace. The surgeon must, however, be familiar with basic radiographic anatomy of the biliary tree and be able to evaluate the images.

Equipment varies from totally dedicated, ceiling mounted units in specialized operating room suites, to the more common and mobile C-arm digital fluoroscope unit found in most hospitals. The image intensifier screen is typically 9/6 inch. This means that under routine operation, the field size is 9 inches, and that additional magnification can be attained by switching to a 6-inch field if needed.

The x-ray tube may be self-rectified or rotating anode. The latter is preferred because the beam penetrates obese patients better. The surgeon and assistants stand behind a mobile lead screen for protection. Use an extension tube on the cholangiogram catheter setup to allow greater distance (see below). Remember the inverse square law which describes radiation intensity: Dose diminishes as the square of the distance from the source; therefore, a small additional distance from the x-ray tube greatly decreases the dose to surgeon and assistants. Radiation exposure is cumulative, and even small doses add up over a professional lifetime (Figs. 13.3.6 to 13.3.8).

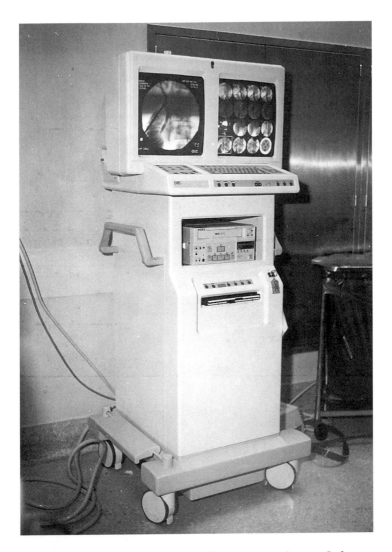

Figure 13.3.6. Mobile digitized C-arm fluoroscopy equipment. Left screen shows real-time full-size fluoroscopic image. Right screen shows stored images (frames) to be selected and printed. VHS is seen below with the full-sized film camera.

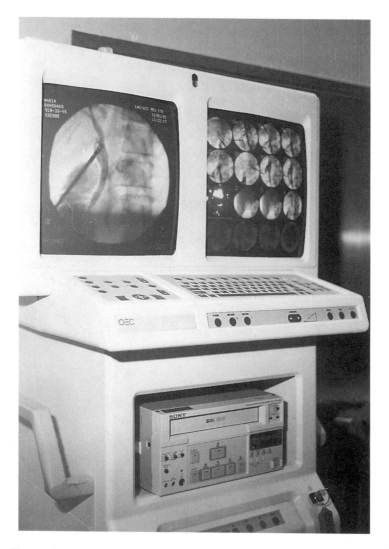

Figure 13.3.7. Close-up view of control panel. The functions for a cholangiogram are preprogrammed and only one button needs to be pushed. Modes are activated by a foot switch, as is VHS record. (OEC Co., Salt Lake City, UT).

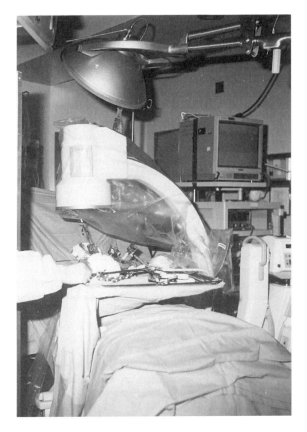

Figure 13.3.8. It is easy to position the sterile covered unit over the abdomen, and the required anatomy is immediately noted and corrected if necessary.

C. Cystic Duct Cholangiography

1. **The easy case.** In the patient with few adhesions, Calot's triangle is easily dissected and the cystic duct identified. It is crucial to see the duct entering the gallbladder, as previously mentioned (Chapter 13.2).

    a. Place a clip or ligature on the cystic duct at or near its termination upon the gallbladder.

    b. Clip the cystic artery as well. This ensures that the cholangiogram will be performed with all crucial structures clipped, minimizing the chance of ductal injury **after** cholangiography.

c.   A large variety of cholangiocatheters are available, and selection is a matter of individual preference. The author prefers a blue 4-French ureteral catheter with black visual markers and an open-end tip. This is easy to manipulate and inexpensive.

d.   Connect the catheter to a long extension tube with a Y connector. At the far end of the extension tube there should be two stopcocks and two syringes (Fig. 13.3.9).

e.   Use a larger syringe for saline, and a smaller one for contrast medium. Have the scrub nurse mark the syringe containing contrast (with sterile marking tape, or a simple ligature of black silk).

f.   Dilute the contrast medium. If you are using 60% contrast, dilute it 1:1. More dilute medium is less likely to obscure small stones within a dense dye column. Conversely, less dilute medium will show fine ductal detail better and may be preferred if stones are not a consideration.

g.   Ensure that all air bubbles are removed from the system. Air bubbles can hide in the stopcocks, the Y connectors, or in the space between the syringe full of contrast and the extension tubing. Therefore, after the saline has been flushed through the system including the catheter, it is worthwhile to open the stopcock from the contrast syringe and push a full milliliter of saline back through the system into the contrast syringe to eliminate any air bubbles.

h.   Make a small incision in the anterior wall of the cystic duct using a sharp pair of fine-tipped scissors. Try to judge the thickness of the duct and enter the lumen with a single cut. The cystic duct is often thicker than expected, and making multiple cuts makes it harder to cannulate (as well as increasing the probability that the duct will be totally transected).

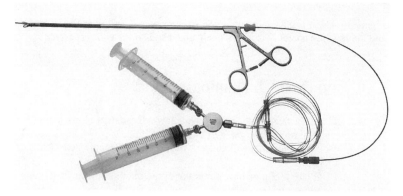

Figure 13.3.9. Cholangiograsper with 4-French ureteral catheter inserted, extension tubing, Y-shaped adapter, and two syringes of different sizes (Karl Storz, Endoscopy-America, Culver City, CA).

i. Use a flat grasper to milk the cystic duct toward the incision, to remove small stones and debris. Clear bile should flow, indicating an unobstructed passage into the proximal biliary tree. If a stone appears, remove it with a stone forceps.

j. Pass the cholangiograsper with its inserted catheter through the fourth trocar site (the one normally used to retract the infundibulum). This is generally done by the assistant, while the surgeon retracts the infundibulum of the gallbladder to provide slide tension on the cystic duct. Do not overstretch the cystic duct, as this will make the lumen collapse and render cannulation much more difficult.

k. The catheter should protude slightly (½ to 1 inch) from the end of the cholangiograsper jaws (Fig. 13.3.10).

l. Advance the catheter into the dochotomy with very small motions. Do not introduce too much of the catheter into the duct (1 to 2 cm is sufficient). Monitor the length of the catheter by watching the markings (one to two markings should go into the duct).

m. Open the cholangiograsper and slide it coaxially over the catheter, without introducing more catheter into the duct. Close the grasper to secure the catheter and secure a watertight closure of the dochotomy. Inject some saline to confirm placement.

n. Secure the grasper on the outside of the abdomen to avoid dislodgment. Remove the laparoscope. The infundibular grasper may be removed or left in situ. Place the fluoroscope in position and confirm that the field is centered. A marker on the abdomen is a great help to surgeon and technician in ensuring the field is approximately centered. Make a scout film without contrast.

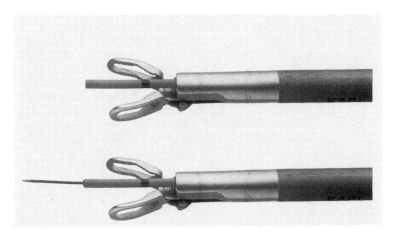

Figure 13.3.10. Cholangiograsper seen in close-up with protruding ureteral catheter (top). In case of difficult introduction, a guide wire is advanced and introduced into the cystic duct, followed by the catheter (bottom).

o. Inject contrast medium very slowly and freeze a frame shortly after the first few drops are injected. Ascertain whether or not the catheter is in a good position. If the catheter is inserted too far, pull it back. Go very slowly with small increments and save several images during the procedure (6–8 films per cholangiogram). Record the images digitally or on tape.

2. **Management of problems**

a. **Inability to cannulate** the cystic duct: Ask the nurse to inject a small amount of saline as cannulation is attempted. This will open the lumen. If the catheter cannot be introduced after repeated attempts, the problem may be the spiral valves of Heister. In this case, introduce a small (0.35 inch) guide wire with a floppy end through the catheter. Slip the soft (floppy) end of the guide wire into the dochotomy and pass the catheter over the guide wire. Remove the guide wire before closing the cholangiograsper.

b. **Flaccid sphincter**. In this case, contrast material immediately passes out of the distal common duct into the duodenum and the upper biliary tree is not filled. Place the patient in the Trendelenburg position and ask the anesthesiologist to administer intravenous morphine to cause the sphincter to go into spasm. Repeat the cholangiogram. Sometimes additional contrast medium must be injected under sufficient pressure to fill the entire biliary tree because of spasm of the sphincter.

c. **Abnormal appearance of the sphincter**: Use the magnification function to observe the sphincter in greater detail (be sufficiently familiar with the equipment to do this!) and observe the sphincter for 5 or 10 seconds. By watching for sphincter motion a "pseudocalculus" may disappear (Fig. 13.3.11).

d. **Rounded lucencies**: stones or air bubbles? Slowly inject 2 to 3 ml of contrast under constant fluoroscopic control. Then withdraw the plunger to create a vacuum. Repeat this maneuver twice and observe the motion and appearance of the lucency. Bubbles move in synchrony with the column of contrast. Stones tend to adhere to the wall of the duct and do not move.

e. **Overfilled ductal system** or excess dye in the duodenum. Too much contrast on the film creates difficulties in interpretation. Wash out the duct with warm saline (to avoid sphincter spasm) and then repeat the cholangiogram (Fig. 13.3.12).

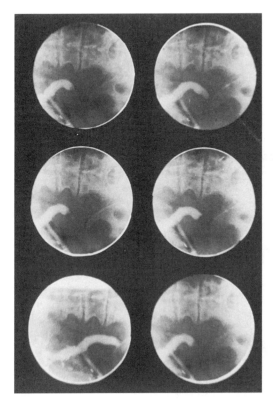

Figure 13.3.11. Sphincter function during the opening and closing cycles. The thumbprint configuration shown in middle figures can easily be misinterpreted as a stone. By observing the sphincter for a few seconds longer, the opening and closing of the sphincter can be easily seen and the image correctly interpreted.

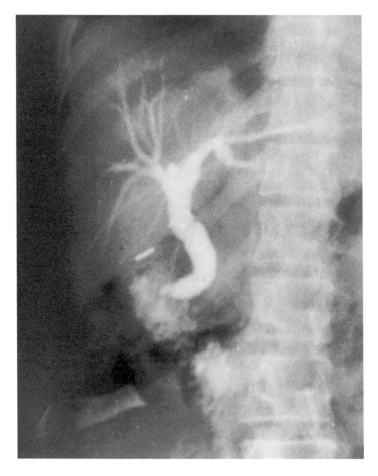

Figure 13.3.12. The ductal system is overfilled with contrast and no early filling stage is seen. The cystic duct drainage into the common duct is obscured by excess contrast.

D. Danger Signs

The surgeon should be able to recognize certain radiographic danger signs, which mandate immediate exploration:

1. Contrast material is seen in the distal common bile duct (CBD) below the cystic duct but contrast extravasation is observed above this site: open the patient up immediately. There is a great probability that there is a **transection of the duct** (Fig. 13.3.13).

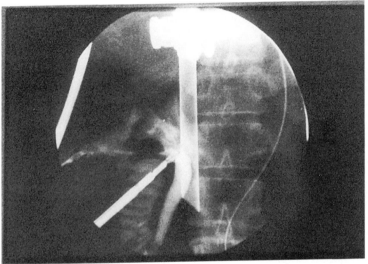

A

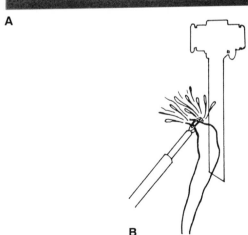

B

Figure 13.3.13. A. The distal duct is well seen but there is obvious extravasation of dye proximal. The duct was found to be transected. The injury was recognized and immediate repair performed. B. Schematic of cholangiogram.

2. The distal duct is well filled with contrast but there is no filling of the proximal ductal system, and the situation does not change with repeated injection and the maneuvers described above. Convert to an open procedure because there is a chance that a clip (what you should see on films) or other manipulations caused the obstruction (Fig. 13.3.14).

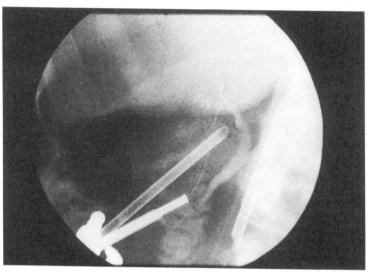

A

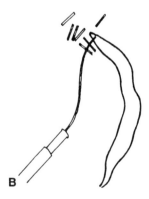

B

Figure 13.3.14. A. Distal duct is seen but no contrast material is seen in the proximal duct. A clip occluded the duct. If the proximal duct cannot be filled with contrast, open the patient immediately. B. Schematic of cholangiogram.

E. Other Difficulties and Their Solution

There are a few additional tricks that every laparoscopic surgeon should be familiar with.

1. **Stone knowingly left behind**: Sometimes a stone is seen in the common duct and the decision is made not to do laparoscopic common duct exploration. If the equipment or expertise to perform laparoscopic common duct exploration are not available, or a stone is difficult or impacted and cannot be removed, insert a guide wire through the cholangiocatheter. Pass the guide wire through into the duodenum under fluoroscopic guidance. Fix the other end of the guide wire at its exit site in the flank. This will greatly facilitate subsequent postoperative ERCP and sphincterotomy.

2. **Alternative methods of cholangiography**: There are other ways to perform a cystic duct cholangiogram. Sometimes these are easier than the method just described, particularly if it is difficult to get the correct alignment to introduce the catheter through one of the existing trocars, or if traction on both the infundibular and fundic graspers must be maintained to expose the cystic duct. In this case, pass a straight or angled needle through the abdominal wall at the desired site and introduce the cholangiocatheter through the needle.

3. **Cholecystocholangiography**: At times, dissection in the cystic duct area is extremely difficult or appears hazardous and a decision must be made whether to convert the case. Cholecystocholangiography is performed by needle puncture and injection of contrast directly into the gallbladder. When successful, it delineates the anatomy of the cystic duct and common duct.

   a. Tilt the patient to the right to avoid a contrast-filled gallbladder obscuring ductal anatomy.

   b. Puncture the gallbladder with the Veress needle connected to an extension tube filled with contrast.

   c. Place a clip near the infundibulum of the gallbladder as a marker.

   d. For this procedure, a large volume of contrast medium is needed. Instruct the nurse to prepare more than the usual 30 ml (100–200 ml may be needed).

   e. Inject slowly under continuous fluroroscopic guidance. Observe the location, relative to the clip on the infundibulum, where the cystic duct joins the gallbladder and then terminates on the common duct (Fig. 13.3.15).

   f. Subsequent decision making (to dissect further or to convert to an open procedure) can then be made rationally and with better information. At the end of the procedure, evacuate some of the contrast medium (now mixed with bile) and close the puncture site with a large clip or pretied ligature.

4. **Laparoscopic Choledocholithotomy (LCL)**: LCL is a logical extension of laparoscopic cholecystectomy. It requires more skill, teamwork, and equipment—but the patient can be treated and cured in one

session. Operative (fluoro) cholangiography is an essential part of LCL (for further details see chapters 14.1 and 14.2 on laparoscopic common duct explorations).

5. **Preoperative ERCP**: If you routinely perform operative (fluoro) cholangiography, the overwhelming number of (negative) ERCPs can be eliminated. ERCP and E. Sphincterotomy are procedures with complications and additional costs involved. The indication for the pre-op ERCP is the high-risk patient with cholangitis, septicemia, and severe underlying disease.

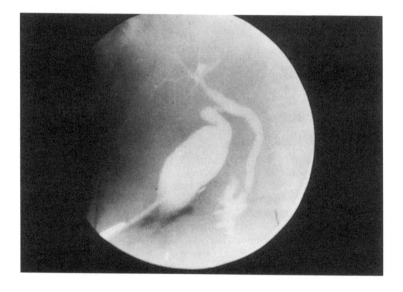

Figure 13.3.15. Cholecystocholangiogram. In the difficult case, direct needle puncture of the gallbladder with contrast injection can display the anatomy. In this example, the cystic duct drains directly into the common hepatic duct.

F. Selected References

Berci G, Hamlin JA, eds. Operative Biliary Radiology. Baltimore: Williams and Wilkins, 1981.

Berci G, Hamlin JA. Operative cholangiography. In: Berci G, Hamlin JA, eds. Operative Biliary Radiology. Baltimore: Williams and Wilkins, 1981.

Berci G, Sackier J. Intraoperative cholangiography. In: Berci G, ed. Problems in General Surgery: Laparoscopic Surgery 1991;8:310–318. Philadelphia: Lippincott.

Berci G, Shore JM, Hamlin JA, Morgenstern L. Operative fluoroscopy and cholangiography. The use of modern radiological techniques during surgery. Am J Surg 1977;135:32–35.

Bergman JG, Vander Mays, Rauw AJ, et al. Long-term follow-up after endoscopic sphincterotomy. G.I. Endoscopy 1996;44:643.

Cohen SA, Siegel JH, Kasmin FE. Complications of diagnostic and therapeutic ERCP. Abdominal Imaging 1996;21:385.

Cotton PB, Lehman G, Vennes J, et al. Endoscopic sphincterotomy complications and their management. Special Report GI End 1991;37:383.

Cullen JJ, Scott-Conner CEH. Surgical anatomy of laparoscopic common duct exploration. In: Berci G, Cushieri A, eds. Ducts and Ductal Stones. Philadelphia: WB Saunders. 1997;20–25.

Cuschieri A, Berci G. Training for laparoscopic surgery. In: Laparoscopic Biliary Surgery. London: Blackwell, 1982;1–17:1–217.

Cushieri A, Berci G. The role of intraoperative fluorocholangiography during laparoscopic cholecystectomy. In: Berci G, Cushieri A, eds. Bile Ducts and Ductal Stones. Philadelphia: WB Saunders, 1997.

Fletcher DR. Laparoscopic cholecystectomy: role of pre-operative and post-operative endoscopic retrograde cholangio-pancreatography and endoscopic sphincterotomy. Gastrointest Endosc Clin North Am 1993;3:249–259.

Freeman ML, Nelson DB, Sherman ST, et al. Complications of endoscopic biliary sphincterotomy. N.J. Med 1996;825–909.

Hamlin, JA. Radiological anatomy and anomalies of the extrahepatic biliary ducts. In: Berci G, Cushieri A, eds. Bile Ducts and Ductal Stones. Philadelphia: Saunders, 1997.

Hicken NF, Best RR, Hunt HB. Cholangiography. Ann Surg 1936;103:210–215.

Katos GS, Tomplins RK, Turnipseed W, Zollinger R. Operative cholangiography. Arch Surg 1972;104:484–490.

Lee KH. Radiation safety considerations in fluoroscopy In: Berci G, Cushieri A, eds. Bile Duct and Ductal Stones. Edit: Philadelphia: WB Saunders, 1997

Lillemoe D, Martin SA, Cameron J, et al. Major bile duct injuries during lapar- cholecystectomy. Ann Surg 1997;225:459–469.

Malley-Guy P. Television radioscopy during operations of the biliary passages. Surg Gynecol Obstet 1958;106:747-751.

Mirizzi, PL. Operative cholangiography. Surg Gynecol Obstet 1932;65:702–710.

Soper NJ, Brunt LM. The case for routine operative cholangiography during laparoscopic cholecystectomy. Surg Clin North Am 1994;74:953–959.

Stewart L, Way LW. Bile duct injuries during laparoscopic cholecystectomy. Arch Surg 1995;130:1123–1133.

Stiegmann G, Goff, Manseur A, et al. Pre-cholecystectomy endoscopic cholangiography. Am J Surg 1992;163:227–232.

Strasberg SM, Hertl M, Soper NJ. An analysis of the problem of biliary injury during laparoscopic cholecystectomy. J Am Coll Surg 1995;180:101–125.

Traverso W, Hargrove K, Kozarek R. A cost effective approach to the treatment of CBD stones with surgical versus endoscopic techniques. In Berci G, Cushieri A, eds. Bile Ducts and Ductal Stones. Edit: Philadelphia: WB Saunders, 1997;154–160.

Woods MS, Traverso W, Kozarek R. Characteristics of Biliary complications during laparoscopic cholecystectomy. Am J Surg 1994;167:27–30.

13.4. Laparoscopic Cholecystectomy: Ultrasound and Doppler

Maurice E. Arregui, M.D., F.A.C.S.

A. Indications and Equipment

Laparoscopic ultrasound is a safe, effective, sensitive, and specific technique to use for detecting choledocholithiasis during laparoscopic cholecystectomy. It is also useful for ruling out ligation or transection of the common bile duct. When sufficient experience is attained, it is an excellent substitute for digital fluorocholangiography. Additional information on other applications of laparoscopic ultrasound is given in Chapter 12, Elective Diagnostic Laparoscopy and Cancer Staging.

For ultrasound of the biliary tree, high-frequency probes in the 7- to 10-MHz range using solid state linear transducers are optimal. The ultrasound probe must fit through a 10-mm trocar. A deflectable tip is useful but a rigid probe will suffice. Curved array or mechanical sector probes are options, but they do not provide the resolution and near-field detail necessary for accurate diagnosis.

Color Doppler is a costly addition. This device can distinguish bile duct from vascular structure. It does not substitute for a surgeon's knowledge of anatomy. Doppler without the dynamic color feature is a useful and much less expensive device. For the most part, Doppler for the examination of the common bile duct is seldom needed.

B. Technique

1. Dissect and clip or ligate the cystic duct before performing laparoscopic ultrasound.
2. The ultrasound probe may be passed through a 10-mm epigastric trocar. From this access, the probe may be placed on the porta hepatis to obtain a transverse view of the biliary tree and portal structures.
3. The author prefers to place the probe through the 10-mm umbilical port. This gives a linear view of the portal structures, which is more useful and easier to interpret.
    a. Place a 5-mm laparoscope through the lateral right upper quadrant trocar to check the position of the ultrasound probe.
    b. Place the probe over segment IV of the liver, directing the ultrasound beam to the liver hilum.

c. Identify the common hepatic duct through the liver parenchyma and follow the left and right hepatic ducts to their secondary and tertiary branchings.

d. Place the probe on the porta hepatis with the tip in the liver hilum. The hepatic duct will be seen longitudinally. The hepatic artery is usually seen in transverse section between the bile duct and portal vein. Posterior to the portal vein is the caudate lobe of the liver, and deep to this is the inferior vena cava.

e. The junction of the cystic duct with the hepatic duct is identified and the common duct distal to this is then measured with acoustic calipers (Fig. 13.4.1).

f. Preliminary ligation or clipping of the cystic duct allows the surgeon to assure that the anatomy has been correctly identified, by correlating the ligated structure with the ultrasound anatomy.

g. Follow the common duct to the head of the pancreas, where overlying fat and omentum often make visualization of the intrapancreatic bile duct difficult (due to poor transmission through the fat).

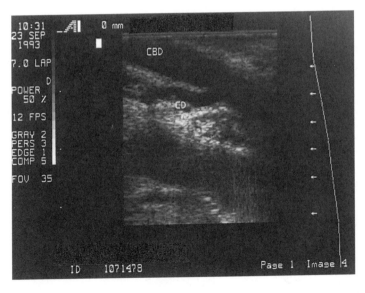

Figure 13.4.1. The cystic duct (CD) is seen to join the hepatic duct to form the common bile duct. A lymph node is seen posterior to the common bile duct. The inferior vena cava is posterior.

h. The duodenum provides a better acoustic window. Position the probe lateral to the duodenum with the ultrasound beam pointing toward the pancreas. From this perspective, the common bile duct is seen transversely. Follow the common duct caudad until the pancreatic duct joins it (Fig. 13.4.2).

i. Follow both ducts to the ampulla (Fig. 13.4.3).

j. If the distal bile duct is poorly seen, insert a cholangiocatheter into the cystic duct and infuse saline to distend the intrapancreatic bile duct, providing a better view.

k. A stone in the bile duct usually appears as a crescent-shaped hyperechoic structure with posterior shadowing.

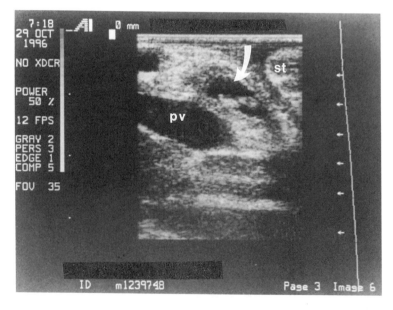

Figure 13.4.2. An oblique view of the common bile duct (arrow) with a thickened wall reveals two small nonshadowing distal common bile duct stones. The stomach (st) and portal vein (pv) are also seen.

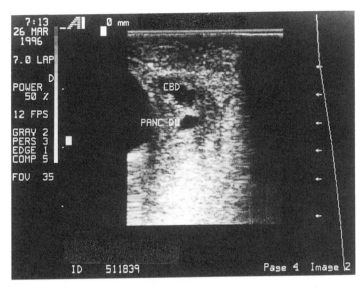

Figure 13.4.3. From a lateral view through the duodenum, the intrapancreatic common bile duct (CBD) and pancreatic duct (PANC DU) are seen transversely.

C. Results in Clinical Practice

The author has compared laparoscopic ultrasound to digital fluorocholangiography in 360 patients. The overall sensitivity and specificity of laparoscopic ultrasound was 90% and 100%, respectively, and that of digital fluorocholangiography, 98.1% and 98.1%. There were a total of five false negatives for ultrasound and one for digital fluorocholangiography. Four of the false negatives on ultrasound were in our first 140 patients. The last false negative was missed by ultrasound and digital fluorocholangiography. In our latest series of 142 patients the sensitivity and specificity of laproscopic ultrasound was 95.7% and 100%, respectively, and that of digital fluorocholangiography, 95.2% and 100%. Rothlin compared laparoscopic ultrasound with static cholangiography and reported sensitivities of 100% and specificities of 98% for ultrasound compared with 75% and 99%, respectively, for static cholangiography. With experience, laparoscopic ultrasound can be as sensitive and specific as digital fluorocholangiography. It is more rapidly performed than either static x-rays or digital fluorocholangiography.

D. Selected References

Jakimowicz JJ, Rutten H. Jurgens PI, Carol EJ. Comparison of operative ultrasound and radiography in screening the common bile duct for calculi. World J Surg 1987;11:628–34.

Machi J, Siegel B. Ultrasound for Surgeons, 1st ed. New York: Igaku-Shoin, 1997.

Rothlin MA, Schlumpf R. Largiader F. Laparoscopic sonography: an alternative to routine intraoperative cholangiography? Arch Surg 1994;129:694–700.

Staren ED, Arregui ME. Ultrasound for the Surgeon, 1st ed. Philadelphia: Lippincott–Raven, 1997.

Thompson DM, Tetik C, Arregui ME. Laparoscopic ultrasound. Probl Gen Surg 1997;14:107–116.

14.1. Laparoscopic Common Bile Duct Exploration: Transcystic Duct Approach

Joseph B. Petelin, M.D., F.A.C.S.

A. Indications, Contraindications, and Choice of Approach

1. **Indications:** The most common indication for laparoscopic common bile duct exploration (LCDE) is an **abnormal intraoperative cholangiogram.** Preoperative abnormalities that suggest a possible need for LCDE are listed in Table 14.1.1.

Table I. Preoperative abnormalities that suggest that LCDE may be required

Clinical history	Jaundice Pancreatitis
Liver function tests	↑ Bilirubin ↑ Alkaline phosphatase ↑ Gamma GTP
Ultrasound	Dilated bile ducts Choledocholithiasis Ductal obstruction
ERCP (or, rarely, transhepatic cholangiography)	Choledocholithiasis

ERCP, endoscopic retrogradecholangiopancreatography; GTP, Glutamyl transpeptidase.

2. **Contraindications:** The most significant contraindication to LCDE is inability of the surgeon to perform the necessary maneuvers. Absence of any of the indications above, instability of the patient, and local conditions in the porta hepatis that would make exploration hazardous are also contraindications.

3. **Choice of approach:** There are two possible routes for LCDE. The **transcystic duct** approach is discussed in this section. LCDE may also be performed by laparoscopic **choledochotomy** (see Chapter 14.2).

a. The transcystic approach is particularly useful when the cystic duct is ample in diameter and enters the common duct via a relatively straight, lateral approach.
b. The factors that influence choice of approach are summarized in Table 14.1.2.

Table 14.1.2. Factors influencing the approach to LCDE. Note that negative factors have a more profound impact on choice of approach than positive or neutral ones.

Factor	Transcystic	Choledochotomy
One stone	+	+
Multiple stones	+	+
Stones ≤ 6 mm diameter	+	+
Stones > 6 mm diameter	−	+
Intrahepatic stones	−	+
Diameter of cystic duct < 4 mm	−	+
Diameter of cystic duct ≥ 4 mm	+	+
Diameter of common duct < 6 mm	+	−
Diameter of common duct ≥ 6 mm	+	+
Cystic duct entrance—lateral	+	+
Cystic duct entrance—posterior	−	+
Cystic duct entrance—distal	−	+
Inflammation—mild	+	+
Inflammation—marked	+	−
Suturing ability—poor	+	−
Suturing ability—good	+	+

c. Transcystic duct exploration is generally attempted before laparoscopic choledochotomy because it is both possible and highly successful in the majority of cases, and because it is less invasive than laparoscopic choledochotomy. In addition, transcystic duct exploration does not require facility with laparoscopic suturing techniques.

B. Patient Positioning, Equipment Needed, Room Setup

1. Position the patient supine with both arms tucked at the sides.
2. Reverse Trendelenburg position and rotation to a slight left lateral decubitus position are often helpful in displaying the porta hepatis; this consideration is more important for laparoscopic common bile duct exploration than for laparoscopic cholecystectomy because access to the cystic duct–common duct junction is often necessary.

3. The standard instruments used for laparoscopic cholecystectomy with intraoperative cholangiography are needed, and include forceps, scissors, dissecting instruments, cholangiographic accessories, and a fluoroscope. Specialized instruments, drugs, and supplies needed to perform common bile duct exploration are listed in Table 14.1.3.

Table 14.1.3. Instruments, drugs, and supplies needed for transcystic duct exploration

Glucagon, 1 to 2 mg (given IV by the anesthetist)
Balloon-tipped catheters
4 French preferred over 3 and 5 French
Segura-type baskets
4-wire, flat, straight in-line configuration
Guide wire (0.035-inch diameter)
Mechanical "over-the-wire" dilators (7 to 12 French)
High-pressure "over-the-wire" pneumatic dilator
IV tubing (for saline instillation through the choledochoscope)
Atraumatic grasping forceps (for choledochoscope manipulation)
Flexible choledochoscope with light source ($\leq$3 mm outside diameter, with $\geq$1.1 mm working channel preferred)
2nd camera
2nd monitor (or picture-in-picture display on the primary laparoscopic monitor)
Video switcher (for simultaneous same monitor display of choledochoscopic and laparoscopic images)
Waterpik, Teledyne Water Pik, Fort Collins Colorado
Electrohydraulic Lithotripter
C-Tube (transcystic)
Stent (straight, 7 French or 10 French)
Sphincterotome (for antegrade sphincterotomy)

4. Keep all this equipment on a separate cart that can be brought into the room for LCDE.
5. Place the specific items that are needed for a particular case on a separate sterile Mayo stand, located to the right of the surgeon near the patient's left shoulder.

C. Trocar Position and Choice of Laparoscope and Choledochoscope

1. Place the trocars in the standard laparoscopic cholecystectomy configuration.
   a. Place a 10-mm port at the umbilicus and insert a laparoscope.
   b. Place 5- to 10-mm ports under direct laparoscopic vision in the epigastrium just to right of the midline, in the right midclavicular line, and in the right anterior axillary line.

     c.   The author routinely performs laparoscopic cholecystectomy with just three ports, and uses the last port mentioned only for laparoscopic common bile duct exploration.

2.   The author prefers a **0-degree, 10-mm laparoscope** for visualization, but others favor a 30-degree, 10-mm laparoscope. The angled laparoscope is especially useful in obese patients where the mesenteric and omental adipose tissue obscures visualization of the porta hepatis.

3.   Many vendors supply flexible choledochoscopes. Several points should be kept in mind:

     a.   Reusable scopes generally perform better than disposable scopes, but are expensive, fragile, and easily damaged.

     b.   Become facile with the gentle maneuvers required for manipulation of the scope.

     c.   Use atraumatic instruments to grasp or position the choledochoscope.

D. Preparation for LCDE

1.   Generally, LCDE is performed in conjunction with laparoscopic cholecystectomy. Elevate the gallbladder and expose the cystic duct in the usual fashion (Chapter 13.3).

2.   Obtain an image of the bile ducts to delineate the anatomy, confirm the presence of choledocholithiasis, and determine the number and location of stones.

     a.   Either standard cystic duct cholangiography with fluoroscopy (see Chapter 13.3.2), or intraoperative ultrasound (see Chapter 13.3.3) may be used.

     b.   Fluoroscopic imaging is the gold standard for intraoperative radiologic evaluation because it is faster than other methods, more detailed, and allows the surgeon to interact with the images in real time (for example, scanning the ductal system by moving the C-arm while injecting contrast material).

3.   Dissect the porta hepatis.

     a.   Start the dissection of the triangle of Calot from just lateral to the neck of the gallbladder and continue this dissection toward the cystic duct–common duct junction as the anatomy is further defined.

     b.   Access to the cystic duct–common duct junction or the anterior surface of the common duct itself is usually necessary for ductal exploration.

     c.   Use the cholangiogram as a guide to the anatomy during this sometimes-tedious dissection.

4.   Determine whether the transcystic approach is appropriate or whether laparoscopic choledochotomy will be required (see Table 14.1.2).

E. Techniques for LCDE

These techniques may be used with either the transcystic or laparoscopic choledochotomy access route.

1. **Irrigation techniques:** When very small stones (≤2-mm diameter), sludge, or sphincter spasm is suspected to be responsible for lack of flow of contrast into the duodenum, transcystic flushing of the duct with saline or contrast material is occasionally successful in clearing the duct.

    a. Intravenous glucagon (1–2 mg), administered by the anesthetist, may relax the sphincter of Oddi and improve the success rate.

    b. Monitor the progress (or lack thereof) fluoroscopically.

    c. This method is unlikely to work for stones 4 mm and larger.

2. **Balloon techniques:** Fogarty-type, low-pressure, balloon-tipped catheters are sometimes useful in clearing the ductal system of stones or debris. The technique described here is used for retrieval of stones from the distal common bile duct. Stones in the upper biliary tree may be retrieved under choledochoscopic guidance.

    a. A long 4-French–sized catheter is passed through the 14-gauge sleeve used for percutaneous cholangiography.

    b. The insertion site for the sleeve is usually located 3 cm medial to the mid-clavicular port.

    c. Use forceps, introduced through the medial epigastric port, to guide the catheter into the cystic duct.

    d. Advance the catheter into the common duct, and pass it into the duodenum. Generally, the 10-cm mark on the catheter will have just entered the cystic duct.

    e. Inflate the balloon and withdraw the catheter slightly until resistance is felt at the papilla. Confirm the location of the papilla by observing motion of the duodenum as the catheter is moved.

    f. Deflate the balloon, withdraw it an additional centimeter, and reinflate.

    g. Withdraw the catheter until the balloon exits the cystic duct orifice.

    h. Repeat this maneuver until no debris or stones exit from the cystic duct orifice.

3. **Basket techniques:** Baskets may be used to retrieve stones under fluoroscopic control, under choledochoscopic control, or freely without either visual monitoring method. Thus these methods are useful in cases where unsuspected stones are encountered (i.e., when the duct exploration equipment is not already prepared), while the nursing team is preparing the choledochoscope. They are also useful in somewhat rare cases in which the patient's common bile duct is of such small diameter < 5 mm) that choledochoscope passage would be difficult or hazardous.

a. In the **fluoroscopic method**, insert the basket through a 14-gauge sleeve (an IV sheath), placed 3 cm medial to the mid-clavicular port.

   i.   Advance the basket through the cystic duct into the common bile duct with forceps inserted through the medial epigastric port (Fig. 14.1.1).

   ii. Under fluoroscopic guidance, identify and capture the stone in the contrast-filled common bile duct.

   iii. If too much contrast has drained from the ductal system after completion of the cholangiograms, then it may need to be instilled again with the cholangiocatheter. This may become cumbersome and time-consuming and is one of the disadvantages of this method.

   iv. Another disadvantage of this method is the increased radiation exposure for the patient and the team during stone capture.

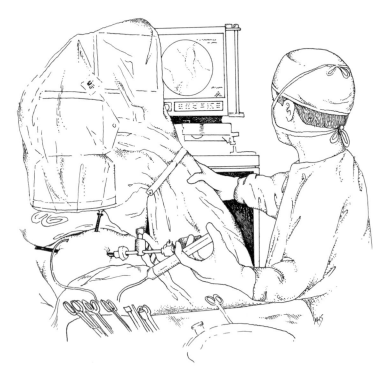

Figure 14.1.1. Cholangiography in preparation for basket retrieval of common bile duct stones under fluoroscopic guidance. Note location of monitors, surgeon, and instruments.

      v. In addition, it is often difficult or impossible to manipulate the forceps controlling the basket while the C-arm is in place, because the fluoroscope impedes movement of the forceps introduced through the medial epigastric port.

  b. When used in conjunction with the **choledochoscope**, insert the basket through the working channel of the scope.

      i. Capture the stone under direct vision.

      ii. Remove the entire ensemble from the cystic duct; deposit the stone on the omentum.

      iii. Grasp and deliver the stone through the medial epigastric or other 10-mm port.

  c. Baskets may also be used without fluoroscopic or choledochoscopic guidance.

      i. Introduce the basket through the 14-gauge sleeve and guide it into the common duct through the cystic duct.

      ii. Open the basket as soon as the tip of the basket passes into the common bile duct.

      iii. Use forceps, introduced through the medial epigastric port, to advance the open basket to the distal portion of the common bile duct. This minimizes the risk of accidental perforation of the duct by the basket tip or accidental capture of the papilla (since it is the rounded contour of the basket, rather than the relatively sharp tip, that forms the leading edge).

      iv. After the basket has reached the distal duct, it is withdrawn proximally as the basket is closed. Incomplete closure of the basket handle usually signals stone capture.

      v. The basket may have to be passed back and forth in the duct several times before the stone is captured.

4. **Choledochoscopic techniques:** Capturing stones under direct vision has always given the greatest sense of safety and accuracy. While the surgeon may choose to look directly into the choledochoscope, it is much simpler to attach a video camera and view the image indirectly. Viewing the video image then either requires a third monitor, replacement of the image on the "slave" or secondary monitor, or, preferentially, use of a video switcher to incorporate the image onto the same monitors used for the laparoscopic camera. This switcher should reside on one of the monitor towers for easy manipulation. Simultaneous visualization of both images allows the surgeon to manipulate the controls of the choledochoscope as well as employing external manipulation with atraumatic forceps. Smaller diameter (<3 mm) flexible choledochoscopes facilitate transcystic choledochoscopy. Even with the smallest scopes, the cystic duct generally must be dilated.

  a. Adequate dilatation is usually possible if the initial cystic duct diameter is greater than 2.5 mm, and unlikely if it is not.

  b. Dilatation may be carried out with either mechanical over-the-wire graduated dilators or pneumatic over-the-wire dilators. The former are inexpensive and found in most urology departments.

    i.   Pass a guide wire through the mid-clavicular port into the cystic duct.

    ii.   Guide a series of successively larger dilators over the guide wire and into the cystic duct and common duct, using forceps inserted through the medial epigastric port. Because these dilators exert a shearing-type force, exercise great care to avoid disruption of the cystic duct–common duct junction.

    iii. In general, **if the duct will not initially accept a 9-Fr**–size dilator easily, then adequate dilatation to the requisite12 Fr is unlikely.

c.   High-pressure, balloon-tipped catheters may be used to dilate the cystic duct.

    i.   Pass a guide wire through the mid-clavicular port into the cystic duct and advance it into the common duct.

    ii.   Advance the balloon catheter over the guide wire.

    iii. Position the balloon catheter in the cystic duct.

    iv.   Inflation of the balloon distends the duct with radially directed force, which may be safer than the graduated dilators (less shear force). Still, both the pressure on the balloon and cystic duct changes must be closely observed in order to avoid injury. This is a more expensive way to dilate the cystic duct.

d.   Insert the flexible choledochoscope through the mid-clavicular port and guide it into the cystic duct with atraumatic forceps inserted through the medial epigastric port. Some authors have suggested the use of a semiflexible sleeve, inserted through the mid-clavicular port into the cystic duct, as a guide for the choledochoscope. In the author's experience, this impedes some of the manipulations necessary for adequate choledochoscopic intervention.

e.   Control the choledochoscope both at its insertion site on the abdominal wall and with the controls on the head of the choledochoscope. This allows rotational movements of the shaft of the scope and deflection movements of the scope tip.

f.   Advance the choledochoscope into the common duct and visualize the stone(s) located. Generally a **stone basket** is the preferred tool for choledochoscopic stone extraction.

    i.   Capture the stone closest to the choledochoscope first to avoid difficulty in removing the stone from the duct.

    ii.   Insert the basket through the working channel of the choledochoscope and advance it to the stone under direct choledochoscopic vision.

    iii. Advance the closed basket beyond the stone. Open the basket and pull back, capturing the stone within the basket. Close the basket gently but firmly to secure the stone.

    iv.   Remove the entire ensemble through the cystic duct, and deposit the stone temporarily on the omentum.

v. Grasp the stone with forceps inserted through the medial epigastric port and remove it.

g. Stones that defy capture with a basket may be removed with a Fogarty-type balloon catheter.

i. Pass the catheter into the ductal system alongside the scope, because the working channel of the scope is too small to admit it.

ii. Advance the catheter beyond the stone under direct vision.

iii. Inflate the balloon beyond the stone, and withdraw the catheter enough to impact the stone against the choledochoscope.

iv. Remove the entire ensemble through the duct. Combined use of these techniques requires either a large-diameter cystic duct or a choledochotomy approach (see Chapter 14.2).

v. In the unlikely event that stones are displaced into the common hepatic duct during balloon manipulations, flush the stones back down into the distal system by altering the position of the table, or retrieve the stones by passing the balloon catheter proximally. In the author's experience this is a rare event, and in no case have other measures been necessary to retrieve common hepatic duct stones.

5. **Lithotripsy:** Intraoperative lithotripsy is primarily indicated for impacted stones that defy less aggressive removal techniques. Both electrohydraulic (EHL) and laser lithotripters are available. The laser lithotripters are far too expensive to encourage widespread implementation, and therefore EHL devices have been used somewhat more frequently. EHL devices must be used with great caution because they may cause unwanted ductal damage if the tip of the EHL probe is not accurately applied to the stone. However, with careful, direct visualization and application of EHL energy to the stone surface, stones may be safely fragmented without undue risk.

6. **Laparoscopic antegrade sphincterotomy:** Laparoscopic antegrade sphincterotomy was first described by DePaula and coworkers in 1993.

a. In this method a sphincterotome is passed through the working channel of the choledochoscope and through the sphincter.

b. Monitor the cutting action by simultaneous side-viewing endoscopy of the duodenum.

c. Gagner has advocated passage of the sphincterotome through the side-viewing scope in this situation, rather than through the choledochoscope.

d. While these techniques achieve excellent results as a drainage procedure, they are logistically quite difficult to accomplish.

i. More equipment and an additional endoscopic team must be present in an already crowded operating room.

ii. It is more difficult to pass the ERCP scope and perform sphincterotomy with the patient supine (rather than in the typical semiprone position).

iii.   Laparoscopic visualization is more difficult due to air in-
       sufflation of the duodenum and small bowel by the endo-
       scopist.
iv.   For all these reasons, laparoscopic antegrade and retrograde
       sphincterotomy has not gained widespread acceptance.
e.   An alternative, when stones cannot be removed using the meth-
     ods detailed above, is to pass a guide wire through the cystic
     duct and advance it into the duodenum. This assists in post-
     procedure ERCP and sphincterotomy.
7.   Biliary bypass procedures may be indicated in patients with an im-
     pacted distal stone, a stone or stones located distal to a stricture, or
     with dramatically dilated ducts (>2 cm) with multiple stones. Cho-
     ledochoenterostomy may be accomplished laparoscopically, but re-
     quires significant advanced laparoscopic suturing skills. These tech-
     niques are described elsewhere in this manual.

F. Selected References

Berci G, Cuschieri A. Bile Ducts and Bile Duct Stones. Philadelphia: WB Saunders,
    1996.
Carroll BJ, Phillips EH, Daykhovsky L, et al. Laparoscopic choledochoscopy: an effec-
    tive approach to the common duct. J Laparoendosc Surg 1992;2:15–21.
DePaula AL, Hashiba K, Bafutto M. Laparoscopic management of choledocholithiasis.
    Surg Endosc 1994;8:1399–1403.
DePaula A, Hashiba K, Bafutto M, Zago R, Machado M. Laparoscopic antegrade
    sphincterotomy. Surg Laparasc Endosc 1993;3(3):157–160.
Fielding GA, O'Rourke NA. Laparoscopic common bile duct exploration. Aust NZ J
    Surg 1993;63:113–115.
Fletcher DR. Common bile duct calculi at laparoscopic cholecystectomy: a technique for
    management. Aust NZ J Surg 1993;63:710–14.
Franklin ME, Pharand D, Rosenthal D. Laparoscopic common bile duct exploration. Surg
    Laparpsc Endosc 1994;(4)2:119–124.
Petelin J. Laparoscopic approach to common duct pathology. Surg Laparosc Endosc
    1991;1:1:33–41.
Petelin JB. Laparoscopic ductal stone clearance: transcystic approach, in bile ducts and
    bile duct stones. Berci G, Cuschieri A, (eds.). Philadelphia: WB Saunders, 1996, pp.
    97–108.
Phillips EH, Rosenthal RJ, Carroll BJ, et. al. Laparoscopic trans-cystic duct common bile
    duct exploration. Surg Endosc 1994;8:1389–1394.
Shapiro SJ, Gordon LA, Daykhovsky L, et al. Laparoscopic exploration of the common
    bile duct: experience in 16 selected patients. J Laparoendosc Surg 1991;(1)6: 333–
    341.
Stoker ME, Leveillee RJ, McCann JC, Maini BS. Laparoscopic common bile duct explo-
    ration. J Laparoendosc Surg 1991;1(5):287–293.

Traverso LW. A cost-effective approach to the treatment of common bile duct stones with surgical versus endoscopic techniques. In: Bile Ducts and Bile Duct Stones. Berci G, Cuschieri A (eds.). Philadelphia: WB Saunders, 1996, pp. 154–160.

Traverso LW, Roush TS, Koo K. Common bile duct stones—outcomes and costs. Surg Endosc 1995;9:1242–1244.

14.2. Common Bile Duct Exploration via Laparoscopic Choledochotomy

Sir Alfred Cuschieri, M.D., Ch.M., F.R.C.S.
Chris Kimber, M.B.B.S., F.R.A.C.S.

A. Indications and Patient Preparation

Laparoscopic common bile duct (CBD) exploration is performed when transcystic duct extraction is not appropriate or has failed. The current **indications** for laparoscopic direct CBD exploration are:

1. Failed transcystic extraction if CBD diameter is > 8 mm.
2. Large single or multiple stones (>1.0 cm), providing the load is not excessive (see below).
3. Unsuccessful attempts at endoscopic stone extraction for large/occluding stones.
4. Intrahepatic stones, which are inaccessible via a transcystic approach.

Under certain circumstances, other procedures are more appropriate; these may be considered **contraindications** to laparoscopic direct CBD exploration, and include:

1. Small-caliber (<8 mm) ducts are best cleared of stone by endoscopic sphincterotomy and stone extraction. Direct exploration of the CBD is inadvisable due to the risk of stricture formation.
2. A grossly dilated duct (>2.5 cm) with multiple stones (usually brown pigment) indicates a relative obstruction at the distal CBD in the region of the ampulla of Vater. Adequate drainage must be established to prevent recurrent stone formation. Laparoscopic choledochoduodenostomy or endoscopic sphincterotomy are options, as are the corresponding open procedures (choledochoduodenostomy, transduodenal sphincteroplasty).

Antibiotic prophylaxis appropriate for the most likely biliary pathogens (generally a cephalosporin) should be routine, as bile spillage is inevitable during the procedure. The remainder of the preparation is similar to that for laparoscopic cholecystectomy and should include prophylaxis against deep-vein thrombosis.

B. Patient Position and Room Setup

The basic equipment and patient positioning (head-up supine) are as for laparoscopic cholecystectomy. The following additional items are essential:

1. Modern image intensifier (fluoroscopy C-arm unit)
2. Cholangiograsper (Olsen), Fr 3,4 ureteric catheters, contrast medium
3. Flexible choledochoscope (3.3 mm or Fr 10, 5.0 mm or Fr 15) with instrument channel large enough (at least 1.2 mm) to enable concomitant irrigation and instrumentation
4. Separate monitor or picture in picture setup (twin video) to enable both the laparoscopic and choledochoscopic views to be simultaneously displayed
5. Selection of retrieval baskets and balloon catheters
6. Sharp scissors
7. Semm's spoon forceps for stone removal
8. T-tube or Cuschieri cystic duct drainage catheter (Wilson Cook) for biliary decompression

C. Trocar Position and Choice of Laparoscope

Begin with the four standard trocars for laparoscopic cholecystectomy, with the laparoscope at the umbilicus. One further port (10.0 mm) is placed high in the right epigastrium, in line with the choledochotomy. This port is used to introduce the choledochoscope and extraction devices. A reducer sleeve is an important adjunct. This guides the choledochoscope and other flexible instruments to the choledochotomy, adds stability, and protects the choledochoscope from being damaged by the trocar valves.

The 30-degree, forward-oblique, 10-mm laparoscope provides the best visualization of the common duct and is recommended in preference to the forward viewing (0 degree) type.

D. Performing the Choledochotomy

In the vast majority of patients, laparoscopic supraduodenal CBD exploration is performed concomitant with laparoscopic cholecystectomy, and a certain amount of dissection in Calot's triangle will precede CBD exploration.

1. Generally the operation has proceeded thus far: Calot's triangle has been dissected, the cystic artery divided, and a clip has been placed on the distal cystic duct (at the junction with the neck of the gallbladder).
2. The cystic duct is opened and an operative cholangiogram obtained. This pre-exploration cholangiogram serves several crucial functions and should be performed even if preoperative studies of the common duct were obtained (Table 14.2.1). Good opacification of both the intra- and extrahepatic portions of the biliary tree must be obtained.

This is particularly important in elderly patients with brown pigment stones, in whom the diagnosis of Klatskin tumor or other pathology may not have been made on preoperative ultrasound examination.

Table 14.2.1. Function of pre-exploration cholangiogram

1.	Confirm presence, size, location, and number of stones
2.	Demonstrate anatomic relationships and diameter of the extrahepatic bile duct
3.	Exclude unsuspected pathology, such as cholangiocarcinoma, in jaundiced patients

3. Maintain the **continuity of the cystic duct with the gallbladder and common bile duct.** This is essential for traction, exposure, and manipulation. Hence, defer transection of the cystic duct and removal of the gallbladder from the liver bed until the CBD exploration is completed. This differs from the usual practice during open cholecystectomy and open CBD exploration.
4. Visualize the supraduodenal CBD. The 30-degree laparoscope is essential for adequate visualization. The CBD is generally readily apparent as a large tubular blue or greenish structure. Visible pulsations in the hepatic artery are a useful landmark.
5. Use curved scissors to **divide the peritoneum** over the CBD. Displace the duodenum inferiorly. A layer of fascia surrounds the CBD. Divide this and expose the anterior wall of the CBD with gentle pledget dissection. Use electrocautery sparingly and limit the dissection to the anterior wall of the CBD. Expose an area approximately 2 cm long and 1 cm wide.
6. Use low-voltage coagulating electrocautery to mark the line of incision on the CBD. The incision should not exceed 1 cm. The authors prefer a lengthwise incision, but some use a transverse orientation.
7. Entry into the CBD is marked by a gush of bile, gas bubbles (after failed endoscopic retrograde cholangiography [ERC]), or even a stone. Suction irrigation is often required to maintain a clear view. Make the choledochotomy with scissors, cutting electrocautery, or a sheathed knife. It is important to keep the choledochotomy **as small as possible.** Because the CBD contains a large amount of elastin, a 1.0-cm choledochotomy can be stretched to deliver a 1.5-cm stone. Avoiding a long choledochotomy reduces the amount of suturing required and minimizes the risk of stricturing due to devascularization of the CBD.

E. Stone Extraction

Stone extraction is accomplished through the choledochotomy using a series of steps:

1. Apply **external compression** to the CBD from below upward, with two atraumatic forceps, gently pushing a stone toward the choledochotomy and milking the stone out through the choledochotomy. This simple maneuver is often successful for floating stones that are then grasped inside the Semm's spoon forceps and removed.

2. If the above fails, insert a **biliary balloon catheter** through the choledochotomy toward the distal end of the CBD. Inflate the balloon and withdraw the catheter slowly toward the choledochotomy. Ease or suction any dislodged stones out through the choledochotomy.

3. Perform visually guided extraction using the choledochoscope if the first two measures fail (as is often the case when the stones are occluding or impacted). Attach the irrigation system to the choledochoscope and insert the scope (using a reducer sleeve) through the extra trocar placed in the right subxiphoid region. (See Chapter 50-51, Diagnostic Choledochoscopy, for additional information.)

    a. Gently guide the choledochoscope into the choledochotomy. Avoid grasping the choledochoscope as it is easy to damage the sheath or fibers.

    b. Once the scope is inside the CBD, use an atraumatic grasper to gather the choledochotomy around the endoscope, creating an adequate seal for distention and visualization of the biliary tree.

    c. Two operators working synchronously are needed for efficient visually guided stone extraction—one manipulates the scope (tip flexion and torque) to obtain the desired view of the stone, and the other is in charge of trapping the stone inside the basket (preferably four wires).

    d. Pass the closed basket and negotiate it beyond the stone. Open the wire basket and trawl it slowly backward under visual guidance.

    e. Once the stone falls inside the wires, close the basket just enough to grasp the stone without crushing it.

    f. Withdraw the entire assembly (scope, basket, and stone) through the choledochotomy.

    g. Release the stone and remove it from the abdomen using a Semm's spoon forceps.

4. After all the stones have been removed, irrigate the biliary tract with warm saline to flush out any small fragments.

5. Perform a **completion check choledochoscopy** by inspecting the proximal and distal sections of the extrahepatic biliary tracts. Remove any debris, stone fragments, or residual calculi.

F. Closure of the Choledochotomy

Although some advocate primary closure without decompression of the extrahepatic biliary tract, the authors feel this is inadvisable for two reasons. First, manipulations at the lower end of the bile duct frequently cause periampullary edema, increasing the risk of bile leakage through the sutured choledochotomy. Second, primary closure precludes completion or postoperative cholangiography.

Drainage may be accomplished by placement of a T-tube or by placement of a drainage catheter through the cystic duct. Both are acceptable, but the authors prefer decompression through the cystic duct for two reasons: first, this method of drainage minimizes the postoperative hospital stay; and second, it allows primary common duct closure. Both methods will be described here.

1. Transcystic decompression requires a 1.0-m-long 8 to 10 Fr, shaped drainage cannula with a terminal S-shaped perforated segment (Cuschieri cystic duct drainage catheter set—Wilson-Cook—Fig. 14.2.1). The set consists of introducer needle, guide wire, dilator tube, and tear-away sheath, and allows percutaneous insertion of the drainage cannula.

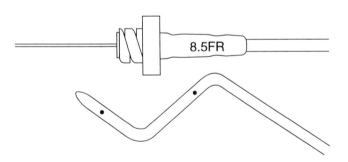

Figure 14.2.1. Cuschieri transcystic biliary decompression set.

Choose an insertion site in the right flank and introduce the catheter using Seldinger technique (Fig. 14.2.2).

a. Use two graspers to thread the cystic duct drainage cannula (with the guide wire projecting for a distance of 2.0 cm beyond its tip) through the cystic duct into the CBD.

b. Advance the cannula until the perforated segment is beyond the junction of the cystic duct with the common hepatic duct.

c. Remove the guide wire. Confirm accurate positioning of the S-shaped segment by inspection through the choledochotomy.

d. Secure the catheter with two chromic catgut Roeder knots to the cystic duct.

e. Anchor the drainage cannula by skin sutures and attach a saline syringe (to flush the biliary tract during suture closure of the choledochotomy) (Fig. 14.2.3).

f. Maintain continuous saline irrigation through the cystic duct cannula during closure. This facilitates visualization of the edges of the wound and helps ensure a leak-proof suture line.

g. Closure is best performed with accurately placed interrupted sutures. Use 4/0 absorbable atraumatic sutures (Polysorb or coated Vicryl). Place the suture bites accurately, 2-mm apart.

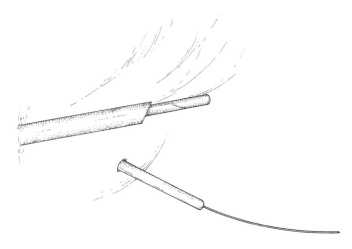

Figure 14.2.2. The drainage cannula is threaded over the guide wire into the peritoneal cavity.

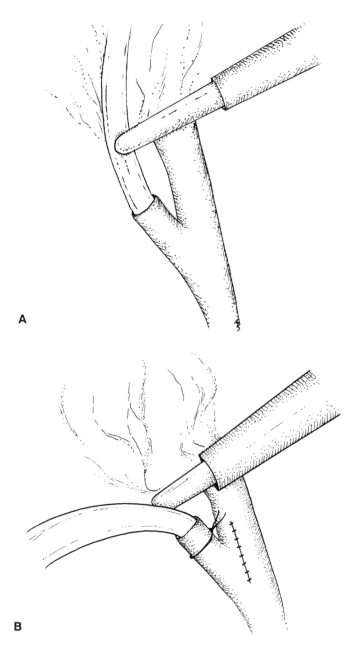

A

B

Figure 14.2.3. Fixation of the biliary decompression cannula to the cystic duct stump by catgut Roeder knots.

2. **Decompression by T-tube**—The practical considerations if this method of decompression is used include appropriate size (Fr 14) and correct exit course of the long limb of the T-tube.

   a. Trim the crossbar of the T (the intracholedochal segment) to twice the length of the choledochotomy (generally 2 cm) and fillet this segment longitudinally.

   b. Fold the two ends together using an atraumatic grasper and introduce the T-tube into the CBD.

   c. Exteriorize the long limb in the right flank.

   d. Close the choledochotomy from above downward (using interrupted 4/0 absorbable sutures, as previously discussed) so that the long limb comes to lie at the lower end of the suture line (Fig. 14.2.4).

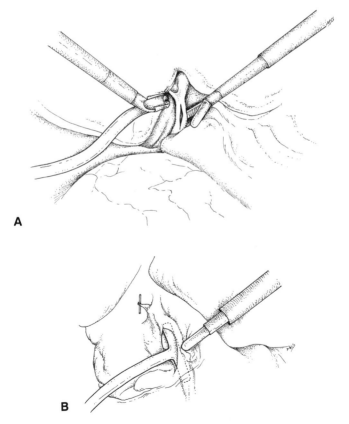

Figure 14.2.4. A. The folded T-tube is inserted into the choledochotomy. B. T-tube in place. The choledochotomy will be closed from above downward. The T-tube will exit from the lower end of the choledochotomy when the sutures are placed.

3. **Completion fluorocholaniogram** is advisable, even when completion choledochoscopy has been normal, as small stone fragments in the ampullary region are easily missed. Begin screening during the early filling phase with slow injection of contrast, as otherwise small calculi may be obscured by the contrast medium (see Chapter 13.2, Cholangiography).

4. Always **insert a subhepatic drain** via the right subcostal trocar and place the tip of the drain near the choledochotomy.

5. If exploration is unsuccessful, consider conversion to an open procedure (Table 14.2.2).

Table 14.2.2. Indications for conversion to open procedure

1.	Failure to progress with the operation (beyond 2 hours); the most common problem is an impacted stone that has excavated a diverticulum; these cases frequently require open transduodenal sphincteroplasty
2.	Large stone load in a grossly dilated bile duct (if the surgeon is not experienced with the performance of laparoscopic choledochoduodenostomy)
3.	Difficult anatomy or unsuspected pathology of the biliopancreatic tract
4.	Uncontrollable bleeding

G. Postoperative Management

1. Continue perioperative antibiotics for 48 hours.

2. **Management of transcystic drainage catheter**: The average output from the 8-Fr cystic duct drainage cannula is 300 ml per day. Perform postoperative transcystic cholangiography on the 2nd postoperative day.
   a. If the cholangiogram is normal with good entry of dye into the duodenum, clamp the drainage catheter and cover it with an occlusive dressing.
   b. Remove the subhepatic drain on the next day (if no bile drainage) and discharge the patient.
   c. Remove the transcystic drainage catheter after a minimum of 7 days (longer if the patient is elderly or diabetic) to assure that a secure tract has formed.

3. Management of T-tube.
   a. Delay performing the cholangiogram until the 7th postoperative day.
   b. If normal, clamp the tube for 6 hours.
   c. If there are no symptoms or bile drainage from the subhepatic drain (and provided the patient is not immunosuppressed, elderly, or diabetic), remove the T-tube.

    d.   Remove the subhepatic drain 12 to 24 hours later.

    e.   Immunosuppressed patients should be sent home with the T-tube clamped. The T-tube may be removed 2 weeks later.

4.   If stones are identified on the postoperative cholangiogram, insert a guide wire into the duodenum under fluoroscopic control for use during the subsequent endoscopic retrograde cholangiopancreatography (ERCP) (see Chapter 60).

H. Selected References

Berci G, Cuschieri A. Bile Ducts and Bile Duct Stones. Philadelphia: WB Saunders, 1997.

Cuschieri A, Croce E, Faggioni A, et al. EAES ductal stone study: preliminary findings of multi-centre prospective randomized trial comparing two staged vs single-stage management. Surg Endosc 1996;10:1130–1135.

Fielding GA, O'Rouke NA. Laparoscopic common bile duct exploration. Aust NZ J Surg 1993;63:113–115.

Hensman C, Crosthwaite G, Cuschieri A. Transcystic biliary decompression after direct laparoscopic exploration of the common bile duct. Surg Endosc 1997;11:1106–1110.

Holdsworth RJ, Sadek SA, Ambikar S, Cuschieri A. Dynamics of bile flow through the choledochal sphincter following exploration of the common bile duct. World J Surg 1989;13:300–304.

Lezoche E, Paganini AM. Single-stage laparoscopic treatment of gallstones and common duct stones in 120 unselected consecutive patients. Surg Endosc 1995;9:1070–1075.

15. Complications of Laparoscopic Cholecystectomy and Laparoscopic Common Duct Exploration

Mark A. Talamini, M.D.
Joseph Petelin, M.D.
Alfred Cuschieri, M.D.

A. Management of Bile Duct Injury

Both the common duct and the right hepatic duct are at risk during laparoscopic biliary surgery.

1. **Cause and prevention:** The major causes are mistaken anatomy or excessive inflammation. Maintain the dissection high on the gallbladder and carefully delineate the anatomy before clipping or ligating any structures (see Chapter 13.1, Avoiding Complications). Cholangiography (see Chapter 13.2) provides an invaluable roadmap. Suspect inflammation when bowel or duodenum is densely adherent to the gallbladder. Bile duct injury can also occur during common duct exploration (see sections B and C below).

2. **Recognition and management**

   a. **Intraoperative:** The danger signs listed in Table 15.1 should prompt the prudent surgeon to prove, at the very least, that a bile duct injury has not occurred. Bowel plastered to the face of the gallbladder is an early warning sign of **excessive inflammation**. Gently attempt to separate the tissues, and consider conversion to formal laparotomy, particularly if the inflammatory process precludes safe identification of structures in Calot's triangle. **Leakage of bile** after all structures have been clipped and divided (and any holes in the gallbladder repaired) should suggest a ductal injury. Cholangiography may confirm or exclude a defect in the biliary tree, but if suspicion remains, it is safest to convert to formal laparotomy. **Dissection** should normally progress several centimeters from the bifurcation of the right and left hepatic ducts. Dissection up under the liver should raise concern. In rare instances this will actually be the appropriate location for dissection. If that is the case, it probably is most safely dissected through an open incision. At the very least, when dissection is close up under the liver, one must be particularly careful about staying close to the gallbladder. Cholangiography is the best way to delineate anatomy. Figure 13.2.14 shows the classic "cholangiogram from hell" in which the distal common duct is seen but no contrast flows proximal. This cholangiogram is a classic sign that the structure that has been identified as the "cystic duct" is actually the common duct and should prompt conversion to laparotomy. **Examination of the removed gallbladder** specimen can be a very reassuring exercise. This is particularly true after a difficult dissection. A careful dissection of the organ will quickly reveal exactly where the cystic duct was clipped and divided, and confirm that no additional tubular structures (such as a segment of common or right hepatic duct) are attached. **Management of bile duct injury** depends on surgeon experience and comfort level with biliary tree reconstruction procedures. These are complex operations, and the best chance for a good, long-term outcome is during the first reconstruction. If the surgeon is uncomfortable or inexperienced, contact should be made with an experienced surgeon. Under some circumstances the best option may be to drain the site of injury and transfer the patient. The appropriate repair will generally be a Roux-en-Y hepaticojejunostomy to the proximal common hepatic duct or to the bifurcation of the right and left hepatic duct if necessary. The author's practice is to stent these anastomoses with Silastic stents passed through the anastomosis and brought out percutaneously. These are left in for months.

Table 15.1. Danger signs during laparoscopic biliary tract surgery

Sign	Significance
Bile in operative field (in the absence of hole in gallbladder)	Bile duct injury
Dense adhesions to gallbladder	Excessive inflammation
Dissection progressing into hilum of liver	Mistaken anatomy
Extra or unexpected tubular structure encountered during dissection	Mistaken anatomy (aberrant right hepatic duct, or transected common duct)
Presumed cystic duct appears unusually large in diameter	Mistaken anatomy ("cystic duct" is actually common or right hepatic duct)
Extra tubular structure attached to resected gallbladder	Portion of common or right hepatic duct excised with specimen

b. **Postoperative:** In the most common pattern of injury, bile leaks into the peritoneal cavity. The classic signs are pain, fever, abdominal distention, and abnormal liver function tests. Nuclear medicine scan will demonstrate leakage (Fig. 15.1).

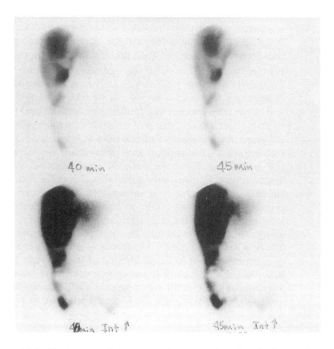

Figure 15.1. Nuclear medicine scan demonstrating free leakage of contrast. This patient had a complete transection of the common duct.

There are three objectives when a bile duct injury is discovered postoperatively: definition and drainage of the biliary tree, control of bile peritonitis, and reconstruction of the biliary tree. **Definition and drainage of the biliary tree** requires an experienced interventional radiology team that can perform complex biliary tree manipulation. Percutaneous transhepatic cholangiography and percutaneous biliary drainage are necessary to delineate biliary defect and to divert the bile away from the area by allowing it to preferentially drain into a gravity bag placed below the level of the bed. **Control of bile peritonitis** often means creating drainage for a biloma in the region of the biliary defect. If the surgeon left a percutaneous drain at the initial operation, this is usually perfectly adequate, and in fact avoids significant peritonitis. **Reconstruction of the biliary tree** usually means construction of a hepaticojejunostomy in an elective setting. Once the biliary tree is diverted and the biloma drained, the pressure is off to move rapidly to the operating room. In fact, it is often advantageous to wait 4 to 6 weeks to allow any existent peritonitis to settle down, improving the likelihood of a good repair. Treatment of patients with laparoscopic bile duct injury requires an experienced multidisciplinary team with specialized equipment. Surgeons without such equipment and personnel at their disposal should consider transfer of the patient to another institution.

B. Complications of Transcystic Duct Exploration

Because laparoscopic common duct exploration (LCDE) is commonly performed in conjunction with laparoscopic cholecystectomy, any of the complications discussed in Chapter 13.3 (or section A above) may occur. Additional complications associated with LCDE include:

1. **Failure to clear the common duct**
   a. **Cause and prevention:** There are numerous reasons for inability to clear the common duct of its obstruction. These include patient instability, intense inflammation in the porta hepatis, obese body habitus, intrahepatic stones, impacted stones, stones distal to a stricture, inadequate equipment, and surgeon inexperience. The most important of these is surgeon inexperience. While it may be difficult to gain actual laparoscopic common bile duct exploration experience, surgeons who practice routine intraoperative cholangiography are using many of the same maneuvers that are used for transcystic ductal exploration, such as catheter and basket insertion into the ductal system. This should serve as useful preparation for LCDE. Additional training may be obtained by participation in a laparoscopic common bile duct exploration course or laparoscopic fellowship.
   b. **Recognition and management:** Completion cholangiography is essential to document the status of the ductal system after LCDE. Intraluminal opacities or failure of contrast to pass into the duodenum is usually indicative of retained intraductal material. After a thorough and careful attempt to clear the ductal system of all stones laparoscopically, decide whether to convert to open common bile duct exploration or resort to postoperative endoscopic retrograde techniques for stone removal.

2. **Bile leak**
   a. **Cause and prevention:** Bile may leak from the gallbladder bed, the cystic duct orifice used for LCDE, the cystic duct–common duct junction, or the common duct itself. This may be the result of dissection and manipulation of these structures during LCDE.
   b. Good visualization and gentle tissue handling techniques may help reduce the incidence of this problem. The cystic duct must be secured adequately after LCDE. Consider suture ligation when the cystic duct is large, thickened, or short. Distal common duct manipulation, recent pancreatitis, or postoperative ERCP may cause temporary elevation of biliary pressure and suture ligation should be considered if any of these conditions apply.

    c.   **Recognition and management:** Postoperative fever, excessive bilious drain output, ileus, and elevated liver function studies may indicate a bile leak. A radionuclide scan may confirm the presence of a leak, and the possibility of a distal obstruction in the common bile duct. Sonography or computed tomography (CT) scanning of the abdomen may help localize a bile collection if there is one.

    d.   If a drain is already in place, and if there is no evidence of distal obstruction of the common bile duct, observation, intravenous fluids, and antibiotic coverage may be all that is necessary. If no drain is in place, and if a bile collection is localized, then radiographically directed placement of a drain may be adequate to allow a period of observation. The surgeon should not wait an excessively long time to intervene if there is no indication that the leak will seal itself or if generalized peritonitis is present.

3. **Abscess**

    a.   **Cause and prevention:** Patients requiring LCDE are often older, with more intense gallbladder inflammation than those requiring laparoscopic cholecystectomy. The bile is frequently colonized with bacteria. Hence, patients may be more prone to the development of postoperative infectious problems at the surgical site. Prophylactic antibiotics are essential here, and when acute or gangrenous cholecystitis or cholangitis is documented therapeutic antibiotic coverage should be continued into the postoperative period.

    b.   Thoroughly cleanse the perihepatic space of debris and stones before completing the case. If there has been severe inflammation or spillage of bile or stones, placement of a closed system suction drain may be prudent.

    c.   **Recognition and management:** Postoperative fever, tachycardia, ileus, and abdominal pain usually signal the presence of a problem at the surgical site. Confirm the presence of an abscess by sonography or CT scanning. Management includes establishing drainage (which can often be accomplished percutaneously under ultrasound or CT guidance) and intravenous antibiotics. Surgical drainage may be needed if the symptoms do not resolve.

4. **Common duct injury**

    a.   **Cause and prevention:** Improper identification of the **anatomy** during dissection may lead to injury to the duct. This may be more likely in cases where there is intense inflammation in the porta hepatis. A thorough knowledge of the anatomy, as seen laparoscopically, is essential. Intraoperative cholangiography via the cystic duct or the gallbladder, if necessary, may provide clues as to the location of the duct.

        During the ductal exploration itself, **aggressive manipulation of instruments** or the duct itself may lead to ductal injury. Pass all instruments gently to avoid ductal injury. Baskets are especially prone to puncture the duct, due to the small size and configuration of the tip. Similarly, **electrohydraulic lithotripsy** must be used under direct visual control, and applied accurately and with care to avoid injury to the duct wall.

    b.   **Recognition and management:** The best time to recognize this injury is at the time of surgery, when it can be either repaired primarily or bypassed if necessary. Unfortunately, most injuries are not recognized at this time and present themselves later with fever, tachycardia, abdominal pain, ileus, and jaundice. At that point, after stabilization of the patient, referral to a center specializing in reconstructive biliary tract surgery is the best option.

5. **Pancreatitis**

    a.   **Cause and prevention:** Pancreatitis may be present before surgery, or exacerbated or induced postoperatively by manipulation of the distal duct. Gentle techniques are the order here in order to minimize the occurrence of this problem. **High-pressure balloon dilatation** of the sphincter of Oddi, advocated by some, commonly causes hyperamylasemia or frank pancreatitis, and is therefore not widely recommended.

       Passage of the **choledochoscope** into the duodenum is similarly a potentially hazardous practice and should only be used when necessary to gently push debris into the duodenum, or when the orifice into the duodenum is widely patent, such as after preoperative sphincterotomy or intraoperative intravenous glucagon administration.

    b.   **Recognition and management:** Pancreatitis may present postoperatively with excessive abdominal or back pain, fever, ileus, anorexia, or failure to thrive. The diagnosis may be confirmed with amylase measurement. CT scanning of the abdomen may be necessary if the patient does not improve with intravenous fluids, NPO status, and nasogastric (NG) suction. Antibiotics may be required if pancreatic abscess is suspected or confirmed with CT scanning.

C. Complications of Laparoscopic Choledochotomy

It is conceptually useful to divide complications of laparoscopic choledochotomy into early and late complications. Many of the complications listed in section A may also occur after laparoscopic choledochotomy.

1. **Early complications** are recognized in the first few days after laparoscopic common bile duct (CBD) exploration. These include:

    a.   **Biloma/bile leakage** through the subhepatic drain. Bile leakage is commoner after T-tube insertion than after transcystic drainage with primary closure. The leakage is usually from the choledochotomy site, but may be from the gallbladder bed.

       i.   Excessive bile leakage indicates probable dislodgment of the T-tube or transcystic cannula.

      ii.   The initial investigations may include ultrasound examination and radionuclide scanning of the biliary tree. The T-tube or transcystic duct cannula provide a convenient route for cholangiography, if needed.

     iii.   Established biliary peritonitis or dislodgment of the T-tube are indications for reintervention laparoscopy/laparotomy.

     iv.   Otherwise percutaneous drainage under radiologic control should suffice (if adequate drainage has not been provided by the closed suction drain placed during surgery).

b. Missed stone

      i.   By definition, these are stones discovered on the postoperative cholangiogram and up to 2 years after the duct exploration.

      ii.   When discovered postoperatively, they should be removed either by endoscopic stone extraction or by removal via the mature T-tube tract (4–6 weeks later).

     iii.   Pressure-controlled flushing with heparinized saline and antispasmodic medication (glucagon, ceruletide) may be effective in some cases.

c. Cholangitis

      i.   Transient cholangitis is common in patients undergoing laparoscopic duct exploration after failed endoscopic sphincterotomy.

      ii.   Postoperative cholangitis often indicates missed stone or other pathology.

     iii.   If adequate drainage of the biliary tract is confirmed by an urgent T-tube/transcystic cholangiogram, the management is by antibiotic therapy. Otherwise endoscopic sphincterotomy or stenting is performed as a matter of urgency.

2. Late complications

a. Abscess formation around a spilled stone. This is especially likely to occur with brown pigment stone (which usually harbor bacteria in the amorphous pits). Open drainage with removal of the stone is required.

b. Recurrent calculi present beyond 2 years after surgery and are managed as new cases either laparoscopically or by endoscopic stone extraction.

c. Stricture of common duct may present several years later.

D. Selected References

Lee VS, Chari RS, Cucchiaro G, Meyers WC. Complications of laparoscopic cholecystectomy. Am J of Surg 1993;165(4):527–532.

Lillemoe KD, Martin SA, Cameron JL, et al. Major bile duct injuries during laparoscopic cholecystectomy: follow-up after combined surgical and radiologic management. Ann Surg, in press.

Ponsky JL. The incidence and management of complications of laparoscopic cholecystectomy. Adv Surg 1994;27:21–41.

Talamini MA. Controversies in laparoscopic cholecystectomy: contraindications, cholangiograpy, pregnancy and avoidance of complications. Baillieres Clin Gastroenterol 1993;7(4):881–896.

Talamini MA. Laparoscopic cholecystectomy. In: Current Surgical Therapy. Cameron JL (ed.). St. Louis: Mosby, 1995.

Wherry DC, Rob CG, Marohn MR, et al. An external audit of laparoscopic cholecystectomy performed in medical yreatment facilities of the Department of Defense. Ann Surg 1994;220:626–634.

16. Laparoscopic Treatment of Gastroesophageal Reflux and Hiatal Hernia

Jeffrey H. Peters, M.D., F.A.C.S.

A. Indications and Preoperative Evaluation

1. **Laparoscopic fundoplication** is indicated for the treatment of objectively documented, relatively severe, gastroesophageal reflux disease. Care in patient selection and preoperative evaluation are essential for good results. Patients with gastroesophageal reflux and any of the following may be considered candidates for the procedure:
    a. Erosive esophagitis, stricture, and/or Barrett's esophagus.
    b. Dependence upon proton pump inhibitors for relief of symptoms in the absence of documented mucosal injury (particularly those less than 50 years of age).
    c. Atypical or respiratory symptoms with a good response to medical treatment.
    d. Risk factors that predict a poor response to medical therapy (Table 16.1).

Table 16.1. Risk factors that predict a poor response to medical therapy

1.	Nocturnal reflux on 24-hour esophageal pH study
2.	Structurally deficient lower esophageal sphincter
3.	Mixed reflux of gastric and duodenal juice
4.	Mucosal injury on presentation

2. **The therapeutic approach** to patients presenting for the first time with symptoms suggestive of gastroesophageal reflux includes an initial trial of H2 blocker therapy. Many patients will already have sought relief with readily-available over the counter agents.
    a. **Failure of H2 blockers** to control the symptoms, or immediate return of symptoms after stopping treatment suggests either that the diagnosis is incorrect, or that the patient has relatively severe disease.
    b. **Endoscopic examination** at this stage of evaluation provides the opportunity for assessing the severity of mucosal damage and the presence of Barrett's esophagus (see Part II, Section II,

Upper Gastrointestinal Endoscopy, Indications). Either finding on initial endoscopy predicts a high risk for medical failure.

3. **Appropriate diagnostic evaluation** should then be undertaken. **The diagnostic approach** to patients suspected of having gastroesophageal reflux disease and being considered for antireflux surgery has three important goals (Table 16.2).

Table 16.2. Goals of diagnostic evaluation for possible antireflux surgery

---

- To determine that gastroesophageal reflux is the underlying cause of the patients symptoms
- To evaluate the status of esophageal body, and occasionally gastric function
- To determine the presence or absence of esophageal shortening

---

Symptoms thought to be indicative of gastroesophageal reflux disease, such as heartburn or acid regurgitation, are very common in the general population, and cannot be used alone to guide therapeutic decisions, particularly when considering antireflux surgery. These symptoms, even when excessive, are not specific for gastroesophageal reflux and are often caused by other diseases (such as achalasia, diffuse spasm, esophageal carcinoma, pyloric stenosis, cholelithiasis, gastritis, gastric or duodenal ulcer, and coronary artery disease).

A common error is to define the presence of gastroesophageal reflux disease by the endoscopic finding of esophagitis. Limiting the diagnosis to patients with endoscopic esophagitis ignores a large population of patients without mucosal injury who may have severe symptoms of gastroesophageal reflux and could be considered for antireflux surgery. The most precise approach to define gastroesophageal reflux disease is to measure the basic pathophysiologic abnormality of the disease, that is, increased exposure of the esophagus to gastric juice. The workup consists of:

a. **24-hour pH monitoring,** to assess the degree and pattern of esophageal exposure to gastric juice.

b. **Manometric examination** of the lower esophageal sphincter and motor function of the body of the esophagus. This will help determine if there is sufficient motor power in the body of the esophagus to propel a bolus of food through a newly reconstructed valve. Patients with normal peristaltic contractions do well with a 360-degree Nissen fundoplication. When peristalsis is absent, severely disordered (greater than 50% simultaneous contractions), or the amplitude of the contraction in one or more of the lower esophageal segment, is below 20 mm Hg, a partial fundoplication may be the procedure of choice.

c. **Assessment of esophageal length to exclude esophageal shortening.** Repetitive injury causes scarring, fibrosis, and ultimately results in anatomic shortening of the esophagus. This compromises the ability to do an adequate repair without tension and lead to an increased incidence of breakdown or thoracic displacement of the repair.

     i.   Esophageal length is best assessed using video roentgeno-graphic contrast studies and endoscopic findings.

     ii. Endoscopically, hernia size is measured as the difference between the diaphragmatic crura, identified by having the patient sniff, and the gastroesophageal junction, identified as the loss of gastric rugal folds. Suspect a short esophagus if there is a large (>5cm) hiatal hernia, particularly if it fails to reduce in the upright position on a video barium esopha-gram. A Collis gastroplasty and partial fundoplication will result in excellent control of reflux in the majority of these patients.

   d. **Selection of a partial versus complete fundoplication,** and an open or laparoscopic approach is based upon on an assessment of esophageal contractility and length. Laparoscopic fundopli-cation is used in the majority of patients who will have normal esophageal contractility and length. Those with weak esophageal contractions (amplitudes of contraction <20 mm Hg) and/or ab-normal wave progression (>20% simultaneous waves) may be treated with a partial fundoplication in order to avoid the in-creased outflow resistance associated with a complete fundopli-cation. If the esophagus is short (>5 cm hiatal hernia on radiog-raphy), a Collis gastroplasty is likely necessary and an open transthoracic approach should be used.

B. Patient Position and Room Setup

1.   Position the patient supine, in a modified lithotomy position. It is im-portant that the knees be only slightly flexed, to avoid limiting mo-bility of the surgeon and the instruments (Fig. 16.1).

2.   The surgeon stands between the legs and works with both hands. This allows the right- and left-handed instruments to approach the hiatus from the respective upper abdominal quadrants.

3.   Use 30–45% of reverse Trendelenburg to displace the transverse co-lon and small bowel inferiorly, keeping them from obstructing the view of the video camera.

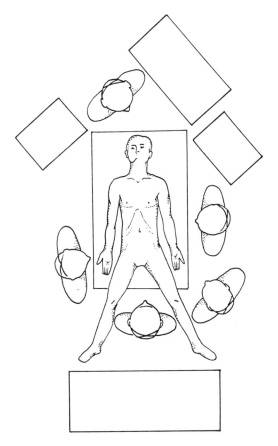

Figure 16.1. Patient positioning and room setup for laparoscopic fundoplication. The patient is placed with the head elevated 45 degrees in the modified
lithotomy position. The surgeon stands between the patient's legs. One assistant, on the surgeon's right, retracts the stomach; and a second assistant, on the
surgeon's left, manipulates the camera.

C. Trocar Position and Principles of Exposure

1. Five 10-mm ports are utilized (Fig. 16.2).
    2. **Place the camera** above the umbilicus, one third of the distance to
        the xiphoid process. In most patients, placement of the camera in the
        umbilicus will be too low to allow adequate visualization of the hiatal
        strictures once dissected.

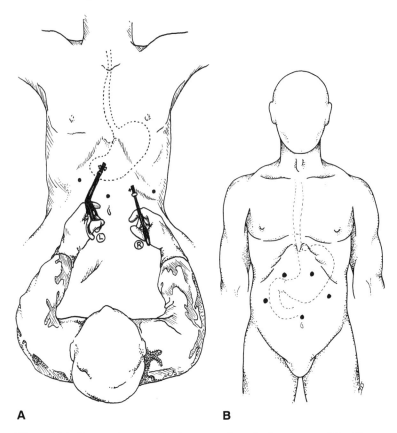

A   **B**

Figure 16.2. Trocar placement for laparoscopic antireflux surgery. Five 10 mm trocars are generally used, but the two lateral retraction ports can be downsized to 5 mm with appropriate instrumentation.

3. **Place two lateral retracting ports** in the right and left anterior axillary lines, respectively. Position the trocar for the liver retractor in the right mid-abdomen (mid-clavicular line), at or slightly below the camera port. This allows the proper angle toward the left lateral segment of the liver and thus the ability to push the instrument toward the operating table, lifting the liver. Place the second retraction port at the level of the umbilicus, in the left anterior axillary line.

4. **Place the operating trocars** in the right and left midclavicular lines, 2–3″ below the costal margin. This allows triangulation between the camera and the two instruments, and avoids the difficulty associated with the instruments being in direct line with the camera. The falciform ligament hangs low in many patients and provides a barrier around which the left-handed instrument must be manipulated.

5. **Initial retraction** is accomplished with exposure of the esophageal hiatus. A fan retractor is placed into the right anterior axillary port, and positioned to hold the left lateral segment of the liver toward the anterior abdominal wall. We prefer to utilize a table retractor to hold this instrument once properly positioned. Trauma to the liver should be meticulously avoided, because subsequent bleeding will obscure the field. Mobilization of the left lateral segment by division of the triangular ligament is not necessary. Place a Babcock clamp into the left anterior axillary port and retract the stomach toward the patient's left foot. This maneuver exposes the esophageal hiatus (Fig. 16.3). Commonly a hiatal hernia will need to be reduced. Use an atraumatic clamp, and take care not to grasp the stomach too vigorously, as gastric perforations can occur.

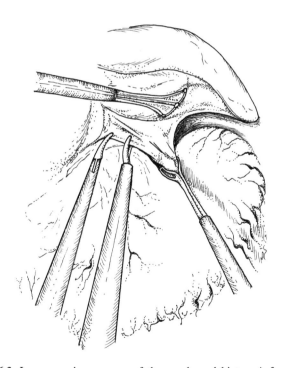

Figure 16.3. Laparoscopic exposure of the esophageal hiatus. A fan-type retractor (placed through the right subcostal port) elevated the left lateral hepatic segment anterolaterally. A Babcock clamp (placed through the left lateral port) retracts the stomach caudad. This places the phrenoesophageal membrane on traction.

D. Technique of Nissen Fundoplication

The critical elements of laparoscopic Nissen fundoplication are enumerated in Table 16.3 and will be discussed in detail here.

Table 16.3. Elements of laparoscopic nissen fundoplication

1.	Crural dissection, identification and preservation of both vagi including the hepatic branch of the anterior vagus
2.	Circumferential dissection of the esophagus
3.	Crural closure
4.	Fundic mobilization by division of short gastric vessels
5.	Creation of a short, loose fundoplication by enveloping the anterior and posterior wall of the fundus around the lower esophagus

1. **Crural dissection** begins with identification of the right crus. Metzenbaum type scissors and fine grasping forceps are preferred for dissection. In all except the most obese patients, there is a very thin portion of the gastrohepatic omentum overlying the caudate lobe of the liver (Fig. 16.4).

   a. Begin the dissection by incising this portion of the gastrohepatic omentum above and below the hepatic branch of the anterior vagal nerve (which the author routinely spares).

   b. A large left hepatic artery arising from the left gastric artery will be present in up to 25% of patients. It should be identified and avoided.

   c. After incising the gastrohepatic omentum, the outside of the right crus will become evident. Incise the peritoneum overlying the anterior aspect of the right crus with scissors and electrocautery, and dissect the right crus from anterior to posterior as far as possible.

   d. The medial portion of the right crus leads into the mediastinum, and is entered by blunt dissection with both instruments.

   e. At this juncture the esophagus usually becomes evident. Retract the right crus laterally and perform a modest dissection of the tissues posterior to the esophagus. Do not attempt to dissect behind the gastroesophageal junction at this time.

   f. Meticulous hemostasis is critical. Blood and fluid tends to pool in the hiatus and is difficult to remove. Irrigation should be kept to a minimum. Take care not to injure the phrenic artery and vein as they course above the hiatus. A large hiatal hernia often makes this portion of the procedure easier as it accentuates the diaphragmatic crura. On the other hand, dissection of a large mediastinal hernia sac can be difficult.

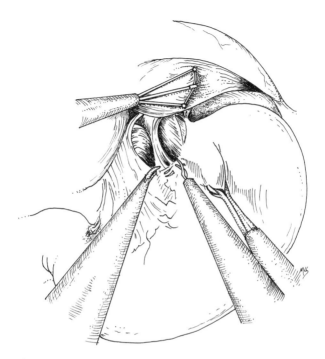

Figure 16.4. Initial dissection of the esophageal hiatus. The right crus is identified and dissected towards its posterior confluence with the left crus.

g. Following dissection of the right crus, attention is turned toward the anterior crural confluence. Use the left-handed grasper to hold up the tissues anterior to the esophagus, and sweep the esophagus downward and to the right, separating it from the left crus.

h. Divide the anterior crural tissues and identify the left crus.

i. Dissect the left crus as completely as possible, including taking down the angle of His and the attachments of the fundus to the left diaphragm (Fig. 16.5). A complete dissection of the lateral and inferior aspect of the left crus and fundus of the stomach is the key maneuver allowing circumferential mobilization of the esophagus. Failure to do so will result in difficulty encircling the esophagus, particularly if approached from the right. Repositioning of the Babcock retractor toward the fundic side of the stomach facilitates retraction for this portion of the procedure.

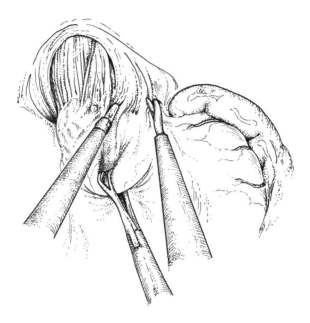

Figure 16.5. Dissection of the left crus. The left crus is dissected as completely as possible and the attachments of the fundus of the stomach to the diaphragm are taken down.

2. **Circumferential dissection of the esophagus** is achieved by careful dissection of the anterior and posterior soft tissues within the hiatus. If the crura have been completely dissected, then dissection posterior to the esophagus to create a window will not be difficult.

    a. From the patient's right side, use the left-handed instrument to retract the esophagus anteriorly. This allows the right hand to perform the dissection behind the esophagus. Reverse this maneuver for the left-sided dissection.

    b. Leave the posterior vagus nerve on the esophagus.

    c. Identify the left crus and keep the dissection caudad to it. There is a tendency to dissect into the mediastinum and left pleura.

    d. In the presence of severe esophagitis, transmural inflammation, esophageal shortening and/or a large posterior fat pad, this dissection may be particularly difficult. If unduly difficult, abandon this route of dissection and approach the hiatus from the left side by dividing the short gastric vessels (see below) at this point in the procedure rather than later.

   e. After completing the posterior dissection, pass a grasper (via the
       surgeon's left-handed port) behind the esophagus and over the
       left crus. Pass a Penrose drain around the esophagus and use this
       as an esophageal retractor for the remainder of the procedure.
3. **Crural closure:** Continue the crural dissection to enlarge the space
   behind the gastroesophageal junction as much as possible.
   a. Holding the esophagus anterior and to the left, approximate the
       crura with three to four (sometimes as many as six) interrupted 0
       silk sutures, starting just above the aortic decussation and
       working anterior (Fig. 16.6).

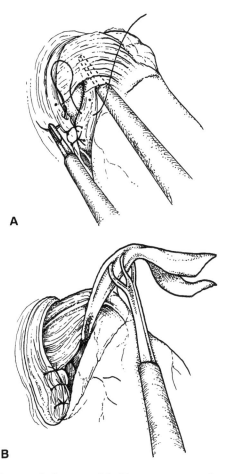

A

B

Figure 16.6. Three to six interrupted 0 silk sutures are used to close the crura.
Exposure of the crura and posterior aspect of the esophagus is facilitated by
traction on a Penrose drain encircling the gastroesophageal junction.

      b.   The author prefers a large needle (CT1) passed down the left upper 10-mm port to facilitate a durable crural closure.

      c.   Because space is limited, it is often necessary to use the surgeon's left-handed (nondominant) instrument as a retractor, facilitating placement of single bites through each crus with the surgeon's right hand.

      d.   The author prefers extracorporeal knot tying using a standard knot pusher, although tying within the abdomen is perfectly appropriate.

4.   **Fundic mobilization:** Complete fundic mobilization allows construction of a tension-free fundoplication.

      a.   Remove the liver retractor and place a second Babcock forceps through the right anterior axillary port to facilitate retraction during division of the short gastric vessels.

      b.   Suspend the gastrosplenic omentum anteroposteriorly, in a clothesline fashion via both Babcock forceps, and enter the lesser sac approximately one third the distance down the greater curvature of the stomach (Fig. 16.7). Sequentially dissect and divide the short gastric vessels with the aid of ultrasonic shears (Ethicon Endosurgery, Cincinnati, OH). An anterior-posterior rather than medial to lateral orientation of the vessels is preferred, with the exception of those close to the spleen. The dissection includes pancreaticogastric branches posterior to the upper stomach and continues until the right crus and caudate lobe can be seen from the left side (Fig. 16.8). With caution and meticulous dissection the fundus can be completely mobilized in virtually all patients.

5.   **Create a short, loose fundoplication** with particular attention to the geometry of the wrap.

      a.   Grasp the posterior fundus and pass it left to right rather than pulling right to left. This assures that the posterior fundus is used for the posterior aspect of the fundoplication. This is accomplished by placing a Babcock clamp through the left lower port, and grasping the mid portion of the posterior fundus (Fig. 16.9). Gently bring the posterior fundus behind the esophagus to the right side with an upward, rightward, and clockwise twisting motion.

      b.   Bring the anterior wall of the fundus anterior to the esophagus above the supporting Penrose drain.

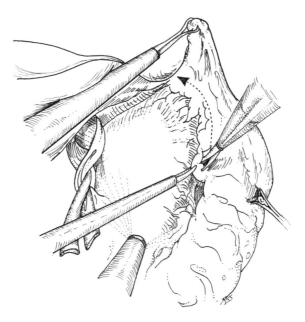

Figure 16.7. Proper retraction of the gastrosplenic omentum facilitates the initial steps of short gastric division.

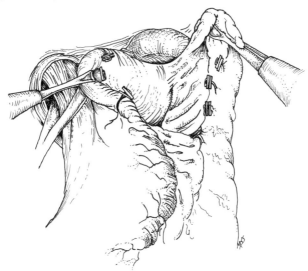

Figure 16.8. Retract the stomach rightward and the spleen and omentum left and downward to complete mobilization of the fundus. These maneuvers open the lesser sac and facilitate division of the high short gastric vessels.

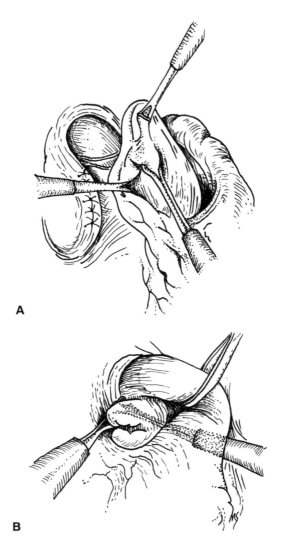

A

B

Figure 16.9. A. Placement of Babcock clamp on the posterior fundus in preparation for passing it behind the esophagus to create the posterior or right lip of the fundoplication. To achieve the proper angle for passage the Babcock is placed through the left lower trocar. B. Pass the posterior fundus from left to right and grasp it from the right with a Babcock clamp (passed through the right upper trocar).

c. Manipulate both the posterior and anterior fundic lips to allow the fundus to envelope the esophagus without twisting (Fig. 16.10). Laparoscopic visualization has a tendency to exaggerate the size of the posterior opening that has been dissected. Consequently, the space for the passage of the fundus behind the esophagus may be tighter than thought and the fundus relatively ischemic when brought around. If the right lip of the fundoplication has a bluish discoloration, the stomach should be returned to its original position and the posterior dissection enlarged.

d. Pass a 60-French bougie to properly size the fundoplication, and suture it utilizing a single U-stitch of 2-0 Prolene buttressed with felt pledgets. The most common error is an attempt to grasp the anterior portion of the stomach to construct the fundoplication rather than the posterior fundus. The esophagus should comfortably lie in the untwisted fundus prior to suturing.

e. Place two anchoring sutures of 2-0 silk above and below the U-stitch to complete the fundoplication. When finished, the suture line of the fundoplication should be facing in a right anterior direction.

f. Irrigate the abdomen, assure hemostasis, and remove the bougie.

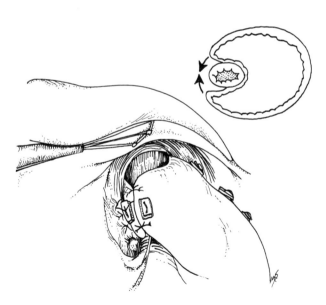

Figure 16.10. The fundoplication is sutured in place with a single U-stitch of 2-0 Prolene pledgeted on the outside. A 60 French mercury weighted bougie is passed through the gastroesophageal junction prior to fixation of the wrap to assure a floppy fundoplication. Inset illustrates the proper orientation of the fundic wrap.

E. Laparoscopic Partial Fundoplication

Although the orientation of partial fundoplication may be either anterior, posterior, or lateral, the most commonly performed laparoscopic partial fundoplication is the modified Toupet procedure, a 270-degree posterior hemifundoplication.

1. **Patient positioning,** trocar placement, hiatal dissection, crural closure, and fundic mobilization are performed exactly as for laparoscopic Nissen fundoplication.

2. **Fixation of the fundoplication** is the only portion of the procedure that differs from that of Nissen fundoplication. The posterior lip of the fundoplication is created as described for Nissen fundoplication.

3. With adequate fundic mobilization the posterior fundus should lie comfortably on the right side of the esophagus prior to suturing it in place.

4. Place a Babcock clamp on the superior aspect of the right lip and suture the posterior fundus to the crural closure with three interrupted sutures of 2-0 silk.

5. Rather than bringing the lips together (as in a Nissen fundoplication), suture the right limb of the fundoplication to the esophageal musculature at the 11 o'clock position and the left at the 1 o'clock position on the esophagus (Fig. 16.11). Three interrupted sutures of 2-0 silk are placed along the lower esophagus just above the gastroesophageal fat pad to fix each limb. (see also Chapter 17, in which Toupet and Dor fundoplications are discussed in the context of laparoscopic cardiomyotomy).

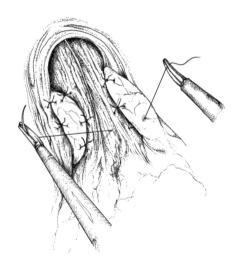

Figure 16.11. Completed 270-degree posterior hemifundoplication (Toupet fundoplication).

F. Postoperative Considerations

Recovery is more rapid than usual after the corresponding open procedure, and several aspects of postoperative management are correspondingly different.

1. **A nasogastric tube** is not necessary.
2. **Pain** is managed with parenteral narcotics or ketorolac for the first 24 hours and oral hydrocodone thereafter as necessary.
3. **A Foley** catheter is placed following induction of anesthesia and left in place until the morning after surgery. The incidence of urinary retention is approximately 10–25% if bladder decompression is not used.
4. **A diet** of clear liquids ad libitum is allowed the morning following surgery. Soft solids are begun on the second postoperative day and continued for 2 weeks. The patient should be instructed to eat slowly, chew carefully, and avoid bread and meats for a minimum of 2 weeks.

G. Complications

The safety of laparoscopic fundoplication has now been established. **Mortality** is rare following an elective antireflux procedure, whether open or closed. The complication rate is similar to that of open fundoplication, averaging 10–15%, but the spectrum of the morbidity has changed. Complications associated with surgical access and postoperative recovery have improved. With the exception of a reduction in the number of splenic injuries and splenectomies performed during laparoscopic fundoplication, intraoperative complications such as gastric or esophageal perforation are slightly higher. Initial concern of the possibility of an increased incidence of pulmonary embolism, has not proven true. Cumulative results suggest an incidence of pulmonary embolism of 0.49%, similar to that of open fundoplication.

Several excellent series of laparoscopic fundoplication have now been published. Three of the best come from Atlanta, Omaha, and Adelaide. These reports document the ability of laparoscopic fundoplication to relieve typical symptoms of gastroesophageal reflux, that is, heartburn, regurgitation, and dysphagia, in over 90% of patients. The average length of follow-up is now about 2 years. These results compare favorably to those of the "modern" era of open fundoplication. Overall, there is a 4.2% conversion rate to open surgery, a 0.5% rate of early reoperation, and excellent to good symptomatic improvement in 91% of patients. Although the incidence of dysphagia was an unacceptably high 9% in early series, it has decreased to the 3–5% range with increasing experience and attention to technical details. Lower esophageal sphincter characteristics and esophageal acid exposure are returned to normal in nearly all patients.

A few complications are particularly noteworthy and are described briefly here.

1. **Pneumothorax and surgical emphysema** have occurred in 1–2% of patients. This is most likely related to excessive hiatal dissection and should decrease with increasing experience of the surgical team.
2. **Unrecognized perforation of esophagus or stomach** are the most life-threatening problems. Perforations of the esophagus and stomach occur during hiatal dissection and are related to operative experience. Intraoperative recognition and repair is the key to preventing life-threatening problems.
3. Although uncommon, **acute paraesophageal herniation** has been noted by a number of authors and usually results in early reoperation.

H. Selected References

Cuschieri A, Hunter J, Wolfe B, Swanstrom LL, Hutson W. Multicenter prospective evaluation of laparoscopic antireflux surgery. Preliminary report. Surg Endosc 1993;7:505–510.

DeMeester TR, Bonavina L, Albertucci M. Nissen fundoplication for gastroesophageal reflux disease—evaluation of primary repair in 100 consecutive patients. Ann Surg 1986;204:9.

Hinder RA, Filipi CJ, Wetscher G, Neary P, DeMeester TR, Perdikis G. Laparoscopic Nissen fundoplication is an effective treatment for gastroesophageal reflux disease. Ann Surg 1994;220(4):472–483.

Hunter JG, Trus TL, Branum GD, Waring JP, Wood WC. A physiologic approach to laparoscopic fundoplication for gastroesophageal reflux disease. Ann Surg 1996;223:673–687.

Jamieson GG, Watson DI, Britten-Jones R, Mitchell PC, Anvari M. Laparoscopic Nissen fundoplication. Ann Surg 1994;220:137–145.

Kauer W, Peters JH, Bremner CG, DeMeester TR. A tailored approach to antireflux surgery. J Thorac Cardiovasc Surg 1995;110:141–147.

Peters JH, Heimbucher J, Kauer WKH, Incarbone R, Bremner CG, DeMeester TR. Clinical and physiologic comparison of laparoscopic and open Nissen. J Am Coll Surg 1995;180:385–93 .

Ratner DW, Brooks DC. Patient satisfaction following laparoscopic and open antireflux surgery. Arch Surg 1995;130:289–294.

Schauer PR, Meyers WC, Eubanks S, Norem RF, Franklin M, Pappas TN. Mechanisms of gastric and esophageal perforations during laparoscopic fundoplication. Ann Surg 1996;223:43–52.

Urschel JD. Complications of antireflux surgery. Am J Surg 1993;165:68–70.

Waring JP, Hunter JG, Oddsdottir M, Wo J, Katz E. The preoperative evaluation of patients considered for laparoscopic antireflux surgery. Am J Gastroenterol 1995;90:35–38.

Watson D, Balgrie RJ, Jamieson GG. A learning curve for laparoscopic fundoplication; definable, avoidable or a waste of time? Ann Surg 1996;224:198–203.

Weerts JM, Dallemagne B, Hamoir E, et al. Laparoscopic Nissen fundoplication; detailed analysis of 132 patients. Surg Laparosc Endosc 1993;3:359–364.

17. Laparoscopic Cardiomyotomy (Heller Myotomy)

Margret Oddsdottir, M.D.

A. Indications and Patient Preparation

Laparoscopic cardiomyotomy (Heller myotomy) is performed for achalasia. The **diagnostic workup** must exclude several diseases that can mimic achalasia (malignant obstruction, gastroesophageal reflux with stricture formation, diffuse esophageal spasm, and nutcracker esophagus), as treatment of these is quite different. A complete diagnostic workup is outlined in Table 17.1.

Table 17.1. Diagnostic workup for laparoscopic cardiomyotomy

Test	Results Consistent with Achalasia
Barium swallow	Dilated esophagus, tapering distally, with a so-called birds beak deformity
Upper GI Endoscopy (EGD) with biopsy if necessary	Smooth mucosa and a tight distal esophageal sphincter which the endoscopist is able to traverse.
Esophageal manometry	Loss of peristalsis in the esophageal body and a normal or hypertensive lower esophageal sphincter that fails to relax upon swallowing
24-hour pH study*	No evidence of gastroesophageal reflux
Computed tomography (CT) scan*	No evidence of malignancy

*Optional tests, depending upon clinical presentation.

There are several therapeutic options once achalasia is definitively diagnosed. Patients who can tolerate general anasethesia are candidates for laparoscopic cardiomyotomy. Pneumatic balloon dilation is an alternative treatment. Botulinum toxin (BOTOX) injection is an alternative that should be reserved for patients who are not candidates for operation or dilatation. Who should be referred for laparoscopic cardiomyotomy?

1. **Young patients**—patients under the age of 40 do not respond well to pneumatic dilation
2. Patients who **fail pneumatic dilations**
3. Patients who are fit for surgery and choose to have surgery

Because patients with achalasia frequently retain food and secretions within the esophagus, preoperative fasting for at least 8 hours is recommended. Some surgeons evacuate the dilated esophagus with an Ewald tube or esophagoscope. Candida albicans frequently colonizes this dilated esophagus and oral antifungal therapy may be warranted. These measures decrease the likelihood of aspiration upon induction of anesthesia, and minimize the consequences of inadvertent mucosal perforation during myotomy.

B. Patient Positioning and Room Setup

1. Position the patient supine on the operating table, with the legs spread apart on leg boards (Fig. 17.1). If possible, tuck both arms at the patient's side. Place the patient in a steep reversed Trendelenburg position.
2. Place an orogastric tube and Foley catheter (optional). Most surgeons use sequential pneumatic compression devices (or perioperative low molecular weight heparin injections) as prophylaxis for deep venous thrombosis.
3. Stand between the patient's legs facing the monitors, maintaining coaxial alignment with the gastroesophageal junction and the laparoscope. The camera operator stands on the patient's right side. The first assistant and scrub nurse stand on the patient's left.

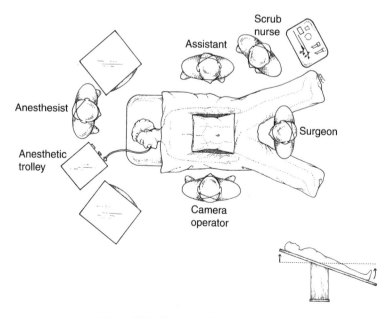

Figure 17.1. The operating room set-up.

C. Trocar Position and Choice of Laparoscope

1. Place the first trocar through the left rectus sheath, medial to the epigastric vessels. This trocar will be used for the laparoscope. It is imperative to use an angled (30- or 45-degree) laparoscope for adequate visualization of the hiatus.
2. Insert the remaining four trocars under direct vision (Fig. 17.2).
3. Pass a liver retractor through the right subcostal trocar and place it under the left liver lobe to expose the hiatus. Several types of self-holding devices are available to hold the liver retractor in place.
4. Place an atraumatic grasper through the 5 mm left flank port. The assistant should use this grasper to retract the epiphrenic fat pad.
5. The left subcostal port and the right epigastric port are the working trocars for the surgeon.

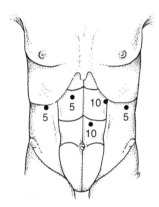

Figure 17.2. Trocar placement. The supraumbilical trocar and the right subcostal trocar are placed 15 cm from the xiphoid, the left subcostal trocar about 10 cm from the xiphoid. The epigastric trocar is placed as high as the liver edge allows and as lateral as the falciform ligament allows. The left flank port is about 7 cm lateral to the left subcostal trocar.

D. Performing the Cardiomyotomy

It is convenient to conceptualize the dissection in three phases: the hiatal dissection, the myotomy, and the antireflux procedure (if desired). The author prefers to add a partial fundoplication (Toupet or Dor procedure) at the completion of the myotomy, and this is described in the last part of this section. The partial fundoplication holds the raw edges of the myotomy open and provides some protection against gastroesophageal reflux, while being sufficiently loose not to obstruct passage of food and liquids (recall that the esophagus lacks normal peristalsis in this disorder).

1. **The hiatal dissection**
   a. Take scissors or a hook electrocautery in the right hand and an atraumatic grasper in the left hand.
   b. Begin by incising the avascular area of the gastrohepatic omentum above the hepatic branch of the vagus. This exposes the caudate lobe of the liver and the right crus.
   c. Continue the dissection across the hiatus, dividing the phrenoesophageal ligament above the epiphrenic fat pad with electrocautery and sharp dissection. The assistant should retract the epiphrenic fat pad down and to the left.
   d. Identify the right and left crura of the diaphragm and dissect these from the esophagus with blunt dissection.
   e. Divide the posterior esophageal attachments under direct vision with blunt and sharp dissection. Retain the posterior vagus with the posterior esophageal wall. Thus far, the dissection is essentially the same as that performed for hiatal hernia repair (see Chapter 16).
   f. Pass the left hand grasper behind the esophagus under direct vision, and place the grasper in front of the left crus. Pull an 8-cm long segment of 1/4″ Penrose drain around the esophagus. Clip the two ends of the drain together and use this sling to retract the esophagus. Special angled or reticulating graspers are available for this purpose.
   g. Complete the periesophageal dissection by dissecting both crura free of all epiphrenic tissue, mobilizing an adequate length of the esophagus and developing a posterior window large enough for a loose partial fundoplication (270 degree). Dissect the epiphrenic fat pad off the anterior surface of the gastroesophageal junction and the cardia.
   h. Divide the short gastric vessels, beginning about one third of the way down the greater curvature using the ultrasonically activated shears or a dissector and clips. Continue the dissection of the gastric fundus, finally taking down the attachments to the diaphragm and left crus. A redundant fundus is thus prepared, and will be used for partial fundoplication at the conclusion of the myotomy.

2. **The myotomy**
   a. Begin the myotomy on the anterior surface of the esophagus, to the left of the anterior vagus nerve, just proximal to the gastroesophageal junction.
   b. Use dissecting scissors and electrocautery to carefully cauterize a longitudinal area of the outer coat. Separate the outer longitudinal fibers using the twin action of the scissors.
   c. Separate the inner circular fibers from the underlying mucosa with blunt dissection, using the scissors or a dissector, then divide these circular fibers with scissors or hook cautery. Tent the fibers away from the mucosa before applying electocautery if a monopolar electrocautery is being used. Once the submucosal

plane is reached, the mucosa bulges up. This is clearly seen in the magnified laparoscopic view.

d. Carry the myotomy proximally for about 5 to 6 cm from the gastroesophageal junction (Fig. 17.3).

e. Distally, carry the myotomy across the gastro-esophageal junction and onto the stomach for about 1 cm. On the stomach site, the separation of the muscle layers from the mucosa is more difficult to achieve, the mucosa becomes thinner, and there are more bridging vessels than on the esophagus. This results in more bleeding than encountered during the esophageal myotomy and increased risk of perforation.

f. Once the myotomy is completed, separate the muscle edges from the underlying mucosa for approximately 40% of the esophageal circumference.

g. Some surgeons place a flexible upper gastrointestinal (UGI) endoscope in the esophagus and visualize the distal esophagus to confirm adequacy of myotomy.

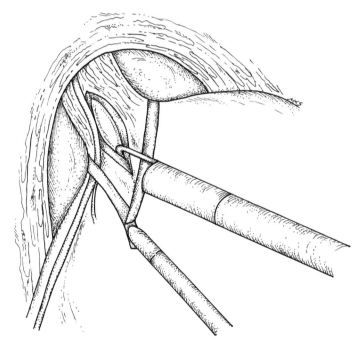

Figure 17.3. The myotomy being carried distally, using hook electrocautery. Care must be taken to elevate the muscle fibers away from the mucosa before the electrocautery is applied. The myotomy extends about 5 to 6 cm proximal to the gastroesophageal junction and about 1 cm onto the stomach. (Reprinted with permission from Oddsdottir M. Laparoscopic management of achalasia. Surg Clin North Am 1996;76:451–457.)

h. Pull the orogastric tube back into the distal esophagus and instill about 100 ml of methylene blue solution (one ampule diluted in 250 ml NaCl) down the tube. This will clearly demonstrate any mucosal perforation. If any perforation is encountered, close it with a stitch (4-D absorbable suture).

3. **Antireflux procedures**

Either a Toupet (a posterior fundoplication) or a Dor (an anterior fundoplication) is recommended in conjunction with the myotomy. If the hiatus is patulous, the crura are approximated with one or two sutures posteriorly.

a. **Toupet procedure**. The first fundoplication sutures anchor the fundic wrap posteriorly to the crural closure using two or three interrupted, nonabsorbable, 2-0 sutures. Suture the right side of the wrap to the right edge of the myotomy with three interrupted sutures. Similarily, suture the fundus on the left to the left edge of the myotomy (Fig. 17.4).

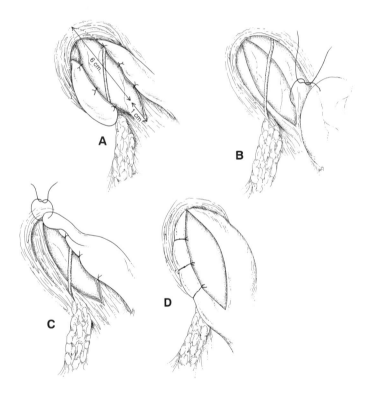

Figure 17.4. A. Completed abdominal myotomy with Toupet posterior fundoplication. B–D. Completed abdominal myotomy with Dor anterior fundoplication. (Reprinted with permission from Hunter et al., Laparoscopic Heller myotomy and fundoplication for achalasia. Ann Surg 1997;225:655–664.)

b. **Dor procedure.** In this partial fundoplication, the redundant fundus is rolled over the exposed mucosa. This may be used to buttress a mucosal repair. Place two or three interrupted sutures between the fundus of the stomach and the left edge of the myotomy. Then place another two or three sutures between the fundus and the anterior crural arch. Finally, suture the fundus to the right edge of the myotomy.

E. Complications

1. **Mucosal perforation**
   a. **Cause and prevention:** This is the most common complication, and the most frequent cause is probably electrosurgical injury. As previously noted, on the gastric side, separation of the muscle layers from the mucosa is more difficult to achieve and the mucosa becomes thinner than on the esophagus. This results in increased risk of perforation. Late perforations are rare, and are probably due to sloughing of a burned mucosa. When performing the myotomy it is very important to tent up the mucosa before applying the electrocautery. The cut edge of the muscularis may bleed, but care should be taken not to apply electrocautery close to the mucosa. Bleeding there usually stops spontaneously.
   b. **Recognition and management:** Mucosal perforations are easily recognized, if not immediately, then during the installation of methylene blue dye into the esophagus. These lacerations are clean and are easily repaired with a stitch. As of today, there are no reports of an infection from a small, recognized mucosal laceration during laparoscopic cardiomyotomy. Late perforations are very rare.

2. **Pneumothorax**
   a. **Cause and prevention:** Pneumothorax is not uncommon during laparoscopic hiatal dissection and esophageal mobilization (5–10%). One can frequently see the pleural edges during these procedures.
   b. **Recognition and management:** These pneumothoraces are usually small and self-limited. They are best recognized on a postoperative chest film. Intervention is rarely needed as the lung reexpands rapidly as carbon dioxide is absorbed. Some surgeons place a small red rubber catheter in the chest and suction the pneumothorax at the conclusion of the procedure, if pleural entry is seen at laparoscopy.

3. **Dysphagia**
   a. **Cause and prevention:** Heller myotomy offers relief of dysphagia in 90–97% of patients. Postoperative dysphagia may be due to either incomplete myotomy or a megaesophagus in "end-stage" achalasia. Incomplete myotomy occurs more commonly

at the distal end of the myotomy, the stomach side. It is important to carry the myotomy across the gastroesophageal junction and onto the stomach for about 1/2 to 1 cm.

b. **Recognition and management:** The magnification during laparoscopic surgery offers excellent view of the myotomy, and of uncut muscle fibers. If incomplete myotomy is not recognized intraoperatively, postoperative dilation can help. If esophageal manometry shows clearly an uncut, high-pressure zone at the gastroesophageal junction, reoperation should be considered. Patients with extremely dilated aperistaltic esophagus generally require esophageal replacement. Workup of postoperative dysphagia requires careful assessment with esophageal manometry and should prompt reconsideration of the underlying diagnosis.

F. Selected References

Abid S, Champion G, Richter JE, et al. Treatment of achalasia: the best of both worlds. Am J Gastroenterol 1994;89:979–985.

Andreollo NA, Earlam RJ. Heller´s myotomy for achaasia: is an added anti-reflux procedure necessary? Br J Surg 1987;74,765–769.

Anselmino M, Zaninotto G, Costantini M, Rossi M, et al. One-year follow-up after laparoscopic Heller-Dor operation for esophageal achalasia. Surg Endosc 1997;11:3–7.

Crookes PF, Wilkinson AJ, Johnston GW. Heller´s myotomy with partial fundoplication. Br J Surg 1989;76:98.

Csendes A, Braghetto I, Henriquez A, et al. Late results of a prospective randomised study comparing forceful dilatation and oephagomyotomy in patients with achalasia. Gut 1989;30:299–304.

Ellis FH. Functional disorders of the esophagus. In Zuidema GD, Orringer MB, eds. Shackelford´s Surgery of the Alimentary Tract, 3rd ed. Philadelphia: WB Saunders, 1991;150–156.

Hunter JG, Trus TL, Branum GD, et al. Laparoscopic Heller myotomy and fundoplication for achalasia. Ann Surg 1997;225:655–664.

Oddsdottir M. Laparoscopic management of achalasia. Surg Clin North Am 1996;76:451–457.

Raiser F, Perdikis G, Hinder RA, et al. Heller myotomy via minimal-access surgery: an evaluation of antireflux procedures. Arch Surg 1996;131:593–597.

Swanstrom LL, Pennings J. Laparoscopic esophagomyotomy for achalasia. Surg Endosc 1995;9:286–292.

18. Laparoscopic Gastrostomy

Thomas R. Gadacz, M.D.

A. Indications

The indications for gastrostomy include access to the stomach for feeding or prolonged gastric decompression. Laparoscopic gastrostomy is indicated when a percutaneous endoscopic gastrostomy (PEG) cannot be performed or is contraindicated (see Chapter 43.2.6, Percutaneous Endoscopic Feeding Tube Placement). Specific situations in which this is likely to occur include:

1. An obstructing oropharyngeal lesion.
2. A lesion in the esophagus when the stomach is not to be used for reconstruction.
3. Concern that the colon or omentum are overlying the stomach, precluding adequate access via a percutaneous blind approach.

Other methods of achieving enteral nutrition (such as Dobhoff tube placement) should be considered, and pyloric obstruction and gastroesophageal reflux should be ruled out. If recurrent aspiration is a problem, a jejunal feeding tube may be more appropriate (but aspiration may still occur).

B. Patient Position and Room Setup

1. Position the patient supine on the operating room table with the arms tucked.
2. As with most upper abdominal procedures, some surgeons prefer a modified lithotomy position and operate between the legs of the patient.
3. The surgeon generally stands on the left side of the patient, and the first assistant and scrub nurse on the right side.
4. The monitors are placed at the head of the bed and as close to the operating room table as the anesthesiologist permits.
5. The general setup is very similar to laparoscopic cholecystectomy in most respects, but less equipment is required.

C. Cannula Position and Choice of Laparoscope

Generally only two cannulas are needed for a laparoscopic gastrostomy (Fig. 18.1).

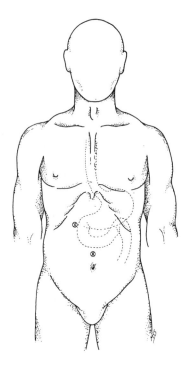

Figure 18.1. Cannula placement for laparoscopic gastrostomy. Consider adequate working distance from anticipated site of gastrostomy placement.

1.   Place the cannula for the 30-degree laparoscope below the umbilicus in short patients and at the umbilicus in tall patients. Estimate the working distance to the probable site of gastrostomy placement. Do not place the laparoscope too close, as a short working distance makes it difficult to proceed.
2.   Place a second 5-mm cannula in the right subcostal region at the midclavicular line.

D. Performing the Gastrostomy

Two methods of laparoscopic gastrostomy have been described. The first method constructs a simple gastrostomy without a mucosa-lined tubed. This is appropriate for most indications. The tract will generally seal without surgical closure when the tube is removed.

An alternative method utilizes the endoscopic stapler to construct a mucosa-lined tube in a fashion analogous to the open Janeway gastrostomy. This provides a permanent stoma that is easily recannulated. Both methods will be described here.

1. **Simple gastrostomy**

    a.   Indentify the anterior wall of the body of the stomach. Avoid the classic error of mistaking colon for stomach by confirming the absence of taeniae.

    b.   Select a location in the left subcostal area for gastrostomy construction.

    c.   Pass an atraumatic grasper from the second cannula and grasp the mid-portion of the selected region. Lift the gastric wall and simultaneously indent the selected region of the abdominal wall with one finger.

    d.   Confirm that the area of the stomach selected for the gastrostomy comfortably reaches the corresponding area selected in the left upper abdominal wall. Reassess and choose different sites if necessary.

    e.   Reduce the pneumoperitoneal pressure to 6 to 8 mm Hg to avoid tension on the stomach.

    f.   Pass the T-fasteners though the skin and abdominal wall, and then through the anterior wall of the stomach (Fig. 18.2).

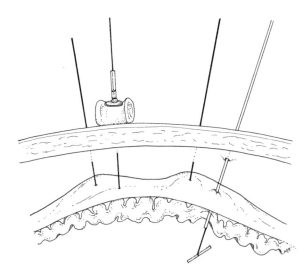

Figure 18.2. T-fasteners through the abdominal wall and anterior gastric wall.

      i.   There is a slight give in resistance as the needle passes thought the gastric wall.

      ii.   Elevate the anterior gastric wall with a grasper to prevent passing the T-fastener through both walls of the stomach.

      iii. Insert the most proximal T-fasteners and pull up slightly to expose the distal sites of the T-fasteners. By pulling on the T-fasteners, the correct placement can usually be determined.

      iv. Place a total of four T-fasteners outlining a 2 to 3 cm square on the abdominal and gastric walls.

g.   Make a 5- to 8-mm stab incision in the skin to adequately accommodate the diameter of the gastrostomy tube.

h.   Pass a 14-gauge needle through the center of the square of the T-fasteners in the abdominal wall and stomach.

i.   Pass a 0.35-mm guide wire through the lumen of the needle and thread at least 25 cm into the stomach.

j.   Enlarge the tract with dilators and pass an 18 Fr gastrostomy tube using Seldinger technique.

k.   Release the pneumoperitoneum and pull up the T-fasteners. Tie these to secure the gastric wall to the abdominal wall.

l.   Pull up the gastrostomy tube to approximate the gastric and abdominal walls. Secure the gastrostomy tube to the skin with sutures or with a Silastic plate.

2. **Construction of gastrostomy with mucosa-lined tube**

a.   Place three cannulas, in addition to the umbilical port for the laparoscope.

      i.   Left upper quadrant (10 mm)—preferably placed at the approximate site of entry of the gastrostomy

      ii.   Right upper quadrant (10 mm)

      iii. Right midabdomen (to right of umbilicus) (12 mm)

b.   Place two endoscopic Babcock clamps through the left and right upper quadrant cannulas and elevate a fold of gastric wall on the anterior surface of the stomach.

c.   Pass the endoscopic linear stapling device through the 12-mm cannula and use it to create a gastric tube. Generally a single application of the stapler will produce a tube of adequate length (Fig. 18.3). Take care to construct a tube with adequate lumen; this is accomplished by placing the stapler 1 cm from the edge of the gastric fold.

d.   Evacuate the pneumoperitoneum.

e.   Pull the cannula, Babcock clamp, and finally the end of the gastric tube out through the left upper quadrant trocar site.

f.   Open the gastric tube and mature the end to the skin with several interrupted absorbable sutures.

g.   Cannulate the gastrostomy with a small diameter Foley catheter. Test the gastrostomy by instilling saline or methylene blue.

h.   Reestablish a limited (6–8 mm Hg) pneumoperitoneum sufficient to visualize the gastric wall with the laparoscope and confirm that the stomach lies comfortably against the anterior abdominal wall and that there is no leakage.

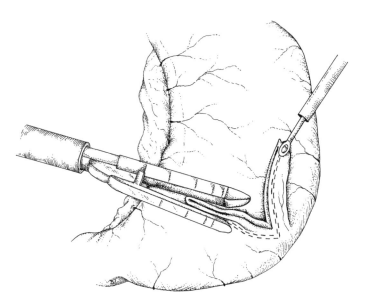

Figure 18.3. Construction of mucosa-lined tube (Janeway-style gastrostomy). A
fold of stomach is elevated and the endoscopic stapler applied. Approximately
1 cm of stomach must be included in the staple line to assure an adequate lumen. The tube is grasped, elevated, and will be pulled out through the left upper quadrant cannula site.

E. Complications

1.   **Leakage of the gastrostomy**
   a.   **Cause and prevention**: The gastrostomy can leak if the gastrostomy tube and T-fasteners are not approximated to the abdominal wall. Prevent this by directly observing the T-fasteners
   being pulled up and ensuring that the gastric wall is adherent to
   the abdominal wall. The balloon of the gastrostomy tube should
   be inflated and pulled with gentle traction to approximate the
   anterior gastric wall to the abdominal wall. This is confirmed by
   visualization though the laparoscope. If a stapled tube is constructed, an incomplete staple line may result in leakage.

   b.   **Recognition and management**: If visualization of the stomach
        to the abdominal wall is unsatisfactory at the time of operation,
        inject methylene blue through the gastrostomy tube while visu-
        alizing the gastric wall. If any dye is seen in the abdominal cav-
        ity, assume inadequate approximation between the stomach and
        abdominal wall. Fix this either by loosening the gastrostomy
        tube and inserting more T-fasteners around the gastrostomy site,
        or by using a gastrostomy tube with a larger balloon and apply-
        ing sufficient retraction to provide a better seal between the
        stomach and abdominal wall.
2. **Gastric perforation**
   a.   **Cause and prevention**: Gastric perforation may occur during
        laparoscopic gastrostomy if there is too much tension on the T-
        fasteners, or if the selected sites cannot be approximated without
        tension. Prevent this by careful site selection and by reducing
        the pressure of the pneumoperitoneum to 6 to 8 mm Hg. Exces-
        sive use of electrocautery may produce a delayed perforation
        and the patient may present with intra-abdominal sepsis 2 to 5
        days after operation.
   b.   **Recognition and management:** Confirm a suspected perfora-
        tion by injecting water-soluble contrast through the gastrostomy
        tube under fluoroscopic observation. If no leak is seen and the
        patient is stable or improving, nasogastric decompression may
        be sufficient. Free leakage of contrast, clinical evidence of peri-
        tonitis, or clinical deterioration mandate exploratory laparotomy.
        Oversew the perforation or convert to a formal gastrostomy.

F. Selected References

Arnaud J-P, Casa C, Manunta A. Laparoscopic continent gastrostomy. Am J Surg
    1995;169:629–630.
Duh Q-Y, Senokozlieff AL, Englehart RN, et al. Prospective evaluation of safety and
    efficacy of laparoscopic gastrostomy. SAGES 1993;poster 28.
Duh Q-Y, Way LW. Laparoscopic gastrostomy using T-fasteners as retractors and an-
    chors. Surg Endosc 1993;7:60–63.
Edelman DS, Unger SW. Laparoscopic gastrostomy. Surg Gynecol Obstret
    1991;173:401.

19. Laparoscopic Vagotomy

Thomas R. Gadacz, M.D.

A. Indications

The indications for a laparoscopic vagotomy (vagectomy) are the same as for an open vagotomy and include permanent gastric acid reduction in patients who have idiosyncratic responses to the H-2 histamine antagonists or the proton-pump inhibitors.

B. Patient Position and Room Setup

1. Position the patient supine on the operating table with the arms tucked at the sides.
2. Some surgeons prefer a modified lithotomy position and operate between the legs of the patient.
3. Place the patient in reverse Trendelenburg position and rotate the right side of the table up slightly.
4. Thoracoscopic vagotomy can also be performed through the left chest (see references at end of this chapter).
5. The surgeon generally stands on the patient's left side and the first assistant and scrub nurse stand on the right.
6. Place the monitors at the head of the table and as close as possible.

C. Trocar Position and Choice of Laparoscope

1. Place the cannula for the laparoscope below the umbilicus in short patients and above the umbilicus in tall patients. Recall that the distance to the esophageal hiatus is farther than generally estimated. A 30-degree laparoscope gives the best visualization (Fig. 19.1).
2. Place four additional cannulas (10- or 12-mm size):
   a. Right subcostal region at the midclavicular line
   b. Right subcostal region at the anterior axillary line
   c. Left subcostal region at the midclavicular line
   d. Epigastric region
3. Additional cannulas may be required to assist in retraction or exposure, and should be placed as needed.

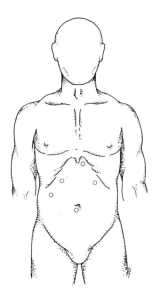

Figure 19.1. Cannula placement for laparoscopic vagotomy.

D. Performing the Vagotomy

Four types of vagotomy, each corresponding to a similar open procedure, may be performed laparoscopically. Each will be discussed here (Fig. 19.2). Thoracoscopic truncal vagotomy represents another option in selected cases, and will be discussed briefly at the conclusion.

1. **Truncal or total abdominal vagotomy** divides the main vagal trunks as they emerge through the hiatus. The dissection at the hiatus and mobilization of the esophagus is the same as if performing a laparoscopic Nissen fundoplication (see Chapter 16, Laparoscopic Treatment of Gastroesophageal Reflux and Hiatal Hernia).

    a. At the esophagogastric junction, incise the peritoneal covering, and isolate a 3- to 4-cm segment of esophagus.

    b. Identify the anterior vagal trunk as it runs over the anterior surface of the esophagus.

    c. Doubly clip the trunk and excise a segment for pathologic confirmation.

    d. Identify the posterior trunk in the space between the esophagus and the right crus of the diaphragm. Doubly clip this trunk, excising a segment for pathologic confirmation.

    e. Seek out small fibers from the main trunks to the stomach or esophagus and divide these.

  f. Truncal vagotomy should be accompanied by a drainage procedure such as pyloroplasty. References at the end of this chapter describe various methods, including laparoscopic stapling and suturing. Some have substituted pyloric dilatation for this procedure, with variable results.

2. A **selective (total gastric) vagotomy** is performed by dissecting the main vagal trunks to the area where the branch to the biliary tree of the anterior trunk divides and transecting a section of vagus distal to the hepatic branch. The celiac branch of the posterior trunk is not easy to identify and a truncal vagotomy may be performed. If a selective vagotomy is performed, a drainage procedure is necessary. A selective laparoscopic vagotomy is rarely indicated or performed (analogous to the open procedure, which is rarely used).

3. A **highly selective** (superselective, parietal cell, or proximal gastric) **vagotomy** (HSV) is the author's vagotomy of choice. It selectively deprives the parietal cell mass of vagal innervation and reduces the sensitivity of the parietal cells to stimulation and the release of acid. It does not require a drainage procedure. The branches of the nerve of Latarjet are divided from the esophagogastric junction to the crow's foot along the lesser curvature of the stomach.

  a. In contrast to the open procedure, the laparoscopic HSV generally begins at the crow's foot and proceeds cephalad. (Some surgeons prefer to begin at the esophagogastric junction and work caudad.)

  b. Retract the stomach caudad and to the left, and identify the crow's foot termination of the nerves of Latarjet on the gastric antrum.

  c. Incise the gastrohepatic ligament and serially divide the branches (beginning at the Crow's foot) between clips. The author prefers the use of the clips rather than cautery to avoid injury to the main nerves of Latarjet.

  d. Continue the dissection superiorly, dividing the anterior leaf of the gastrohepatic ligament.

  e. Once the anterior leaf of the gastrohepatic ligament is divided, the posterior branches are divided in a similar fashion. Magnification with the laparoscope makes visualization of the neurovascular bundles easier than during an open operation.

Figure 19.2 (see following page). Four types of vagotomy. A. Truncal vagotomy produces total abdominal vagal denervation and requires a drainage procedure to prevent gastric stasis. B. Selective vagotomy spares the vagal branches to the liver and small intestine, but produces a total gastric vagotomy. A drainage procedure is required. This vagotomy is rarely performed. C. Highly selective vagotomy (HSV) produces selective denervation of the parietal cell mass. No drainage procedure is needed, as antral innervation is preserved. D. Posterior truncal vagotomy with anterior seromyotomy (Taylor operation) preserves the anterior vagal trunk. No drainage procedure is required.

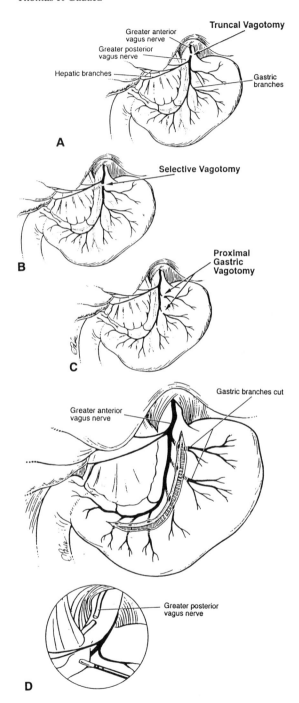

      f.   The nerve of Latarjet appears as a silvery thin thread; it must be identified and must not be injured. It is important to isolate the branches.

      g.   Isolate the vagal trunks for a 3- to-4 cm segment along the esophagus. Posterior branches (nerve of Grassi) to the cardia of the stomach must be identified and divided. These fine branches can usually be cauterized provided they are away from the main trunk.

4.   Posterior truncal vagotomy with anterior seromyotomy (Taylor procedure) is a modification that is technically easier. The corresponding open procedure has been used in Europe for a long time, but there was limited interest in this modification in the United States prior to laparoscopic surgery.

      a.   Perform a posterior truncal vagotomy as previously described.

      b.   Perform an anterior seromyotomy by creating a partial-thickness incision along the lesser curvature of the stomach. The mucosa should be exposed but not entered (Fig. 19.2D). Oversew the area with a continuous suture to prevent a postoperative leak. No drainage procedure is required.

5.   **A thoracoscopic vagotomy** is performed through the third, sixth, and seventh left intercostal spaces. Using a double-lumen endotracheal tube, the left lung is deflated and a cannula inserted in the left sixth midaxillary space. The other cannulas are inserted and the lung retracted anteriorly and cephalad away from the esophagus. The inferior pulmonary ligament usually needs to be divided. If there is difficulty identifying the esophagus, a flexible endoscope can be passed into the esophagus and the light will illuminate the esophagus. The pleura over the distal third of the esophagus is incised and the anterior vagal trunk is identified, clipped, and a segment excised. The esophagus requires mobilization to gain access to the posterior vagal trunk. If a flexible endoscope was inserted, it should be withdrawn to prevent injury to the esophagus. The posterior trunk is isolated, clipped, and a segment excised. A chest tube (28 Fr) is inserted and the thoracoscopy incisions closed.

E. Complications

1.   **Gastric or esophageal perforation**

      a.   **Cause and prevention:** Gastric perforation may occur from electrocautery injury or by clipping the branch of the nerve of Latarjet on the serosa of the lesser curvature. Prevent this by careful dissection and isolation of the branches of the nerve of Latarjet as well as by avoiding the use of electrocautery. The power setting of the electrocautery should be low but sufficient to coagulate tissue. If a seromyotomy vagotomy is performed, the area should be oversewn with a continuous suture. Esophageal perforation may occur during hiatal dissection, particularly if manipulations are performed blindly.

b. **Recognition and management:** Bleeding on the lesser curvature of the stomach should be controlled by low-power electrocautery or suture ligation. Excessive use of cautery may produce a delayed perforation and the patient may present with intraabdominal sepsis 2 to 5 days after operation. The perforation can be confirmed by a Gastrografin study. If no leak is seen and the patient is stable or improving, nasogastric decompression may be sufficient. If a leak is demonstrated or a leak suspected and the patient has evidence of peritonitis and is not improving, then exploratory laparotomy is recommended with oversewing of the area of perforation. If the area is too inflamed to close or if distal obstruction is present, a gastric resection and gastrojejunostomy is usually needed.

2. **Delayed gastric emptying**

a. **Cause and prevention:** This complication is more common after truncal and selective vagotomy, particularly if a drainage procedure is not performed. If inadvertent truncal vagotomy is performed during HSV (for example, by injury to the main nerves of Latarjet), gastric stasis may also occur. Loss of parasympathetic innervation to the antrum disrupts normal pyloric function. This can be prevented by performing a drainage procedure with truncal and selective vagotomy or by performing the preferred highly selective vagotomy, with care to avoid injury to nerves of Latarjet.

b. **Recognition and management:** The patient complains of fullness, bloating, nausea, or vomiting. An upper gastrointestinal barium series usually shows a large stomach with little or no emptying. This is best managed by nasogastric decompressions and parenteral nutrition for several days and restudying the stomach with another barium series. Prokinetic agents such a Propulsid (Jansseu Pharmaceutica, Inc., Titusville, NJ) and other drugs such as erythromycin may also be effective. If the patient does not empty the stomach well and chronic problems persist, endoscopic balloon dilatation of the pylorus or surgical drainage procedure (pyloroplasty or gastrojejunostomy) may be required.

F. Selected References

Katkhouda N, Mouiel J. A new technique of surgical treatment of chronic duodenal ulcer without laparotomy by videocoelioscopy. Am J Surg 1991;161:361–364.

Laws HL, Naughton MJ, McKernan JB. Thoracoscopic vagectomy for recurrent peptic ulcer disease. Surg Laparosc Endosc 1992;2:24–28.

Legrand M, Detroz B, Honore P, Jacquet N. Laparoscopic highly selective vagotomy. Surg Endosc 1992;6:90.

20. Laparoscopic Plication of Perforated Ulcer

Thomas R. Gadacz, M.D.

A. Indications

Laparoscopic plication of perforated ulcer is indicated in patients with a suspected or confirmed duodenal ulcer when laparoscopic access to the perforation is possible. It is an alternative to the standard open Graham patch plication, and is appropriate whenever this procedure would be considered.

B. Patient Position and Room Setup

Laparoscopic exposure for treatment of a perforated duodenal ulcer is analogous to that used for laparoscopic cholecystectomy. Some surgeons prefer to stand between the legs of the patient for all upper abdominal laparoscopic procedures. (See Chapters 18 and 19 for additional positioning information.)

C. Cannula Position and Choice of Laparoscope

The cannula position and laparoscope are the same as described for laparoscopic vagotomy (see Chapter 19).

D. Performing the Laparoscopic Plication

1. Perfom a careful, thorough exploration and lavage the abdominal cavity. If the liver has sealed the perforation, leave this seal undisturbed until the remainder of the abdomen has been explored and lavaged. This minimizes contamination.
2. Pass a dissecting instrument into the right cannula and a Babcock instrument in the left cannula and irrigate any fibrin away to expose the site of perforation.
3. If the liver is adherent to the site of perforation, a fan-type retractor passed through an additional trocar may be necessary.
4. Assess the size, location, and probable cause of perforation. Large perforations, particularly those for which all borders cannot be clearly

identified (for example, large duodenal perforations that extend onto the back wall of the duodenum) are difficult to plicate. Always consider the possibility of gastric malignancy or gastric lymphoma if the perforation is on the stomach. Exercise good judgment and convert to an open surgical procedure if the situation is not conducive to simple Graham patch closure (Fig. 20.1).

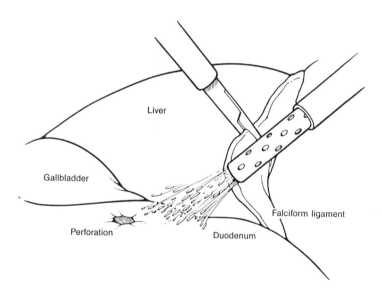

Figure 20.1. Exposure of a typical perforated duodenal ulcer using the suction irrigator to wash away fibrin.

5. Close the perforation with three or four sutures placed 8 to 10 mm from the edge of the perforation.
6. Tie these sutures as they are placed.
7. Place omentum over the plication, if possible. The author prefers to close the perforation first and then overlay omentum, rather than placing omentum in the perforation (Fig. 20.2).
8. Irrigate the area with saline to dilute and remove as much of the gastric contents as possible.

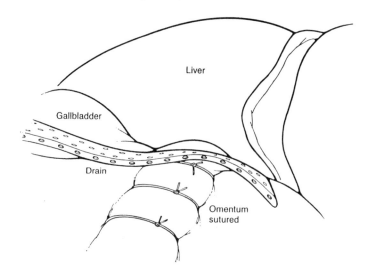

Figure 20.2. Completed plication buttressed with omentum. A drain may be placed if desired.

E. Complications

1. In general, the complications of laparoscopic plication are similar to those previously described for laparoscopic gastrostomy and vagotomy (Chapters 18 and 19) and recognition, prevention, and management are similar.
2. Additional problems with this procedure are incorrect diagnosis (which can be avoided if the laparoscopist is scrupulously careful to visualize the site of perforation), recurrent ulcer (which is likely to occur in 30% if treatment of the underlying ulcer diathesis is not followed), and inadvertent plication of a malignancy or lymphoma. These complications can be avoided by exercising good surgical judgment and converting to formal laparotomy if the diagnosis is unclear or plication does not appear feasible.
3. Gastric outlet obstruction may result if the plicating sutures are placed too deep, or if the ulcer has produced significant pyloric stenosis.

F. Selected Reference

Mouret P, Francois Y, Vignal J, Barth X, Lombard-Platet R. Laparoscopic treatment of perforated peptic ulcer. Br J Surg 1990;77:1006.

21. Gastric Resections

Sir Alfred Cuschieri MD ChM FRCS

A. Indications for Laparoscopic Gastric Surgery

The indications for laparoscopic gastrectomy (in the author's practice) are:

1. **Intractable peptic ulceration** that fails to heal on medical treatment. Successful medical management (including treatment for *Helicobacter pylori*) has made this a rare indication. In the author's experience, the peptic ulcers that require resection are prepyloric ulcers (antectomy and truncal vagotomy) and gastric ulcers.

2. **Smooth muscle tumors of the stomach** (leiomyomas and leimyosarcomas): These usually present with bleeding, less often perforation. The distinction between benign and malignant is size dependent and can be difficult even on pathologic examination.

3. **Some gastric cancers**: Case selection is important here, and the indications are still evolving. Early gastric cancer not involving the submucosa may be suitable for laparoscopic or endoluminal local resection. Early gastric cancer involving the submucosa requires gastrectomy with removal of greater omentum and level 1 lymph nodes. This can be performed safely laparoscopically. Advanced gastric cancer (involving the muscularis propria, T2 and T3) requires a more extensive regional dissection with the gastrectomy. Although this can and has been performed laparoscopically, there is concern on the adequacy of the omental bursectomy/omentectomy and node clearance by the laparoscopic approach and thus the laparoscopic approach cannot be regarded as standard practice. **Incurable (distant metastasis, peritoneal deposits) but resectable disease** is a good indication for laparoscopic palliative resection.

4. **Gastric lymphoma** (from gut-associated lymphoid tissue [GALT lymphoma]) is suitable for laparoscopic gastric resection.

5. **Polyps and other benign lesions:** These are suitable for a laparoendogastric approach.

B. Approaches

The techniques of minimal access gastric resection may be categorized as follows:

1. **Interventional flexible endoscopic approach:** suitable for superficial gastric cancer not involving the submucosa on endoluminal ultra-

sound scanning (even if caught early, tumors with significant involvement of the submucosa have a 15–20% incidence of regional node spread). These approaches include submucosal resection after adrenaline/saline instillation in the submucosal layer, and laser ablation (see Chapter 42, Diagnostic Upper Gastrointestinal Endoscopy).

2. **Laparo-endoluminal resection:** this is an alternative to the interventional flexible endoscopic approach and is suitable for small superficial lesions.

3. **Laparoscopic partial or total gastrectomy** with internal reconstruction of the upper gastrointestinal tract.

4. **Laparoscopic-assisted partial or total gastrectomy** with reconstruction through a midline 5.0 cm minilaparotomy, used for both specimen extraction and reconstruction.

C. Patient Position and Setup

Two options are available for both laparo-endoluminal gastric resection and laparoscopic gastrectomy:

1. Patient in the supine head-up tilt position with the surgeon operating from the right side of the operating table and the main video monitor facing the surgeon.

2. Patient in the supine position with head-up tilt and abduction of the lower limbs with the surgeon operating between the legs of the patient. The main monitor should go at the head of the table. This is easier and more comfortable for the surgeon but may increase calf vein compression trauma and the risk of deep venous thrombosis (DVT), especially if leg stirrups are used.

Irrespective of position, DVT prophylaxis with subcutaneous heparin and graduated compression stockings is recommended as is antibiotic prophylaxis.

D. Endoluminal Gastric Surgery

The technique described here works well for lesions on the posterior wall, fundus, and esophagogastric junction. An experienced laparoscopic surgeon and a skilled endoscopist (working at the head of the table, outside the sterile field) work together.

1. Place a laparoscope through an **umbilical port** and perform a thorough laparoscopic inspection of the peritoneal cavity and stomach.

2. The assistant then passes a flexible upper gastrointestinal endoscope with a large (3.4-mm) instrument channel and inflates the stomach. An instrument passed through this endoscope will provide additional manipulation and assistance during the surgery.

3. Choose the appropriate point for intragastric entry, usually halfway between the greater and lesser curvature in the proximal half of the stomach (Fig. 21.1). The exact site is dictated by the topography of

the intragastric lesion. After evaluating various types of trocar/cannulae systems, the author's preference is for the Innerdyne (Innerdyne, Inc., Sunnyvale, CA) system. This is ideal for endoluminal work.

a. Make a small gastric perforation with a straight electrosurgical needle in the cutting mode.

b. Place a Veress needle through the abdominal wall of the left upper quadrant and into the stomach via the small perforation.

c. Insert the nonexpanded polymer sheath over the Veress needle (Fig. 21.2).

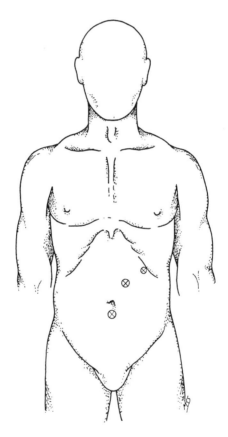

Figure 21.1. Trocar sites for endoluminal gastric surgery. The laparoscope is first placed through an umbilical port and initial inspection of the peritoneal cavity performed. The two additional left upper quadrant trocars are placed under direct vision and an operating laparoscope passed into the stomach via the 11-mm port. The 5-mm port is an additional intragastric operating port.

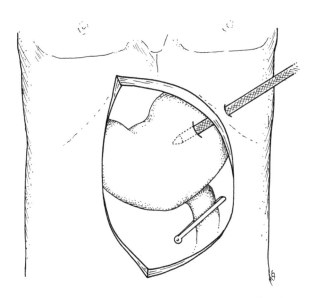

Figure 21.2. Insertion of the Innerdyne gastric cannula into inflated stomach. Thereafter, the radially expandable polymer sheath is stretched by an 11.0-mm port for intragastric insertion of the operating laparoscope.

4. Place a second 5.0-mm cannula, more lateral and cephalad than the operating laparoscope port.
5. The 'second' assisting instrument is provided by the instruments passed through the channel of the flexible endoscope, operated by a trained flexible endoscopist. The completed setup is shown in Fig. 21.3.

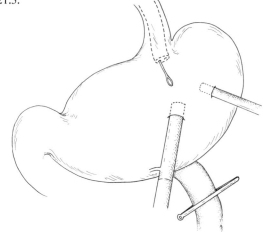

Figure 21.3. Access for endoluminal gastric surgery.

6. Surgery is then performed within the lumen of the stomach. Instruments passed through the operating channel of the laparoscope and the second port are used to elevate, resect, and suture as needed. At the conclusion of the case, instruments are withdrawn and the two holes in the stomach are closed.

E. Laparoscopic Gastric Resection

1. Place the laparoscope through an umbilical trocar. The author favors a 30-degree forward-oblique viewing laparoscope; others prefer a 0-degree laparoscope.
2. Place three additional ports as shown in Fig. 21.4.

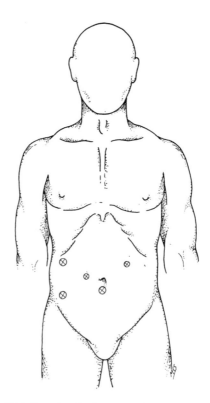

Figure 21.4. Port sites for laparoscopic gastric resections.

3. If the resection is planned for gastric cancer, first **assess resectability**. Fixation of the tumor to the pancreas and celiac axis indicates inoperability. Hepatic metastases or peritoneal deposits confirm incurability, but do not preclude palliative resection unless there is extensive involvement.

4. **Laparoscopic distal partial gastrectomy** is performed for intractable ulcer disease and for early distal gastric cancer. In the latter instance the duodenal bulb, greater omentum, and level 1 lymph nodes (lesser and greater curvature, infra- and suprapyloric nodes) are included in the resection.

    a. Begin **mobilizing the greater curvature** by proximal stapler transection of the gastroepiploic vessels. Continue the mobilization toward the duodenum.

    b. Divide adhesions between stomach and lesser sac with scissors.

    c. The author prefers to **ligate the right gastroepiploic** artery as it comes off the gastroduodenal, but some double clip this vessel before division.

    d. In cancer cases, the mobilization is different and consists of detachment of the greater omentum from the transverse colon and mesocolon until the greater curvature of the stomach is reached. This detachment requires traction of the transverse colon by an atraumatic grasper by the assistant and is performed either with electrocautery scissors or with the harmonic scalpel. The right gastroepiploic artery is secured as outlined previously.

    e. Next pass a **vascular sling** along the posterior aspect of the stomach and then through an avascular window in the lesser omentum. Use this sling to pull the stomach up and away from the lesser sac and pancreas (Fig. 21.5).

    f. Dissect and expose the **right gastric artery** from behind the stomach and secure it high up at the origin from the hepatic artery (especially in cancer cases, to ensure removal of the suprapyloric nodes). The author prefers ligature with an external slipknot but others clip the artery before division.

    g. Mobilization of the **duodenal bulb** is needed in cancer cases. Secure the paraduodenal veins and divide fibrous attachments between the first part of the duodenum and the head of the pancreas.

        i. **Billroth II:** Divide the duodenum with an endoscopic linear stapler well beyond the pylorus. Carefully inspect the staple line and reinforce it with interrupted sutures when necessary.

        ii. **Billroth I:** Maintain duodenal continuity until the stomach is ready for resection.

    h. **Ligation of the left gastric vessels in continuity.** The easiest and safest technique is to visualize the fold of the left gastric vessels as the stomach is pulled away from the retroperitoneum, and then to under-run this fold containing the vessels with a 0 suture, which is then tied intracorporeally in continuity. This completes the devascularization of the stomach.

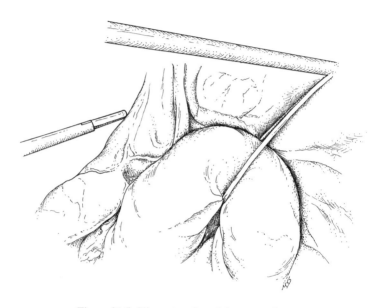

Figure 21.5. Sling retraction of the stomach.

   i.   **Gastric resection:** Select the proximal transection site. Clear the appropriate sites on the greater and lesser curves of fat and blood vessels.

      i.   **Billroth II:** Transect the stomach vertically from the greater to the lesser curvature, using the endoscopic linear stapler. Usually, three applications of the 3.0-cm endoscopic linear stapler (blue cartridge) are necessary. Remove the specimen through a protected upper midline minilaparotomy.

      ii.   **Billroth I:** Make the first application of the endoscopic stapler vertically from the lesser curvature. The second and third applications are at an angle to the first application so that the transection line reaches the lesser curvature more proximally (Fig. 21.6). Divide the duodenum just beyond the pylorus with cutting electrocautery. Remove the specimen through a small midline laparotomy.

5. **Laparoscopic total gastrectomy** (total R1 gastrectomy) is usually performed for early cancers in the middle and upper third of the stomach and for gastric lymphomas. The technique is similar to that for laparoscopic distal gastrectomy with these important differences:

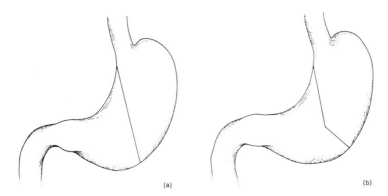

Figure 21.6. Stapler transection of proximal stomach for (a) Billroth II and (b) Billroth I gastrectomy.

a. **Mobilization of the greater curvature:** This involves detachment of the entire greater omentum from the transverse colon/mesocolon and is the most laborious part of the procedure.
   i. Apply downward traction on the transverse colon with a large atraumatic forceps. This is crucial.
   ii. Separate the greater omentum along a line extending from the right side (duodenum and hepatic flexure) to the inferior pole of the spleen and adjacent left paracolic gutter.
   iii. Transect the short gastric vessels using an endoscopic linear stapler (vascular cartridges) with preservation of the spleen.
   iv. On the right side, the right gastroepiploic vessels and the right gastric artery are ligated or clipped as described in the section on distal gastric resection.
b. **Division of lesser omentum** should be as cephalad as possible, and extends from the divided right gastric vessels up to the left gastric vessels. Some small vessels in the lesser omentum may need to be coagulated.
c. **Elevate the stomach with a vascular sling** as previously described.
d. **Hiatal dissection with mobilization of the abdominal esophagus and bilateral truncal vagotomy:**
   i. Begin this dissection on the left with division of the gastrophrenic peritoneal reflection and blunt separation of the posterior aspect of the esophagogastric junction from the left crus until the hiatal canal is entered from the left side.

      ii.   Then move to the right side, medial to the left gastric vessels with separation of the right crus from the esophagus to access the hiatal canal and mediastinum from the right side.

     iii.   Identify the plane between the posterior wall of the esophagus and the preaortic fascia and dissect bluntly behind the esophagus until the left crus is reached.

     iv.   Pass a sling around the mobilized esophagus and pull the esophagus away from the mediastinum. Complete the posterior separation of the esophagogastric junction.

     v.   Identify and divide the posterior vagus between the lower end of the right crus and the right edge of the esophagus. Similarly, identify and divide the anterior vagal trunk. Vagal division allows the surgeon to pull more of the mediastinal esophagus into the peritoneal cavity.

e. **Dissection of the celiac axis with division of the left gastric artery at its origin and division of the left gastric (coronary) vein**:

     i.   Use the sling to retract the esophagogastric junction downward and to the left, and gently depress the superior margin of the pancreas.

     ii.   Dissect carefully with scissors until the origin of the left gastric artery is identified without any doubt. The safest method of securing the left gastric artery is double ligation with external slip knots (using braided 1/0 ligatures) in continuity before the artery is divided (proximal to any lymph node mass). Other surgeons clip the artery but the author does not consider this to be safe. Often, there is insufficient space behind the artery to introduce the limb of the endoscopic linear stapler.

f. **Ligature (or clipping) of the right gastric artery:** This step is identical to that used in distal gastric resections.

g. **Duodenal mobilization and transection:** This step is identical to that used in distal gastric resections. At this stage the completely mobilized stomach (with greater omentum) is only attached to the esophagus.

h. **Proximal transection, removal of specimen and reconstruction through upper midline minilaparotomy:** After the creation of the minilaparotomy, a noncrushing clamp is placed over the esophagus, some 2.5 cm proximal to the transection site, the esophagus is divided, and the specimen removed through the protected wound.

i. **Reconstruction** after laparoscopic gastrectomy can be performed intracoporeally (by staplers, suturing, or both) or through an upper midline minilaparotomy following the completed mobilization (open). In the latter instance, the protected minilaparotomy serves as the route for extraction of the resected specimen. The author rarely performs intracorporeal reconstruction except in palliative distal gastrectomy for incurable cancer with closure of duodenal stump and an antecolic stapled gastrojejunostomy. The reason for this change in practice is the poor functional results after intracorporeal reconstruction of the upper gastrointestinal tract, with open revision for postgastric symptoms being required in 5 out of 19 patients. Open reconstruction saves time and permits a more functional anastomosis.

6. **Reconstruction after distal gastrectomy for cancer (Billroth II)** is best performed with an open Roux-en-Y anastomosis through the minilaparotomy.

7. **Reconstruction after distal gastrectomy for benign disease (Billroth I):** the author's preference is for a sutured gastroduodenostomy through a minilaparotomy.

8. **Reconstruction after total gastrectomy for cancer:** place a pursestring suture (2-0 prolene) at the cut end of the esophagus. Introduce the anvil of the circular stapler into the lumen of the esophagus and tie the purse string over the stem. A classical Hunt-Lawrence Roux-en-Y is created from the upper jejunum using established open surgical technique for this procedure. The pouch is then stapled to the esophagus in standard fashion.

F. Complications

1. **Laparo-endoluminal resections**
   a. **Bleeding** requiring transfusion occurred in one case (out of 10) in the author's experience.
   b. Other possible complications include unrecognized or delayed gastric perforation (excessive electrocutting/coagulation with collateral damage) at the site of local submucosal excision. In full-thickness local resections, suture line leakage is also possible.

2. **Laparoscopic partial or total gastrectomy**
   a. **Pneumothorax** can occur if the pleura is damaged during mobilization of the mediastinal esophagus. Carbon dioxide then insufflates into the pleural space and tension pneumothorax results. Placement of a chest tube corrects the cardiopulmonary compromise but may cause desufflation of the pneumoperitoneum through the chest drain. If this happens, intermittent occlusion of the chest drain allows completion of the operation.
   b. **Bleeding from suture line:** in our experience postoperative oozing from intracorporeally stapled gastrojejunal anastomosis is not uncommon (18%), may require transfusion, and generally stops. It is less frequent (5%) after hand-sutured anastomosis.
   c. **Anastomotic leak** results in a localized collection in the supracolic compartment with fever and leukocytosis. Drainage is required (open or percutaneous) and is often followed by an external fistula. Intravenous hyperalimentation is needed until closure of the fistula.

d. **Pancreatic injury:** this usually declares itself in the postoperative period with ileus, pain, and hyperamylasemia. The pancreatitis may be severe and necrotizing.

e. **Poor functional result** is common (25%) after intracorporeal reconstruction. The most common problems are vomiting and bile reflux.

G. Selected References

Cuschieri A. Gastric resections. In: Operative Manual of Endoscopic Surgery. Cuschieri A, Buess G, Perissat J (eds.). New York: Springer-Verlag, 1993

Goh PMY, Alpont A, Mak K, Kum CK. Early international results of laparoscopic gastrectomy. Surg Endosc 1997;11:650–652.

Goh P. Laparoscopic Billroth II gastrectomy. Semin Laparosc Surg 1994;1:171-181.

Kitano S, Iso Y, Moriyama M, Sugimacki K. Laparoscopic assisted Billroth I gastrectomy. Surg Laparosc Endosc 1994;4:146–148.

Lorente J. Laparoscopic gastric resection for gastric leiomyoma. Surg Endosc 1994;8:887–889.

Uyama I, Pgiwara H, Takahara T, Kato Y, Kikuchi K, Iida S. Laparoscopic and minilaparotomy Billroth I gastrectomy for gastric ulcer using an abdominal wall-lifting method. J Laparoendosc Surg 1994;4:441–445.

22. Laparoscopic Bariatric Surgery

James W. Maher, M.D., F.A.C.S.
Cornelius Doherty, M.D., F.A.C.S.

A. Introduction

The 1991 National Institutes of Health Consensus Conference on Surgery for Severe Obesity concluded that vertical banded gastroplasty (VBG) and Roux-en-Y gastric bypass (RGB) were both safe and effective therapies in producing sustained weight loss. The advantages of adapting minimally invasive surgical techniques to surgery for severe obesity are many; however, the technical challenges in severely obese individuals are formidable. Increased resting intra-abdominal pressure, difficulty in establishing adequate working space, inability to work with standard length instruments, and fat deposits that obscure anatomic landmarks all contribute to the challenge. While Chapter 10.1, Massive Obesity, gives some technical advice for performing laparoscopic surgery in the morbidly obese patient, laparoscopic surgery for severe obesity is currently in the developmental stages and will undoubtedly evolve further as problems are recognized and solved.

At present, laparoscopic surgery for severe obesity is limited to three operations: laparoscopic VBG, laparoscopic RGB, and the laparoscopic adjustable gastric band. The laparoscopic gastric band is an investigational device and will not be addressed in this chapter. None of these operations has published long-term results, and it is not justified to assume that the results of these laparoscopic adaptations will be similar to the results of open surgery until long-term follow-up is published in peer-reviewed journals. The technique of laparoscopic VBG and RGB will be briefly described, as they are currently performed in bariatric surgery centers. These procedures are presently investigative. The instrumentation for laparoscopic bariatric surgery needs improvement. The complication rates and efficacy of these procedures awaits the accumulation of prospective data by experienced bariatric surgeons.

B. Technique of Laparoscopic Vertical Banded Gastroplasty

1. Five trocars are used:
   a. Right subcostal
   b. Left subcostal
   c. Left upper quadrant, just to the left of xiphoid
   d. Right upper quadrant, just to right of linea alba

e.   Midline, approximately one third of the distance from umbilicus to xiphoid

2.   Place a liver retractor through the right subcostal port. Expose the esophageal hiatus and the esophagogastric junction.

3.   Place the patient in reverse Trendelenburg position to allow gravity to aid in retraction of the fatty omentum from the left upper quadrant. Retract the omentum downward with forceps introduced through the left subcostal port.

4.   Begin the dissection by opening the gastrophrenic ligament at the angle of His. Bluntly dissect the fundus downward.

5.   Open the gastrohepatic ligament at the bare area near the caudate lobe of the liver and obtain access to the lesser sac.

6.   Beginning immediately below the left gastric vessels, create a tunnel behind the stomach, through the lesser sac, to communicate with the opening in the gastrophrenic ligament.

7.   Mark a spot on the anterior gastric wall 4 cm down from the angle of His and 3 cm from the lesser curvature, using electrocautery. This point will be the center of the window through the anterior and posterior walls of the stomach.

8.   Make an opening in the gastrohepatic ligament 4 cm down from the esophagogastric junction at the lesser curvature, medial to the nerve of Latarjet. Secure the dissected tract for later identification using a polypropylene mesh band 7.5 cm long and 1.5 cm wide.

9.   Replace the left upper quadrant port with a 33-mm port. Pass a straight Keith needle attached to a heavy suture through both anterior and posterior stomach at the site previously marked for the center of the circular staple line. Thread the portion of the suture posterior to the stomach through the hole in the conical end of the shaft of the stapler. This is then used to deliver the 25 mm wide anvil of the circular stapler into the peritoneal cavity.

10. Hold the anvil with a modified Allis clamp entering through the midline port. Use a Babcock forceps, introduced through the right upper quadrant port, to elevate the stomach for better visualization and access to the lesser sac.

11. Push the plastic trocar with the attached anvil through both gastric walls to exit through the previously marked spot on the anterior surface of the stomach using the attached suture to ensure passage of the shaft at the correct point (Fig. 22.1). Secure the shaft of the anvil, at the point where it penetrates the anterior gastric wall, with a modified Allis clamp. Remove the plastic trocar from the anvil.

12. Pass the circular stapler into the abdomen through the left upper quadrant port and mate it with the anvil.

13. Have the anesthesiologist pass a 9-mm bougie through the mouth into the stomach. Direct this bougie along the lesser curvature to secure the outlet channel before firing the circular stapler.

14. Withdraw the circular stapler and inspect the window. Ligate any bleeding vessels with absorbable sutures.

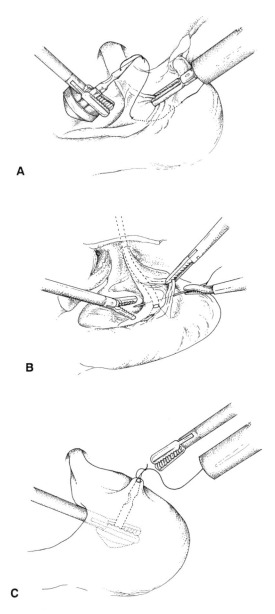

Figure 22.1. A. A Keith needle with attached suture is passed through the anterior and posterior stomach walls at the previously marked spots. B. The anvil of the circular stapling device is passed behind the stomach and guided into position using the suture. C. The suture is pulled through the stomach and the anvil follows the path of the suture.

15. Replace the 10-mm left subcostal port with an 18-mm port for delivery of the 60-mm noncutting linear stapler. Introduce a Babcock forceps through the midline port and direct it through the circular window, lesser sac, and angle of His to define the tract for passage of the linear stapler. The jaws of the linear stapler must extend beyond the stomach at the angle of His. The vertical partition must be at the angle of His and include minimal fundus. This prevents pouch dilatation and reflux. Fire the stapler to create a partition of four rows of staples.

16. Suture the polypropylene mesh band to itself with three nonabsorbable 2-0 sutures. Trim any excess band. The outlet stoma should be 11 mm in diameter. Cover the band with omentum to prevent adhesions to the underside of the liver, which can obstruct the outlet channel (Fig. 22.2).

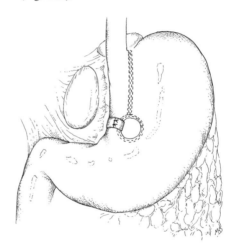

Figure 22.2. Completed vertical banded gastroplasty.

C. Laparoscopic Vertical Roux-en-Y Gastric Bypass

Gastric bypass introduces the variable of malabsorption to the concept of solid food restriction. **Advantages** of this procedure over vertical banded gastroplasty include a 10–20% greater sustained weight loss, increased cosmetic benefit, and less difficult in eating solid food. The **disadvantages** include a higher mortality, interference with absorption of iron, calcium, and vitamin B_{12} (imposing a lifelong requirement that these essential nutrients be supplemented), difficult accessibility for radiographic and endoscopic examinations, and an increased lifelong risk of peptic ulceration and closed segment bowel obstruction.

Performance criteria include a 15- to 30-ml pouch along the lesser curvature with inclusion of minimal fundus, a Roux limb 40 to 60 cm long, and a gastrojejunostomy stoma diameter of 8 to 10 mm.

1. Place trocars and begin the dissection by opening the gastrophrenic ligament at the angle of His and dissecting the fundus downward in the manner previously described for VBG.

2. Pass a Baker tube into the stomach and evacuate the stomach. Inflate the balloon with 15 ml of air. Pull the balloon back against the esophageal hiatus.

3. Create an opening through the gastrohepatic omentum at the lesser curvature, medial to the nerves of Latarjet, 5 cm down from the cardioesophageal junction. The assistant should elevate the stomach to facilitate this maneuver.

4. Transect the stomach with a series of applications of the EndoPath ELC 60-mm linear stapler directed cephalad to form a curvilinear staple line. Prior to transecting the stomach at the angle of His, remove the Baker tube and pass perorally a 27 Fr Maloney dilator to maintain the patency of the cardioesophageal junction. The vertical pouch should be sufficiently large to accommodate the anvil of the Stealth 21-mm circular stapler.

5. Change the operating table to Trendelenburg position to retract the transverse colon and greater omentum toward the upper abdomen. Identify the proximal jejunum at the ligament of Treitz and transect it at a distance 12 cm distal to the ligament (with the ELC 60). Mark the proximal end with clips for easy identification.

6. Make an anastomosis between the proximal duodenal limb and the enteral limb approximately 40 cm distal to the planned gastrojejunostomy with two applications of the ELC 35 linear stapler. Close the stapler defect with the ELC 60.

7. Create an opening in an avascular portion of the transverse mesocolon just anterior to the ligament of Treitz and slightly to the right, thus entering the lesser sac. Pass an Articulating Dissector (Automated Medical Products, New York, NY), loaded with a 6″ silicone drain, behind the colon and stomach into the lesser sac.

8. Suture the distal end of a Jackson-Pratt drain drain to the proximal end of the enteral limb, and use the drain to pull the small bowel through the mesocolon into the lesser sac.

9. Place a 21-mm Stealth stapler anvil into the proximal end of a specially prepared nasogastric tube. Pass the distal end of the nasogastric (NG) tube through the mouth and into the gastric pouch. When the nasogastric tube reaches the staple line of the gastric pouch, make a small gastrotomy and pull the tip of the NG tube into the abdomen. Slowly advance the NG tube out of the abdomen via one of the trocars while the anvil is guided through the oropharynx under direct vision. It is usually necessary to momentarily deflate the endotracheal tube balloon to allow the anvil to pass. Disconnect the nasogastric tube from the anvil.

10. Convert the left lateral port to a 33-mm port. Make an enterotomy in the jejunum and introduce the Stealth stapler. Maintain proper orientation of the bowel as the stapler is closed and discharged.

11. Withdraw the circular stapler and close the enterotomy with the linear stapler. Suture the anterior layer of the gastrojejunostomy with 2-0 absorbable suture to decrease tension on the stapled anastomosis. Return the small bowel below the mesocolon without excess tension (Fig. 22.3).

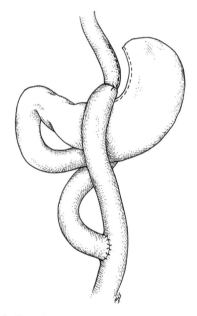

Figure 22.3. Completed Laparoscopic Roux-en-Y gastric bypass.

D. References

Henniford BT, Iannitti DA, Arca MJ, Garcia-Ruiz A, Shibuya K, Gagner M. Laparoscopic isolated gastric bypass using a transoral/transesophageal technique for a stapled anastomosis. Scientific exhibit, 83rd Annual Clinical Congress, American College of Surgeons, Chicago, Illinois, October 12–17, 1997.

Lonroth H, Dalenback J, Haglind E. Vertical banded gastroplasty by laparoscopic technique in the treatment of morbid obesity. Surg Laparosc Endosc 1996;6:102–107.

Mason EE. Gastric surgery for morbid obesity. Surg Clin North Am 1992;72:501–513.

Pories WJ, Swanson MS, MacDonald KG. Who would have thought it? An operation proves to be the most effective therapy for adult onset diabetes mellitus. Ann Surg 1995;222:339–352.

Sugerman HJ. Surgery for morbid obesity. Surgery 1993;114:865-867.

Wittgrove AC, Clark GW, Tremblay LJ. Laparoscopic gastric bypass, Roux-en-Y technique and results in 75 patients with 3–30 months' follow-up. Obesity Surg 1996;6:500–504.

23. Small Bowel Resection, Enterolysis, and Enteroenterostomy

Bruce David Schirmer, M.D., F.A.C.S.

A. Indications

Laparoscopic small bowel resection has been used for essentially all situations for which a small bowel resection might otherwise be done via celiotomy, where circumstances allow the favorable technical performance of the procedure using a laparoscopic approach. Specific indications include:
1. Inflammatory bowel disease (Crohn's disease)
2. Diverticula
3. Ischemia or gangrenous segment of bowel
4. Obstructing lesions
5. Stricture (postradiation, postischemic, etc.)
6. Neoplasms (some controversy exists due to the concern about the appropriateness of laparoscopy for maximizing oncologic principles of resection of potentially curable malignant neoplasms, as with current concerns for colon carcinoma; these concerns stem from reports of port site tumor recurrences using this approach)

Nonresectional laparoscopic small bowel procedures and their indications include **laparoscopic enterolysis** for acute small bowel obstruction, **"Second look" diagnostic laparoscopy** for possible ischemic bowel, and **laparoscopic palliative enteroenterostomy** for bypassing obstructing nonresectable tumors.

B. Patient Positioning and Room Setup

1. Position the patient supine. Tuck the arms, if possible, to create more space for surgeon and camera operator.
2. The surgeon should stand facing the lesion:
   a. on the patient's right for lesions in the patient's left abdominal cavity or those involving the proximal bowel
   b. on the patient's left for lesions in the patient's right abdominal cavity, or those involving the terminal ileum.
3. The camera operator stands on the same side as the surgeon.
4. The assistant stands on the opposite side as the surgeon.
5. Two monitors should be set up if lesion location is in doubt or there is likelihood the lesion may be manipulated from side to side within the peritoneal cavity. Monitors should be near the left shoulder and

near either the right shoulder or right hip. Under some circumstances a single monitor, placed opposite the surgeon, will suffice.

6. Follow the basic principles of laparoscopic surgery setup: the surgeon should stand in line with the view of the laparoscope, and have within comfortable reach a port for each hand. The monitor should be directly opposite the surgeon and facing the line of view of the telescope.

7. An ultrasound machine with laparoscopic probe should be available for use if a condition such as intestinal ischemia or neoplasm (requiring hepatic assessment) is encountered.

C. Trocar Position and Instrumentation

1. Place the initial trocar in the umbilical region and insert the laparoscope. See Chapters 4, Access to Abdomen, and 10.3, Previous Abdominal Surgery for tips on gaining access in the previously operated or difficult abdomen. Look at the intestine and determine whether the lesion is proximal or distal in the small bowel, and which is the best position from which to perform the resection.

2. **For distal intestinal lesions:**
    a. Place the monitor by the patient's right hip.
    b. Place additional trocars in the right upper quadrant and lower midline (10–12 mm), and left abdomen just below the level of the umbilicus and near the cecum (5 mm or larger, depending upon instruments) (Fig. 23.1A).

3. **For proximal intestinal lesions:**
    a. Place the monitor near the left shoulder.
    b. The surgeon stands near the right hip.
    c. Place large (10–12 mm) trocars in the right upper and left lower quadrants. Additional trocars are placed in the left upper quadrant and right mid abdomen, slightly above the level of the umbilicus, as needed (Fig. 23.1B).

4. An angled (30 or 45 degree) laparoscope gives the best view of the small bowel mesentery and is much preferred over a 0 degree scope.

5. Other essential equipment includes atraumatic graspers for safely handling the bowel. Laparoscopic intestinal staplers, both linear dividing [gastrointestinal anastomosis (GIA)-type] and linear closing (TA-type) greatly facilitate anastomosis. Mesenteric division may be accomplished using a combination of vascular endoscopic staplers, clips, and Roeder loops, or using the ultrasonic scalpel. The latter is also quite helpful for initial dissection of the mesentery and division of the nonmajor mesenteric vessels. Laparoscopic scissors with attachment to monopolar cautery are also useful in performing enterolysis when that is required.

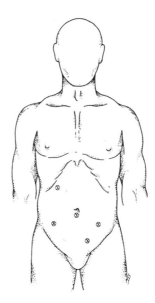

Figure 23.1. Suggested trocar placement for resection of distal small bowel lesions. Trocars #4 and 5 are per the surgeon's preference. For a more proximal lesion, move the left lower quadrant trocar to the left upper quadrant. Once again, trocars #4 and 5 are per the surgeon's preference.

D. Technique of Small Bowel Resection

Because of the potential for multifocal lesions or unsuspected disease in other segments, small bowel resection should be preceeded by a thorough exploration and visualization of the entire small bowel, where this is feasible. If preoperative studies localize a lesion well, and there are extensive adhesions which preclude "running" the entire small bowel, then this rule may not apply.

1. **Laparoscopic-assisted small bowel resection**
   a. Let gravity assist in visualizing the bowel.
      i. Use initial Trendelenburg position. Locate and grasp the transverse colon and maintain upward traction.
      ii. While maintaining upward traction, change the position to reverse Trendelenburg. The small intestine will slip down, away from the transverse colon, allowing identification of the ligament of Treitz.
   b. Run the small intestine between a pair of atraumatic bowel clamps or endoscopic Babcock clamps. Identify the segment to be resected. Lyse adhesions to surrounding loops of bowel (see Chapter 10.3, Previous Abdominal Surgery).

c. Mark and suspend the section of bowel by placing traction sutures through the mesentery just below the mesenteric side of the bowel at the proximal and distal points of intended resection.

   i. These sutures are most easily placed by using large straight needles passed through the abdominal wall, through the mesentery, and back through the same area of abdominal wall, thereby suspending the bowel near the anterior abdominal wall.

   ii. This suspends the segment of small bowel like a curtain (Fig. 23.2).

   iii. Silastic vessel loops may be used if preferred, but must be passed through trocars.

   iv. Choose the site for suspension near one of the large size trocars, which will be enlarged for extracorporeal anastomosis.

d. Score the peritoneum overlying the mesentery, on the side facing the surgeon, with scissors or ultrasonic scalpel along the line of intended resection. This outlines the V-shaped part of small bowel and mesentery that will be resected. Make the V just deep enough for the intended purpose (for example, wide mesenteric excision is appropriate when operating for cancer, but unnecessary when a resection is performed for a benign stricture).

e. Next, divide the mesentery along one vertical limb using the ultrasonic scalpel, placing additional clips or ligatures if needed to control bleeding, or for added security for large transverse crossing vessels.

f. Divide the vascular pedicle between ligatures, using the endoscopic linear stapler, or with the ultrasonic scalpel (for vessels less than 4 mm in size).

g. Divide the bowel at the site of mesenteric division using the endoscopic stapler with the intestinal size (usually 3.5 mm) staples. The end of the bowel is now free for removal through the abdominal wall.

h. Grasp the divided bowel end just proximal to the stapled division with an atraumatic grasper, for easy subsequent identification. Do the same with the distal end.

i. Enlarge the adjacent trocar site (usually to around 4 cm) to allow removal of both ends of bowel. Eliminate the pneumoperitoneum and pull the end of the segment to resected (and associated mesentery) out through the incision. Use wound protection if neoplasm is suspected (Fig. 23.3).

j. Divide the remaining portion of scored mesentery extracorporeally using a standard technique. Divide the bowel extracorporeally using an intestinal stapler.

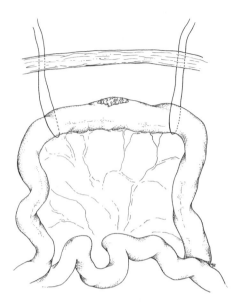

Figure 23.2. The small bowel segment chosen for resection has been suspended by traction sutures passed through the anterior abdominal wall. This facilitates subsequent dissection of mesenteric vessels and provides retraction without additional graspers or trocars.

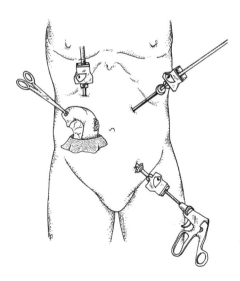

Figure 23.3. External view of exteriorized segment of small intestine prior to resection. Note wound protector.

     k.   Remore the other end of the bowel through the incision and perform an extracorporeal anastomosis with a stapler (functional end-to-end, Fig. 23.4) or by hand suturing.

     l.   Close the mesenteric defect extracorporeally (if possible) or intracorporeally after reestablishment of pneumoperitoneum (see below).

     m. Return the reanastomosed bowel to the peritoneal cavity. Close the small incision in layers, and then reestablish the pneumoperitoneum, confirm hemostasis, and inspect the bowel anastomosis. Perform any additional mesenteric suturing needed at this time.

2. **Laparoscopic small bowel resection**. The totally laparoscopic technique uses an intracorporeal anastomosis. Begin as outlined in Steps 1.a. through 1.d. above.

     a.   Divide the remaining mesentery to completely devascularize the segment to be resected.

     b.   Use a laparoscopic stapler loaded with the 3.5-mm staples to divide the bowel at the proximal and distal points of resection.

     c.   Enlarge a trocar site, using wound protection as needed, and remove the specimen. Close the trocar site and re-establish pneumoperitoneum.

     d.   Align the divided bowel ends with stay sutures placed through the antimesenteric surface of the bowel just proximal and distal to the intended anastomosis.

     e.   Cut off a corner from the staple line of each segment, then pass one limb of the endoscopic gastrointestinal stapler into each enterotomy, approximating the segments. Close the stapler and verify correct alignment.

     f.   Fire the stapler and remove it.

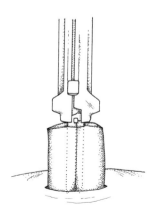

Figure 23.4. Construction of an extracorporeal stapled anastomosis using a linear endoscopic stapler. The jaws of the stapler are being advanced into small enterotomies. Traction sutures help steady the bowel in position.

g. Use the traction sutures to inspect the anastomotic staple line for bleeding. Control any bleeding sites with intracorporeally placed figure-of-8 sutures of absorbable suture material along the staple line.

h. Close the enterotomies with an endoscopic linear stapler.
    i.   Place three traction sutures (one at each end and one in the middle) to approximate the enterotomy and elevate the edges.
    ii. Place the endoscopic TA stapler just beneath the cut edges. Be careful to ensure that both edges are completely enclosed within the stapler, but avoid including excessive amounts of the bowel (which can narrow the enteroenterostomy).
    iii. Fire the stapler and remove excess tissue from the staple line using scissors.
    iv. Alternatively, the defect from the stapler may be closed using one or two layers of interrupted sutures. These sutures are best placed and tied in an intracorporeal fashion, since extracorporeal tying may place excessive tension on the suture as the knot pusher is being advanced.
    v.   A running suture line may be used as an alternative, but the surgeon must take great care to maintain the appropriate degree of tension on the suture line as subsequent sutures are placed. This also requires an intracorporeal technique.

i. Close the mesenteric defect with interrupted sutures, carefully placed in a superficial fashion (so as not to injure the blood supply).

E. Technique of Enterolysis

Enterolysis is performed for acute small bowel obstruction or as an initial step in performing any intra-abdominal laparoscopic procedure where previous adhesions preclude adequate visualization or access to abdominal organs. Each procedure is different, but here are some general rules, followed by details of the technique for enterolysis in the presence of small bowel obstruction. Additional information is given in Chapter 10.3, Previous Abdominal Surgery.

1. Use laparoscopic scissors to sharply lyse adhesions between the intestine, omentum, other viscera, and abdominal wall.
2. Use atraumatic graspers to carefully grasp the viscera or omentum, providing traction and assisting in division. Do not rely simply on traction to tear adhesions, as damage to viscera or bleeding may result.
3. The main precaution to take against visceral damage is adequate visualization of all surfaces to be cut before actual division with the scissors.
4. It may be necessary to reposition the laparoscope to begin work in an area of limited adhesions, then move into others areas as exposure is obtained.

5. **Enterolysis for acute small bowel obstruction**
    a. The usual limiting factor is bowel distention. A laparoscopic approach is feasible only if distension is not excessive.
    b. Use the Hasson technique to place the first trocar.
    c. Trace the bowel from the area of proximal distention to the transition point, identifying the site of obstruction and the distal decompressed bowel.
    d. Sometimes it is easier to work retrograde from the decompressed area. In any case, a clear transition point should be identified and freed, if possible.
    e. Finally, perform full examination of the entire small intestine if at all possible.

F. Technique of Enteroenterostomy

The performance of an enteroenterostomy essentially mimics the anastomotic portion of small bowel resection. In most cases, the anastomosis will need to be performed intracorporeally, since mobilization of both bowel segments proximal and distal to the obstructing point will usually be technically difficult. In addition, the proximal bowel is often dilated and not amenable to exteriorization through a limited size incision. The anastomosis may be performed using a stapled or a sutured technique.

1. **Stapled enteroenterostomy**
    a. Define the segments of bowel proximal and distal to the obstruction point and mobilize these sufficiently to approximate without tension.
    b. Place traction sutures to maintain alignment. Do not tie these, as bowel mobility facilitates insertion of the endoscopic linear stapler.
    c. Make an enterotomy in each segment of bowel. Suction enteric contents and contain spillage as much as possible.
    d. Insert one limb of the endoscopic linear stapler into each enterotomy. Close the stapler and verify good alignment. Fire the stapler to create the anastomosis. Inspect the inside of the staple line for hemostasis, and close the enterotomies as previously outlined.
    e. Reinforce the corners of the GIA staple line, if necessary, with seromuscular interrupted sutures placed and tied intracorporeally.

2. **Hand-sewn enteroenterostomy**
    a. Approximate the bowel as described above for stapled anastomosis.
    b. Perform a one- or two-layer anastomosis as per surgeon's preference. A standard two layer closure is feasible. All sutures should be placed and tied intracorporeally. (See Chapter 7, Principles of Tissue Approximation.)

G. Complications

1. **Anastomotic leak**
   a. **Cause and prevention:** Anastomotic leak most frequently re-
      sults from technical error, excess tension on the anastomosis, or
      poor blood supply to the anastomosis. A number of technical er-
      rors can occur:
      i.   Incomplete closure of the enterostomies with the linear sta-
           pler. This is particularly likely if the two ends of the staple
           lines are apposed in the center rather than at the end points
           (resulting in poor tissue approximation at the double staple
           site). Prevent this by always placing these two staple lines
           at the two ends of the stapled enterotomy closure.
      ii. Similar technical problems can occur if the enterostomy is
           hand-sewn and the sutures are not placed carefully.
      iii. Take care that the anastomosed ends have adequate blood
           supply and are not under tension. Evidence of ischemia
           mandates   further   resection   back   to   clearly   well-
           vascularized intestine. Excessive tension requires mobili-
           zation of additional length of bowel.
      iv. Edematous bowel is best approximated by a hand-sewn,
           rather than a stapled, anastomosis. This may require an ex-
           tracorporeal technique
   b. **Recognition and management:** Maintain a high index of suspi-
      cion. A small leak may seal and present with minimal symp-
      toms. The more classic presentation includes postoperative fe-
      ver, abdominal tenderness, and leukocytosis. Treatment is based
      on the clinical condition of the patient. Small leaks occasionally
      seal, or manifest as low volume enterocutaneous fistulae through
      an abdominal wound. Favorable conditions (absence of distal
      obstruction, intravenous antibiotics, limiting oral intakes) may
      allow the situation to resolve without surgery.

      Clinical deterioration, sepsis, persistence of the fistula, high-
      volume or proximal location of the fistula, or the presence of
      conditions likely to prevent fistula closure (such as distal obstruc-
      tion, foreign body, or neoplasm) are all indications for reoperation
      as treatment for anastomotic leak.

      In general, suture closure of the leak will not work as the tissues are
      too edematous and friable to hold suture, and there is an intense lo-
      cal inflammatory reaction. Recurrence of the fistula is the norm
      when this is the treatment. Give strong consideration to proximal
      diversion of the enteric stream (through creation of an ileostomy or
      jejunostomy), or repair plus drainage of the fistula to control any
      likely postoperative leak. The former is more definitive and hence
      greatly preferred unless precluded by condition of the intestinal tis-
      sue itself (for example, intestinal loops virtually "frozen" by severe
      intra-abdominal adhesions). Proximal diversion may require
      placement of a feeding tube for administration of an elemental

formula or even total parenteral nutrition. Occasionally bypass of the leaking anastomosis may be feasible; adequate diversion of the enteric stream should be assured by this technique to prevent likely releakage. Do not attempt to restore intestinal continuity for at least 3 months. It is prudent to wait longer if severe inflammation and adhesions were encountered at the second operation. These management principles are no different from those followed when an open small bowel resection results in leak.

2. **Anastomotic stricture**
   a. **Cause and prevention:** Anastomotic stricture is usually caused by one of three factors—technical error, ischemia, or tension on the anastomosis—probably in that order of frequency.
      i. The technical errors that most frequently result in anastomotic stricture include creation of an inadequate size opening, including the opposite side of the bowel wall in a suture (thereby effectively closing the opening at that point), turning in too much bowel wall, incorporating excess bowel wall in a staple enterotomy closure (hence narrowing the outflow), and creation of a hematoma at the anastomotic site (which may produce transient stenosis).
      ii. Prevent these errors through diligence and careful visualization of tissues as sutures are placed.
      iii. In some situations it is possible to pass a dilator through the anastomosis to prevent inadvertent inclusion of the back wall in a suture when the front walls are being approximated to complete the anastomosis.
      iv. Remember, during intracorporeal anastomosis it is not possible to palpate the anastomosis to confirm patency. Exercise vigilance and inspect the anastomosis carefully.
      v. Ischemia results from resecting excess mesentery relative to the length of bowel wall resected, or from sutures placed in the mesentery to reapproximate it or control hemorrhage.
      vi. In situations where low flow states or thromboembolic events resulted in bowel ischemia requiring resection, the potential for anastomotic ischemia postoperatively remains high due to persistence of the conditions causing thromboembolic events or low-flow status. Prevention of this low flow state is often impossible as it usually results from intrinsic cardiovascular disease and its complications.
      vii. Tension on the anastomosis will often result in leakage or complete disruption. When it does not, it may result in excessive scarring and narrowing of the anastomotic lumen.
   b. **Recognition and management:** Recognize intraoperative technical errors by vigilance and by testing the anastomosis for patency afterward (milk succus or intestinal gas across the anastomosis and observe the result). If an error is recognized, redo the anastomosis.
      i. When anastomotic strictures are recognized during the postoperative period, the severity of obstructive symptoms

dictates whether reoperation and revision of the anastomosis is indicated.

ii. Usually in this situation, a picture of mechanical postoperative bowel obstruction arises. Confirm the site with contrast studies such as barium small bowel follow-through, but take care to avoid vomiting and aspiration. Confirmation of postoperative obstruction at the anastomotic site demands reoperation and anastomotic revision.

Intestinal ischemia, if recognized at the time of the original procedure, must be addressed by further resection of ischemic intestine and performance of an anastomosis only in well-vascularized bowel if the ischemia resulted from a technical error. Ischemia from low flow mandates careful correction of the underlying hemodynamic abnormality with optimization of cardiopulmonary status to prevent recurrence. A second-look procedure should be performed 24 hours later. Depending on the severity of the condition and the potential for rethrombosis, primary anastomosis may be contraindicated and the patient better served by anastomosis at the time of second look. Alternatively, if a primary anastomosis was performed, the integrity can be assessed at the second look.

Anastomotic tension is often appreciated at the time of anastomotic construction. If present, the anastomosis should be abandoned until adequate mobilization has been performed to allow construction without tension. If tension is unrecognized and anastomotic stricture results, reoperation is indicated if obstructive symptoms of significant severity arise, since they almost always will persist or worsen.

3. **Small bowel obstruction**

   a. **Cause and prevention:** The majority of small bowel obstructions occur as a result of postoperative adhesions. There is no certain way to avoid this problem, but limiting the amount of dissection and hemorrhage intraoperatively will usually limit the extent of postoperative adhesions. On occasion, a technical error will result in obstruction, such as failure to close a mesenteric defect with resultant internal herniation of bowel and obstruction.

   b. **Recognition and management:** Bowel obstruction presents with the typical picture of nausea, vomiting, distention, and cramping abdominal pain. Radiographic confirmation is helpful. Partial small bowel obstruction, particularly in the early postoperative period, is usually successfully managed with bowel rest, decompression, and intravenous fluid support until spontaneous resolution. In cases of significant mechanical small bowel obstruction, surgical intervention is indicated. Reoperation should be done emergently if there is any concern that tissue compromise (strangulation obstruction) exists.

4. **Prolonged postoperative ileus**

   a. **Cause and prevention:** Postoperative ileus is a normal response after abdominal surgery. While its severity is often lessened using a laparoscopic approach, it nevertheless does occur, even if subtle enough to have few clinical manifestations. The etiology of postoperative ileus is unknown, as are factors that govern its usual spontaneous reversal. Postoperative ileus is particularly likely in settings of ongoing intra-abdominal sepsis and inflammation, and should raise the suspicion of a postoperative infection, particularly an anastomotic leak.

b. **Recognition and management:** The signs and symptoms of postoperative ileus typically include lack of signs of intestinal peristalsis, abdominal bloating and distention, nausea, and vomiting. The condition must be differentiated from mechanical obstruction. Treatment for ileus is nonoperative and consists of intravenous fluids and bowel rest until peristalsis begins. Prokinetic agents may, on occasion, be of some help in treatment.

5. **Hemorrhage**

a. **Cause and prevention:** Intra-abdominal hemorrhage almost always arises as a result of technical error from inadequately securing vascular structures as they are divided. Less frequently it may arise as a result of delayed trocar-site bleeding. On occasion, it results from postoperative anticoagulation. Prevention of this problem relies on careful assessment of vascular structures for hemostasis intraoperatively, and use of appropriate ligature or hemostatic measures for vascular structures. Cautery is an inadequate means of dividing significant-sized vessels. Instead, vascular staples, clips, or ligatures are required. The ultrasonically activated scissors may be used to safely divide vessels up to 3 mm in diameter; larger ones require the above measures. Trocar sites should be checked for hemostasis as the pneumoperitoneum is being decompressed and the trocars are being removed. Postoperative anticoagulation is rarely indicated for the first few days. If it is, care should be taken to administer heparin or Coumadin in conservative doses with careful monitoring of clotting parameters.

b. **Recognition and management:** A drop in hematocrit, abdominal distention, and hemodynamic instability with hypotension and tachycardia are the symptoms, either singularly or in combination, that suggest postoperative hemorrhage. An abdominal wall hematoma may also be detected for trocar-site bleeding. Management is based on the severity of the problem: hemorrhage of a significant enough quantity to cause hemodynamic instability requires reoperation, while a simple drop in hematocrit of five points may be best treated conservatively with fluids and, if necessary, transfusions. The time course is also important: the earlier the problem arises after surgery, the more likely significant-sized vessels are involved and the more urgent the need for reoperation.

Bleeding arising as a result of excessive anticoagulation should be treated by correcting the clotting factors, transfusion, and then determination if hemorrhage is ongoing. If it is not, nonoperative treatment is indicated.

6. **Inadvertent enterotomy (during enterolysis)**
   a. **Cause and prevention:** Most enterotomies result from technical errors and are more likely in the previously operated abdomen or when extensive tumor is present (for example, carcinomatosis). Prevention involves careful sharp dissection in the proper plane. When extremely difficult dissection is encountered, consider converting to open laparotomy.
   b. **Recognition and management:** Usually a full-thickness enterotomy is recognized at the time of surgery. Sutured repair is immediately indicated. When tissue quality precludes adequate repair and closure, a diverting ostomy or tube drainage via the site to create a controlled fistula may be the only options. When partial-thickness violation of the bowel wall has occurred but an enterotomy has not been done, attempt to ascertain the likelihood of the injured area converting to a full-thickness injury in the postoperative period. Many partial-thickness injures require suture reinforcement. Small deserosalized segments usually do not require such repair, and overzealous reinforcement of such areas may do more harm than good. This is no different than the open situation, but the laparoscopic surgeon may have greater difficulty judging the degree of injury. Delayed recognition of an enterotomy (in the postoperative period) is treated in the same manner as an anastomotic leak.

H. Selected References

Adams S, Wilson T, Brown AR. Laparoscopic management of acute small bowel obstruction. Aust NZ J Surg 1993;63:39–41.

Duh QY. Laparoscopic procedures for small bowel disease, Baillieres Clin Gastroenterol 1993;7:833–50.

Ibrahim IM, Wolodiger F, Sussman B, et al. Laparoscopic management of acute small-bowel obstruction. Surg Endosc 1996;10:1012–5.

Lange V, Meyer G, Schardey HM, et al. Different techniques of laparoscopic end-to-end small-bowel anastomoses. Surg Endosc 1995;9:82–7.

Nehzat C, Nezhat F, Ambroze W, Pennington E. Laparoscopic repair of small bowel and colon. A report of 26 cases. Surg Endosc 1993;7:88–9.

Schlinkert RT, Sarr MG, Donohue JH, Thompson GB. General surgical laparoscopic procedures for the "nonlaparologist." Mayo Clin Proc 1995;70:1142–7.

Scoggin SD, Frazee RC, Snyder SK, et al. Laparoscopic-assisted bowel surgery. Dis Colon Rectum 1993;36:747–50.

Soper NJ, Brunt LM, Fleshman J Jr, et al. Laparoscopic small bowel resection and anastomosis. Surg Laparosc Endosc 1993;3:6–12.

Waninger J, Salm R, Imdahl A, et al. Comparison of laparoscopic handsewn suture techniques for experimental small-bowel anastomoses. Surg Laparosc Endosc 1996;6:282–9.

24. Placement of Jejunostomy Tube

Bruce David Schirmer, M.D., F.A.C.S.

A. Indications

Placement of a jejunostomy tube is indicated in situations where the proximal gastrointestinal system is unable to be used safely as a route for delivery of enteral nutrition, but intestinal function is otherwise unimpaired. Tube placement may be the sole indication for the operation, or may accompany another procedure. Where tube placement is the sole procedure, the indications include:

1. Documented gastroparesis with nutritional compromise
2. Proximal gastrointestinal obstruction precluding percutaneous gastrostomy placement
3. Specific requirements for a jejunostomy rather than a gastrostomy, such as for the delivery of L-dopa to treat Parkinson's disease (where the medication is less effective if exposed to an acid environment).

Jejunostomy tube placement may also be incorporated as part of a larger operation. Common indications for its placement regardless of using celiotomy or laparoscopic approaches include:

1. Major upper gastrointestinal reconstruction where postoperative anastomotic problem, if present, will preclude enteral feeding. Examples include esophagogastrostomy, total gastrectomy, and pancreaticoduodenectomy.
2. Operations to treat pancreatic or duodenal trauma, and severe pancreatitis.

B. Patient Positioning and Room Setup

1. Position the patient supine. Place a monitor near the patient's left shoulder.
2. The surgeon stands by the patient's right hip, with the camera operator on the same side. The assistant may stand on the opposite side.

C. Trocar Position and Instrumentation

1. Place the initial trocar in the infraumbilical region. Where jejunostomy accompanies another procedure, this may already have occurred.

2. Place a second trocar in the left lower quadrant. This must be of sufficient size to allow intracorporeal suturing (10–12 mm, or smaller depending upon instrumentation and needle size.

3. Place the final trocar in the right upper quadrant, not far from the midline, in a comfortable position for use by the surgeon's left hand (Fig. 24.1).

4. In addition to standard laparoscopic instruments, a 30-degree laparoscope, two needle holders, and a pair of atraumatic bowel graspers are needed.

5. A commercially available gastrostomy or jejunostomy kit is helpful. These consist of a Silastic catheter with an inflatable balloon, separate channels for decompression and feeding, and an outer bolster to secure it to the skin. Serial dilators and a percutaneous needle and guide wire for tube insertion via a Seldinger technique are also required using the technique described here.

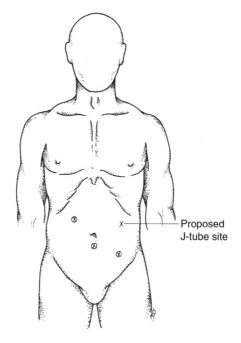

Proposed J-tube site

Figure 24.1. Trocar placement for laparoscopic jejunostomy.

D. Technique of Jejunostomy Tube Placement

1. As described in Chapter 23, initial Trendelenburg positioning with retraction of the transverse colon helps visualize the ligament of

Treitz. It is essential that clear identification of the proximal jejunum occur.

2. Once the ligament of Treitz is seen, place the patient in slight reverse Trendelenburg to allow easier tracing of the bowel and the remainder of the distal intestine to fall away. Trace the proximal jejunum to a convenient point, usually 1 to 2 feet beyond the ligament, where the bowel can be elevated to touch the left upper quadrant abdominal wall.

3. Determine the location for the tube site in the left upper quadrant (See Chapter 18, Laparoscopic Gastrostomy, for more information about tube siting.)

4. Place four anchoring sutures in a diamond configuration around this site. The author uses 3-0 nylon suture on a straight needle to pierce the abdominal wall, and a laparoscopic needle holder to then pull the needle into the abdominal cavity.

5. Take a seromuscular bite of the antimesenteric border of the intestine, in a position corresponding to the diamond configuration proposed for the suture placement (Fig. 24.2).

6. Pass the needle out through the abdominal wall adjacent to its entry site. Do not tie these sutures at this point.

7. Additional absorbable 3-0 braided sutures may be placed (and subsequently tied intracorporeally) to anchor the bowel wall to the underside of the abdominal wall and safeguard against leakage if desired.

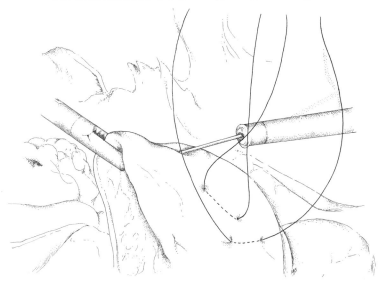

Figure 24.2. The anchoring sutures are being placed. The suture is passed through the abdominal wall, a seromuscular bite of intestine is taken, and the suture is then passed out of the abdomen. Four sutures are placed in a diamond-shaped configuration, providing both retraction and anchoring.

8. Insert the jejunostomy tube via a Seldinger technique.

   a. Pass the percutaneous needle through the abdominal wall in the center of the diamond configuration of anchoring sutures.

   b. Take care to position the bowel and advance the needle only far enough to penetrate into the lumen. Do not allow the needle to pierce the back wall.

   c. Pass the guidewire through the needle, into the lumen of the jejunum. Laparoscopic visualization of intestinal movement from wire manipulation is used to confirm the wire's position within the lumen of the bowel. Turn the bowel and inspect it to confirm that penetration or injury to the back wall has not occurred. Repositioning the laparoscope to the left lower quadrant trocar facilitates this maneuver.

   d. With the guide wire in place, enlarge the skin site with a knife and pass serial dilators percutaneously to dilate the track for the tube (Fig. 24.3). Take care to avoid excessive passage of the stiff dilators into the jejunum; posterior bowel wall perforation may result.

9. Once the largest of the dilators has been passed and withdrawn, pass the tube into the jejunum under laparoscopic vision, using the stent available in the kit (Fig. 24.4). Remove the stent.

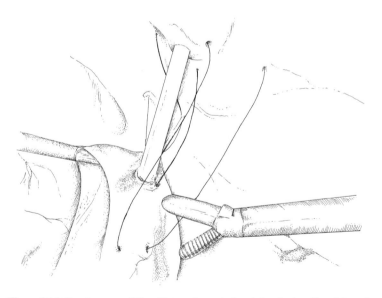

Figure 24.3. Passing one of the dilators through the abdominal wall and into the lumen of the jejunum. Care is taken to pass the dilator just into the lumen of the bowel (under visual laparoscopic control), and not so far as to risk posterior intestinal wall perforation.

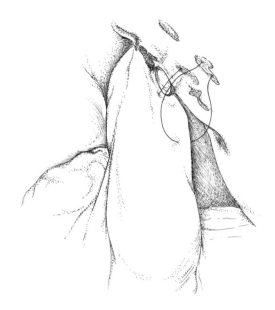

Figure 24.4. Passing the Silastic feeding jejunostomy tube into the lumen of the jejunum and tying the sutures.

10. Tie the anchoring sutures. If additional intracorporeal sutures are needed, these may be placed and tied at this point rather than earlier.
11. Inflate the balloon with 3 ml of saline. Overdistention of the balloon may cause intestinal obstruction. Position the catheter so that the balloon is snug against the abdominal wall within the lumen of the jejunum.
12. Adjust the outer bolster to the skin level and secure it with nylon skin sutures.
13. Test the catheter for ease of gravitational flow of saline into the jejunum, and observe the resulting flow into the bowel with the laparoscope. Methylene blue may be used if there is concern about leakage.
14. Secure the four anchoring sutures without excessive skin trauma by passing the needle through a small cotton dissector roll, both before entering and after exiting the abdominal wall. This roll serves as a bolster to prevent skin damage from the suture (Fig. 24.5).

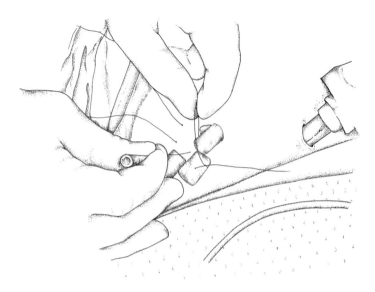

Figure 24.5. The abdominal wall upon completion of the procedure. The externals and anchoring sutures are secured to the skin.

E. Complications

1. **Intestinal perforation**
   a. **Cause and prevention:** Intestinal perforation may result if the guide wire or dilator are passed too far, injuring the back wall. Careful attention to technique as described should prevent this complication.
   b. **Recognition and management:** Intraoperative recognition is the goal; this requires careful intraoperative inspection of the posterior intestinal wall. Any injuries that are recognized need immediate suture repair and confirmation that the repair is watertight. Absence of leakage of methylene blue from the repaired site provides good reassurance that the repair is sound.
2. **Intestinal obstruction**
   a. **Cause and prevention:** The most common cause of postoperative intestinal obstruction is overinflation of the intraluminal balloon. Do not use more than 3 (or at most 4) ml of saline to prevent this problem.
   b. **Recognition and management:** Maintain a high index of suspicion for this problem. Balloon deflation is both diagnostic and therapeutic.

3. **Leakage from balloon site**
   a. **Cause and prevention:** The most likely causes are inadequate fixation of the bowel to the abdominal wall or an unrecognized perforation. Prevention is through careful technique.
   b. **Recognition and management:** A high index of suspicion for this problem should occur when signs and symptoms of peritonitis result postoperatively. A water-soluble contrast study through the tube is indicated to help determine if a leak is present. If the study is negative and strong suspicion still exists that the tube is the source of the peritonitis, reexploration is indicated.

      If a tube site leak is identified, it must be repaired operatively with sutures or even reconstruction if needed. On occasion, the leak may result from balloon deflation, and balloon reinflation to the appropriate size should be performed and the contrast study repeated to determine if the leak has been corrected.

4. **Dislodgment of catheter**
   a. **Cause and prevention:** Most often this results when a disoriented patient pulls on the tube. When the patient's condition predisposes to such action, protect all but the very end of the tube under an occlusive dressing or abdominal binder. Make connections to external feeding or drainage tubes **loose** so that a pull on the tube results in disruption of the external connection rather than tube dislodgment. Careful intraoperative securing of the tube and postoperative protective dressing should prevent this problem.
   b. **Recognition and management:** Recognition is usually obvious clinically. Management depends on the time course after surgery and after tube dislodgment. In all cases, an attempt to replace the tube into the intestinal lumen should be made immediately. If this is felt to be successful, radiographic confirmation of correct tube positioning and absence of tube site leak is mandatory in the first 10 days after surgery or if question as to tube position remains at any time thereafter. If the tube cannot be replaced, and the patient is less than 10 days from tube placement, emergent reoperation for tube replacement and to prevent potential intraperitoneal contamination is indicated. If the tube has been in place for more than 10 days, elective reoperation to replace it may be performed.

F. Selected References

Duh QY, Senokozlieff-Englehart AL, Siperstein AE, et al. Prospective evaluation of the safety and efficacy of laparoscopic jejunostomy. West J Med 1995;162:117–22.

Edelman DS, Unger SW. Laparoscopic gastrostomy and jejunostomy: review of 22 cases. Surg Laparosc Endosc 1994;4:297–300.

Hotokezaka M, Adams RB, Miller AD, et al. Laparoscopic percutaneous jejunostomy for long term enteral access. Surg Endosc 1996;10:1008–11.

Murayama KM, Johnson TJ, Thompson JS. Laparoscopic gastrostomy and jejunostomy are safe and effective for obtaining enteral access. Am J Surg 1996;172:591–4.

Saiz AA, Willis IH, Alvarado A, Sivina M. Laparoscopic feeding jejunostomy: a new technique. J Laparoendosc Surg 1995;5:241–4.

Sangster W, Swanstrom L. Laparoscopic-guided feeding jejunostomy. Surg Endosc 1993;7:308–10.

25. Laparoscopic Appendectomy

Keith N. Apelgren, M.D.

A. Indications

1. Laparoscopic appendectomy is indicated when acute appendicitis is suspected. It is especially helpful in the obese patient, in young women, or when the diagnosis is in doubt.
2. Laparoscopic removal of the normal appendix is indicated if the indication for the procedure was right lower quadrant pain.
3. Incidental laparoscopic appendectomy (i.e., as part of laparoscopic cholecystectomy) is not generally indicated.

B. Patient Position and Room Setup

1. Position the patient supine.
2. Some surgeons prefer to use the lithotomy position in women. This allows access to the perineum so that a cervical manipulator may be used to elevate and provide better visualization of the pelvic organs.
3. Tuck the patient's arms at the sides. This is **extremely important** to allow sufficient room for the assistant and camera operator to move cephalad as required.
4. The surgeon stands on the patient's left side.
5. Place the monitors at the patient's hip on the right and left.

C. Trocar Position and Choice of Laparoscope

1. Place the initial 10-mm trocar at the umbilicus. Use a 0-degree telescope for visualization.
2. Place the second 5-mm trocar in the right upper quadrant. (RUQ) to accommodate a grasping instrument. A 10-mm trocar may be needed to accommodate an endoscopic Babcock clamp. This trocar must be placed far enough from the appendix to allow sufficient working distance. Occasionally it will need to be placed in the right mid-abdomen or even right lower quadrant.
3. The third trocar is usually a 12-mm trocar inserted in the left lower quadrant, if the endoscopic linear stapler is to be used, or a 5- or 10-mm trocar if clips or ultrasonic scalpel will be employed. Place this trocar lateral to the rectus muscle to avoid injury to the inferior epi-

gastric vessels. Placement in the midline suprapubic area may not allow enough working space for the endoscopic stapler.

4. A fourth trocar may be necessary to assist in grasping or dissecting the appendix (Fig. 25.1).

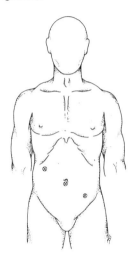

Figure 25.1. Trocar placement for laparoscopic appendectomy. The laparoscope is inserted through an umbilical port. A second trocar (5 or 10 mm) is placed in the right upper quadrant and used to elevate the appendix. The third trocar is the working port and should be placed on the left side, beyond the border of the rectus muscle. Placement through the rectus muscle risks injury to the inferior epigastric vessels with subsequent bleeding, and should be avoided.

D. Performing the Appendectomy

1. Place the patient in steep Trendelenburg position to allow the intestines to slide out of the pelvis and perform a thorough exploration to confirm the diagnosis.
2. If the appendix is normal, seek other sources for abdominal pain. If no other source is found, it is reasonable to proceed with appendectomy. In many cases a fecalith or other evidence of pathology will be found.
3. Identify the appendix by blunt dissection at the base of the cecum. Elevate the cecum or terminal ileum with an endoscopic Babcock clamp, placed through the RUQ trocar. Generally the base of the appendix will come into view first.
4. Grasp the appendix with an atraumatic grasper or Babcock clamp placed through the RUQ trocar. An extremely inflamed appendix may be lassoed with a pretied suture ligature, which provides a handy way to elevate it with minimal trauma (Fig. 25.2).

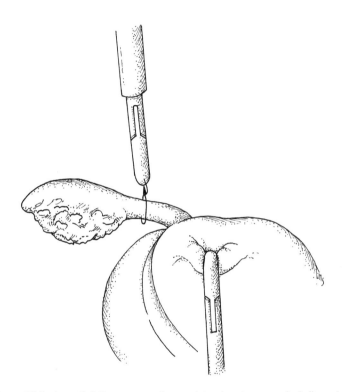

Figure 25.2. A pretied ligature may be used to elevate a grossly inflamed appendix with minimal trauma.

5. Depending upon how the appendix presents, it may be simplest to divide the base before the mesentery. In general, dividing the mesentery first provides the greatest assurance that the dissection of the appendix is carried all the way to the base.
6. Divide the mesoappendix serially with clips, cautery, ultrasonic scalpel, or endoscopic stapler (Fig. 25.3).

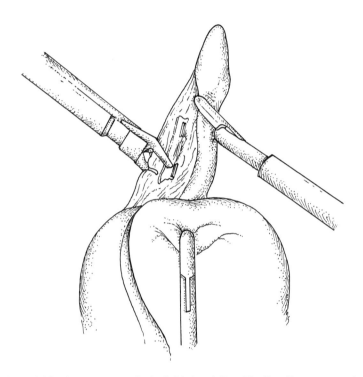

Figure 25.3. The mesoappendix is divided serially with clips, ligatures, or other hemostatic devices. Both the endoscopic stapler and the ultrasonic scalpel may also be used for this purpose.

7.   Divide the base of the appendix. Ligatures or the endoscopic stapling device may be used (Fig. 25.4). The endoscopic stapling device saves time but is more costly than using two pretied sutures. If the appendix is normal, both the appendiceal base and mesoappendix may be divided by a single application of the stapler.

8.   Remove the appendix by pulling it into the 12-mm trocar and removing trocar and appendix together, thus protecting the abdominal wall from contamination. An extremely bulky or contaminated appendix may be placed in a specimen bag to facilitate removal (see Chapter 8, Principles of Specimen Removal).

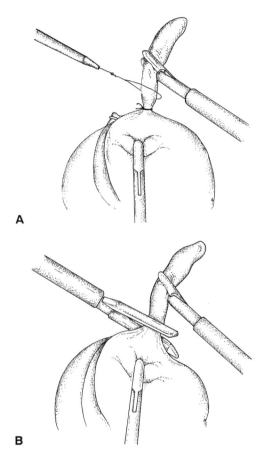

A

B

Figure 25.4. A. Division of the appendiceal base using pretied sutures. B. Division of the base using the endoscopic stapling device.

E. Complications

1. **Bleeding**
   a. **Cause and prevention:** Aggressive dissection of the mesoappendix may lead to troublesome bleeding. Likewise, bleeding from omental vessels or the retroperitoneum may occur as the inflamed appendix is dissected out. Careful dissection with early control of the mesoappendix with minimal dissection should prevent this complication.

    b. **Recognition and management:** Bleeding is not difficult to recognize. Suction, adequate lighting, and pressure will aid in identifying the bleeding site. An additional trocar may be needed to allow retraction around the field or grasping of the vessel. Control with an endoloop or clip seems more certain than the application of cautery.

2. **Leakage of appendiceal pus or fecalith**
    a. **Cause and prevention:** This problem may occur in the situation of a tensely distended, but not yet perforated, inflamed appendix. Careful dissection with the use of a sterile specimen bag for extraction may prevent it.
    b. **Recognition and management:** This complication is easy to recognize and quite distressing. Irrigate the field and suction carefully after removal of the specimen. Retrieve any dropped fecaliths immediately, while still visible. It is easy for a small object like a fecalith to become lost in the pelvis or between loops of bowel. Continue antibiotic coverage for several days after surgery, at least until the patient is afebrile with a normal WBC count.

3. **Incomplete appendectomy**
    a. **Cause and prevention:** This problem, although rare, may lead to recurrent appendicitis. It is caused by ligation of the appendix too far from the cecum. It may be prevented by carefully identifying the junction of the base of the appendix with the cecum before ligating and dividing the appendix.
    b. **Recognition and management:** See above. The surgeon must be aware that a patient who has had a laparoscopic or open appendectomy may later present with signs and symptoms of appendicitis due to this complication.

F. Selected References

Apelgren KN. Laparoscopic appendectomy. In: Brooks DC, ed. Current Review of Laparoscopy. Philadelphia: Current Medicine, 1995.

Apelgren KN, Cowan BD, Metcalf AM, Scott-Connor CEH. Laparoscopic appendectomy and the management of gynecologic pathologic conditions found at laparoscopy for presumed appendicitis. Surg Clin North Am 1996;76:469–482.

Macarulla E, Vallet J, Abad JM et al. Laparoscopic versus open appendectomy: a prospective randomized trial. Surg Laparosc Endosc 1997;7:335–339.

Milne AA, Bradbury AW. Residual appendicitis following laparoscopic appendectomy. Br J Surg 1996;83:217.

Scott-Conner CEH, Hall TJ, Anglin BL et al. Laparoscopic appendectomy. Am Surg 1992;215:660–667.

Troidl H, Gaitzsch A, Winkler-Wilforth A, et al. Fehler und Gafahren bei der laparoskopischen appendektomie. Chirurg 1993,64:212–220.

26. Laparoscopic Colostomy

Anne T. Mancino, M.D., F.A.C.S.

A. Indications

1. Laparoscopic colostomy is an effective tool for management of unresectable cancer and severe perianal disease, whenever proximal fecal diversion is required. The ability to perform a thorough exploration of the rest of the abdomen, with biopsy of any suspicious areas (staging), to mobilize a loop, and to create a stoma with minimal adhesion formation makes it an attractive option for obstructing anorectal cancers (prior to neoadjuvant therapy). Laparoscopic colostomy formation is indicated in the following circumstances:
   a. Unresectable pelvic cancer
   b. Rectovaginal fistula
   c. Complex fistula-in-ano
   d. Perianal sepsis
   e. Fecal incontinence
   f. Obstructing cancers of the anus or rectum, prior to neoadjuvant therapy
2. In cases of a proximal obstruction or an immobile colon from carcinomatosis, a **laparoscopic loop ileostomy** can be formed in a similar manner, with similar advantages.

B. Patient Position and Room Setup

1. Position the patient supine on the operating table with the right arm tucked to the side. The modified lithotomy position (low stirrups) may also be used.
2. Place the patient in the Trendelenburg position and rotate the table to left side up, to move the small intestine out of the pelvis and expose the desired segment of colon.
3. The surgeon stands on the patient's right with the first assistant on the left.
4. Monitors are positioned toward the foot of the bed.
5. If an ileostomy is planned, the left arm is tucked and the surgeon stands on the patient's left.

C. Trocar Placement and Choice of a Laparoscope

1. The first trocar is placed at or just inferior to the umbilicus (Fig. 26.1). A 0-degree (straight-viewing) laparoscope is used to explore the abdomen and verify that the planned ostomy site is free of adhesions.
2. The second trocar is a 10/12-mm port placed at the planned ostomy site. This site should be identified and marked by an enterostomal therapist or surgeon prior to the procedure.
3. Further trocars can be positioned in the opposite iliac fossa lateral to the rectus muscle, in the midline suprapubic area or in the ipsilateral upper quadrant to allow for better mobilization of the bowel. If an end stoma is planned, one of these ports should be 12 mm to accommodate an endoscopic stapler. Otherwise 5-mm ports are in order.

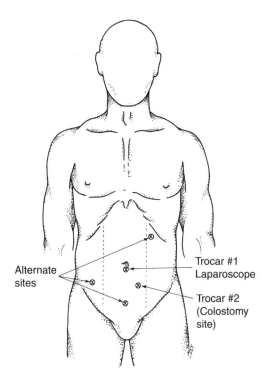

Figure 26.1. Trocar placement for colostomy. The laparoscope should be placed through trocar #1 and the site for trocar #2 inspected for suitability prior to port insertion. The other trocar sites should be used as needed to facilitate exposure and mobilization. If a loop ileostomy is planned, the port sites will be reversed in a mirror image.

D. Technique of Colostomy

1. Insert the laparoscope through the umbilical port and perform a thorough inspection of the abdominal contents and perform any needed biopsies (see Chapter 12, Elective Diagnostic Laparoscopy and Cancer Staging).

2. Assess the suitability of the predetermined stoma site and ascertain that a proximal loop of sigmoid colon will reach without tension.

3. If the site is acceptable, excise a disk of skin and subcutaneous tissue down to the anterior fascia and insert a 10/12-mm port through the center of the incision.

4. Pass an atraumatic clamp such as a Babcock into the port, grasp the sigmoid colon, and pull it toward the abdominal wall to assess mobility.

5. If there are adhesions or mesenteric attachments to the paracolic gutters, a third trocar is inserted to allow countertraction. The lateral attachments can be dissected through the left lower quadrant port using coagulating scissors.

6. Once the colon is mobilized it is again grasped with the Babcock clamp (Fig. 26.2A).

7. Back the trocar out over the clamp, withdraw the laparoscope into its trocar, and remove other instruments (with the exception of the Babcock) from the abdomen.

8. Enlarge the fascial defect to allow the colon to be exteriorized. At this point, pneumoperitoneum will be lost.

9. Construct an end colostomy by dividing the colon with a linear stapler, either extracorporeally, which is the simplest method, or under laparoscopic vision using a linear stapling device.

10. Place the distal colon back into the peritoneal cavity and fashion an end stoma in the usual manner (Fig. 26.2B).

11. If an end stoma is not desired, the loop of colon may be matured as a loop colostomy.

12. Do not fully mature the stoma at this point.

13. Reestablish pneumoperitoneum and inspect the intestine to verify:
    a. Absence of any tension or twist
    b. Adequacy of hemostasis
    c. Correct identification of proximal and distal segments

14. Remove the trocars, close the fascial defects, and mature the ostomy.

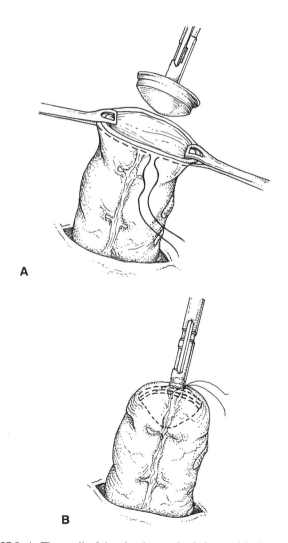

A

B

Figure 27.8. A. The anvil of the circular stapler is inserted in the proximal end of the bowel (which has been drawn out of the abdomen through an enlarged trocar site). B. The purse-string suture is tied. The bowel is then returned to the abdomen.

20. Insert a circular stapler transanally and advance it to the distal staple line. Under direct laparoscopic visual control, extend the spike of the stapler through the distal staple line. Attach the anvil (Fig. 27.9).
21. Move the laparoscope to the right or left lower quadrant port to best visualize the anvil and stapler head coming together. Once satisfied, close, fire, and remove the stapler. Inspect the two donuts for completeness.
22. Test the anastomosis by placing an atraumatic Dennis-type clamp across the bowel proximal to the anastomosis. Use the suction-irrigator to fill the pelvis with saline and immerse the anastomosis. Insufflate the rectum with air, using a bulb syringe, proctoscope, or flexible sigmoidoscope, and observe for air bubbles.
23. Irrigate the abdomen, obtain hemostasis, and close the trocar sites. Close the 33-mm port site with interrupted absorbable sutures.

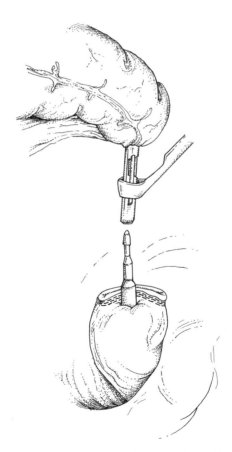

Figure 27.9. The anvil is attached to the circular stapler (which has been passed transanally) and the stapler will be closed and fired in the usual fashion.

E. Performing the Laparoscopic Anterior Resection

1. Patient position is similar to that described in section D.
2. Place the first three (10–12 mm) trocars in the supraumbilical region (laparoscope) and right upper and right lower quadrants, lateral to the rectus muscle.
3. Place a fourth (10–12 mm) trocar in the left upper quadrant lateral to the rectus muscle. This will be exchanged for a 33-mm trocar later. Additional (10–12 mm) trocars may be needed for retraction.
4. After mobilizing the left colon (see section D), grasp the rectosigmoid junction using an endoscopic Babcock clamp and retract it anteriorly toward the abdominal wall.
5. Enter the presacral plane posteriorly with ultrasonic or cautery scissors. Dissect posteriorly to well below the level of the pathology, using sharp dissection.
6. Intraoperative rigid proctoscopy is often helpful to confirm the exact level of the lesion. Mark the site with clips.
7. Continue the dissection laterally and finally anteriorly to circumferentially free the mesorectum at least 5 cm distal to the distal edge of the tumor.
8. Serially divide and ligate the mesorectum (at right angles to the rectum) with a series of clips, vascular stapler, or ultrasonically activated scissors. Bare rectum should be demonstrated circumferentially. Perform a total mesorectum excision for tumors in the lower two thirds of the rectum, to obtain adequate tumor control.
9. The remainder of the procedure is analagous to that described above for a sigmoid or left colectomy (section D).

F. Performing a Laparoscopic Abdominoperineal Resection

1. The patient position and trocar sites are as previously described, except that the third 10- to 12-mm trocar should be placed at the site of the proposed colostomy (which will have been marked by the enterostomal therapist prior to surgery). This mark will typically overlie the rectus muscle. Insert this trocar with great care to avoid laceration of the inferior epigastric vessels.
2. The initial mobilization is similar to that already described for a sigmoid colectomy, left colectomy, or anterior resection.
   a. It may not be necessary to mobilize the splenic flexure depending on the length and mobility of the sigmoid colon.
   b. The level of vascular ligation may vary based on the same considerations.

3. Choose a point at which to divide the bowel. Serially divide the mesentery at this level using ultrasonically activated scissors, ligatures, clips, or vascular stapler. At this site, the mesentery is serially divided to this level using either the ultrasonically activated scissors, vessel loops, ligaclips, or vascular stapler.

4. Transect the bowel as previously described for sigmoid and left colectomy.

5. Grasp the distal colonic staple line and retract it anteriorly or inferiorly to expose the presacral space. The presacral space is entered posteriorly using either cautery scissors or an ultrasonic scalpel.

6. Dissect the presacral space posteriorly to the level of Waldeyer's fascia. Open this fascia to expose the levator muscles.

7. Continue this dissection laterally on both sides.

8. Perform the anterior dissection last.
    a. Retract the rectum superiorly and posteriorly. In the female, retract the uterus (if present) anteriorly and inferiorly.
    b. Dissect the rectum from vagina or seminal vesicles and prostate.

9. At this point, with the rectum fully mobilized intracorporeally, the perineal dissection is made.
    a. Make an elliptical incision around the external sphincter.
    b. Deepen this incision into the ischiorectal fat to expose the levator muscles. Posteriorly, place the levator plate at the level of the tip of the coccyx. Introduce a finger into the pelvis posteriorly and visualize it with the laparoscope.
    c. Divide the levators laterally and posteriorly.
    d. Insert a ring forceps into the pelvis from below. Under laparoscopic control, the tip of the rectum/sigmoid colon is handed to the perineal operator via the ring forceps. The rectosigmoid colon is then extracted from below.
    e. Complete the remaining dissection from the perineal aspect in the usual fashion.

10. Pass an endoscopic Babcock clamp via the trocar at the stoma site, and grasp the remaining end of sigmoid colon. Excise a 2-cm disk of skin around the trocar site and enlarge the trocar site. Bring out the end of the colon as a colostomy. Mature this in the usual fashion.

11. From the perineal wound, pass an endoscopic Babcock clamp into the abdomen and guide it up retrograde through the right lower quadrant trocar site. Grasp and pull an irrigation sump catheter through the trocar site and position it just above the levators. Close the levators and perineum, and complete the operation in the usual fashion.

G. Complications

1. **Anastomotic leak**
    a. **Cause and prevention:** A well-vascularized, tension-free, circumferentially intact anastomosis is necessary to prevent such

problems. If any of the above requirements are not present during a laparoscopic-assisted colectomy, then the anastomosis must be revised. It is often prudent, if not mandatory, to convert to a laparotomy at this point. Identification of ischemia may be difficult and the aid of intravenous fluorescine should be used. One ampule of fluorescine given intravenously followed by inspection with a Wood's lamp allows for identification of ischemic bowel. Resection proximally to viable colon will alleviate this problem. Intraoperative testing of the anastomosis is mandatory as described above. Any leak requires, at minimum, reinforcement if not complete revision. The use of only a diverting stoma to protect such an anastomosis is inadequate.

b. **Recognition and management:** Postoperative fevers, prolonged ileus, elevated leukocyte counts, and abdominal pain are all hallmarks of postoperative anastomotic leak. Aggressive detection and delineation will often allow conservative therapy to be employed. Perform prompt radiologic evaluation of the anastomosis using a water-soluble contrast enema [perhaps in concert with a computed tomography (CT) scan of the abdomen and pelvis]. If a small leak or a leak associated with a localized abscess is identified, percutaneous drainage, antibiotics, bowel rest, and total parenteral nutrition often allow for spontaneous closure. If a large, free leak is identified, prompt laparotomy with stoma creation is necessary.

2. **Postoperative small bowel obstruction**

a. **Cause and prevention:** Postoperative small bowel obstruction is almost universally caused by adhesion formation. Postoperative adhesions may be less common with the laparoscopic approach. However, internal hernias or port site hernias may still occur. Closing mesenteric defects and closing all port sites of 10 mm or greater should help minimize this problem.

b. **Recognition and management:** Abdominal distention, cessation or no passage of flatus, and the inability to tolerate oral intake associated with nausea or vomiting are all common signs and symptoms of small bowel obstruction. When these symptoms occur early in the postoperative course (3–10 days), it is often difficult to distinguish a bowel obstruction from a normal postoperative ileus. Initial management is similar in both cases with nasogastric tube decompression, intravenous fluids, and possibly nutritional support. This conservative management may continue in the absence of fevers, rising white blood counts, or peritonitis (which would indicate leak, see above). Consider evaluation of the port sites via CT scan or ultrasound in any patient who develops a bowel obstruction after a laparoscopic procedure. Failure to resolve mandates reexploration (usually via laparotomy) for lysis of adhesions and possible bowel resection. If possible, the addition of an anti-adhesion product should be employed to prevent further postoperative adhesions.

H. Selected References

Bernstein MA, Dawson JW, Reissman PR, Weiss EG, et al. Is complete laparoscopic colectomy superior to laparoscopic assisted colectomy? Am Surg 1996;62:507–511.

Cohen SM, Wexner SD. Laparoscopic right hemicolectomy. In: Lezoche E, Paganini AM, Cuschieri A (eds). Minimally invasive surgery. Documento Editoriale Srl; Milan, Italy; 1994:23–26.

Darzi A, Lewis C, Menzies-Gow, Guillou PJ et al. Laparoscopic abdominoperineal excision of the rectum. Surg Endosc 1995;9:414–417.

Fine AP, Lanasa S, Gannon MP, Cline CW, et al. Laparoscopic colon surgery: report of a series. Am Surg 1995;61:412–416.

Franklin ME. Laparoscopic low anterior resection and abdominoperineal resections. Seminars Colon Rectal Surg 1994;5:258–266.

Jacobs M, Verdeja JC, Goldstein MD. Minimally invasive colon resection (laparoscopic colectomy). Surg Laparosc Endosc 1991;1:144–150.

Lacy AM, Garcia-Valdercasas JC, Delgado S, Grande L, et al. Postoperative complications of laparoscopic assisted colectomy. Surg Endosc 1997;11:119–122.

Larach SW, Salomon MC, Williamson PR, Goldstein E. Laparoscopic assisted abdominoperineal resection. Surg Laparosc Endosc 1993;3:115–118.

Ludwig KA, Milsom JW, Church JM, Fazio VW. Preliminary experience with laparoscopic intestinal surgery for Crohn's disease. Am J Surg 1996;171:52–56.

Phillips EH, Franklin M, Carroll BJ, Fallas MJ, et al. Advances in surgical technique: laparoscopic colectomy. Ann Surg 1992;216:703–707.

Quattlebaum JK, Flanders D, Usher CH. Laparoscopically assisted colectomy. Surg Laparosc Endosc 1993;3:81–86.

Reissman P, Salky BA, Pfeifer J, Edye M, et al. Laparoscopic surgery in the management of inflammatory bowel disease. Am J Surg 1996;171:47-51.

Sackier JM, Berci G, Hiatt JR, Hartunian S. Laparoscopic abdominoperineal resection of the rectum. Br J Surg 1992;1207-1208.

Tate JJT, Kwok S, Dawson JW, Lau WY, et al. Prospective comparison of laparoscopic and conventional anterior resections. Br J Surg 1993;80:1396–1398.

Zucker KA, Pitcher DE, Martin DT, Ford RS. Laparoscopic assisted colon resection. Surg Endosc 1994;8:12–18.

28. Laparoscopic-Assisted Proctocolectomy with Ileal-Pouch-Anal Anastomosis

Amanda Metcalf, M.D., F.A.C.S.

A. Indications

Laparoscopic assisted proctocolectomy with ileal-pouch anastomosis is indicated for young patients with ulcerative colitis or familial polyposis.

1. In patients with **ulcerative colitis**, the most common indication is intractible disease or carcinoma prophylaxis in patients who wish a continences preserving procedure. It is **not indicated** in the surgical management of toxic megacolon.
2. The procedure is indicated for patients with **familial polyposis**, when multiple adenomatous colonic polyps are detected on surveillance endoscopy.

B. Patient Position and Room Setup

1. Place the patient in the dorsolithotomy position, with arms extended, and legs in Allen stirrups (Allen Medical Co., Bedford Heights, OH), with minimal hip flexion, (i.e., with the upper legs almost parallel to the floor). This position allows the surgeon and assistants to manipulate instruments from between the legs with full mobility.
2. Prep and drape both the abdominal wall and perineum to allow full access to both areas.
3. The surgeon usually stands on the side opposite to the site of dissection; on the left side during mobilization of the right colon, between the legs for the transverse colon, and on the right side for the left colon.
4. The camera operator should stand adjacent to the surgeon, ensuring that the camera view of the operative field is parallel to the surgeon's view.
5. Other assistants usually stand on the opposite side of the table.
6. Place the monitors on each side, toward the head of the patient for the abdominal portions of the procedure, and then toward the feet if the pelvic dissection is performed laparoscopically.

C. Trocar Position and Choice of Laparoscope

1. Place the first trocar just inferior to the umbilicus.
2. A 30 degree angled laparoscope is useful during the majority of the procedure.
3. In general, four additional port sites will be placed, one in each quadrant of the abdomen (Fig. 28.1). The exact number and location depends upon the habitus of the patient and the location and mobility of the colon.
4. All trocar sites should be at least 10 mm in size, and those in the lower abdomen optimally should be 12 mm in size, to allow use of the Multifire Endo-GIA stapler (United States Surgical Corp., Norwalk, CT).
5. Use of a 12-mm site in all quadrants will add versatility in the application of the endostapler on all the major mesenteric pedicles.
6. Port sites are ideally placed lateral to the rectus sheath but modification of placement locations can allow one to "hide" a site in, for example, the proposed right lower quadrant ostomy site, or to the left of the midline in the anticipated site of a Pfannenstiel incision. This incision is made after full laparoscopic mobilization of the colon, for specimen delivery and construction of the ileal pouch. Threaded cannula oversleeves are useful in each port site to prevent accidental dislodgment of cannulas during manipulation.

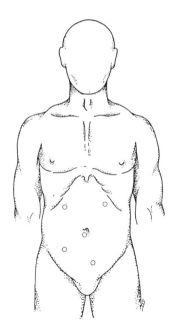

Figure 28.1. Suggested port sites for laparoscopic proctocolectomy.

D. Performing the Abdominal Colectomy

1. The dissection **begins in the right lower quadrant** and follows the colon around to the sigmoid.

2. **Mobilization of the right colon**

    a. Rotate the operating table to the left, and place the patient in the Trendelenburg position to facilitate displacement of small bowel loops from the right lower quadrant. Place the laparoscope through the infraumbilical or the left upper quadrant port.

    b. The assistant retracts the ascending colon medially using an atraumatic bowel grasper. Babcock forceps may be used instead, but tend to cause serosal tears that can convert to inadvertent enterotomies.

    c. The surgeon will generally work through the lower abdominal cannula sites, using a bowel-grasping instrument through one cannula, and the dissecting instrument through the other site (Fig. 28.2).

    d. Incise the peritoneum along the white line of Toldt using Endoshears with electrocautery or the Harmonic Scalpel (Ethicon Endosurgery, Cincinnati, OH) to minimizes bleeding, which can quickly obscure the operative field.

    e. As dissection is performed in this areolar plane, apply increasing traction to the right colon to facilitate complete dissection of even flimsy attachments.

    f. Recognize complete dissection of all attachments by clear identification of Gerota's fascia overlying the right kidney and the duodenal sweep.

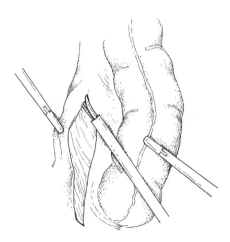

Figure 28.2. With the patient rotated to the left in steep Trendelenburg, the surgeon retracts the peritoneum laterally while the assistant retracts the right colon medially.

g. Incomplete dissection will make intracorporeal ligation of the vascular pedicles extremely difficult.

3. **Mobilization of Transverse Colon**

a. Place the patient in reverse Trendelenburg during this portion of the procedure, with traction applied in a caudad direction to either the omentum overlying the transverse colon or the transverse colon itself.

b. Stand between the patient's legs or on either side of the patient as preferred.

c. As the dissection progresses around the hepatic flexure, divide the greater omentum and expose the lesser sac with the Harmonic Scalpel (The omental vessels are too larger to be reliably controlled with cautery, and endoclips are tedious to apply to each omental vessel).

d. Retract the stomach cephalad by grasping it opposite the colonic retractor (Fig. 28.3).

e. After division of several omental vessels the defect in the omentum will allow the use of a fan-shaped retractor to either the colon or the stomach.

f. As in all portions of this procedure, application of the appropriate amount of traction and countertraction greatly facilitates the dissection.

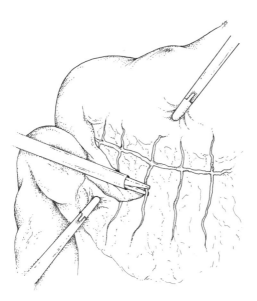

Figure 28.3. The stomach is retracted cephalad as the transverse colon is retracted caudad while the omentum is divided with the Harmonic Scalpel.

ine. Minimize the risk of this complication by clearly identificating the ureter during dissection, and convert to an open procedure if this is not possible. Recognition of a ureteral injury usually mandates conversion to an open procedure for repair.

4. **Pressure injuries**: The length of the procedure with frequent operating table position changes increases the risk of pressure injuries to the ulnar, peroneal, and brachial plexus nerves. Careful patient positioning with padding of pressure points is imperative, as is securing the patient to the table. Use sequential compression devices to minimize the incidence of deep venous thrombosis.

G. Selected References

Bruce CJ, Coller MA, Murray JJ, Schoetz DJ, Roberts PL, Rusin LC. Laparoscopic resection for diverticular disease. Dis Colon Rectum 1996;39(10 suppl):S1–10.

Franklin ME Jr, Rosenthal D, Abrego-Medina D, et al. Prospective comparison of open vs. laparoscopic colon surgery for carcinoma. Five year results. Dis Colon Rectum 1996;39(10 suppl):S35–46.

Jacobs M, Plasencia G. Laparoscopic colon surgery: some helpful hints. Int Surg 1994;79:233–234.

Jager RM, Wexner SD. Laparoscopic Colorectal Surgery New York: Churchill-Livingstone, 1996.

Liu MD, Rolandelli R, Ashley SW, Evans B, Shin M, McFadden DW. Laparoscopic surgery for inflammatory bowel disease. Am Surg 1995;61:1054–1056.

Lointier PH, Lautard M, Massoni C, Ferrier C, Dapoigny M. Laparoscopically assisted subtotal colectomy. J Laparoendosc Surg 1993;3:439–453.

Mathis CR, MacFayden BV Jr. Laparoscopic colorectal resection: a review of the current experience. Int Surg 1994;79:221–225.

29. Distal Pancreatectomy

Barry Salky, M.D., F.A.C.S.

A. Indications

1. Laparoscopic **distal pancreatectomy with splenectomy** is indicated for tumors of the tail and distal body of the pancreas. The procedure is most commonly applied to benign tumors in which the splenic vein or artery cannot be separated from the pancreatic lesion. It can also be used in palliative resection of the distal pancreas for malignant disease. Conditions in which this may be appropriate include:
   a. Cystadenoma
   b. Neuroendocrine tumors
   c. Cysts
   d. Carcinoma of the pancreatic tail
2. When the splenic vein and artery are uninvolved by the disease process, laparoscopic distal pancreatectomy **with splenic salvage** may be considered. This is more common with cysts and small cystadenomas.

B. Patient Position and Room Setup

1. Position the patient in the modified lithotomy position with both arms tucked to the side. As with other advanced upper abdominal procedures, this enhances access and facilitates a two-handed suturing and knot-tying technique.
2. The thighs must be parallel to the floor (rather than flexed at hip and knee) so as not to impede movements of the instruments.
3. If an arm needs to be out for anesthesia access, it should be the left one.
4. Place a bolster beneath the left thoracic cage to elevate the left side 15 to 20 degrees.
5. Place the camera operator to the left and the first assistant to the patient's right.
6. Place the video monitor above the head of the patient in the midline. A suitable alternative position is to place the monitor opposite the patient's left shoulder.
7. A Foley catheter is optional.

C. Trocar Position and Choice of Laparoscope

1. Place the first trocar just above and to the left of the umbilicus. This should be a 10/11-mm trocar. Use an angled laparoscope (30-45 degree) to facilitate visualization of the left upper quadrant structures.
2. Place a 5-mm trocar in the epigastric midline just below the xiphoid.
3. Place a 10/12-mm trocar in the left midclavicular line. This will be used for dissection and placement of an endoscopic linear stapler for pancreatic transection. This trocar must be low enough in the abdomen to allow the jaws of the stapler to open completely. Usually, placement at the level of the umbilicus is sufficient.
4. Place the fourth trocar in the anterior axillary line. This site will be used for retraction, suction and irrigation. Although the size of this trocar (5 versus 10/11 mm) depends upon the instrumentation, use of the larger trocar allows the laparoscope to be repositioned if needed to enhance visualization (Fig. 29.1).

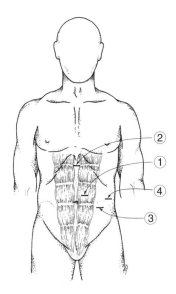

Figure 29.1. Trocar placements for distal pancreatectomy. These sites are proper for both splenic salvage and with splenectomy. There should be at least a hand's breadth distance between trocars 1, 3, and 4. The trocar for the laparoscope should be above the umbilicus, or visualization of the upper short gastric vessels and splenic attachments will be difficult. The #3 trocar must be of sufficient size for placement of the gastrointestinal anastomosis (GIA) stapler (12 mm). On occasion, replacement of the laparoscope into trocar #3 or #4 will be helpful in delineating the anatomy. Suturing and knot tying are prerequisites for advanced laparoscopic surgery. The angle of attack should be at about 90 degrees, which explains the placement of trocars #2 and #3.

D. Initial Dissection and Mobilization of Pancreas

1. First explore the abdomen for other pathology before commencing the pancreatic dissection.
2. Position the angled laparoscope to look down on the abdominal structures.
3. **Enter the lesser sac** by dividing the gastrocolic omentum.
    a. This is facilitated by superior retraction of the stomach (trocar #2) and lateral traction of the ligament (trocar #4).
    b. The operating port is trocar #3.
    c. The dissection can be accomplished with the Harmonic Scalpel (Ultracision, Ethicon Endo-Surgery, Cincinnati, OH) scissors, monopolar electrocautery, and titanium clips.
    d. It is easier to stay outside the gastroepiploic vessels.
    e. Wide mobilization of the gastrocolic omentum is required to fully visualize the pancreas.
4. Incise the posterior peritoneum at the inferior border of the pancreas. Identify the inferior mesenteric vein and avoid it. With that exception, the plane is fairly avascular.
5. Mobilize medial to lateral. Divide the splenocolic ligament and visualize the splenorenal attachments.
6. Dissect the posterior aspect of the pancreas to ascertain involvement of the splenic vein and/or artery. **The decision to remove or salvage the spleen is made now.** Each procedure will be described separately in the sections that follow.

E. Distal Pancreatectomy with Splenectomy

1. Identify the splenic artery beneath the posterior peritoneum at the superior border of the pancreas.
2. It may be advantageous to divide the short gastric vessels at this stage (Fig. 29.2). Clips or the LCS work well here. (See Chapter 31, Laparoscopic Splenectomy.)
3. Dissect the splenic artery by staying in the adventitial plane next to it. The site of division should be at the planned line of pancreatic transection. Doubly clip the and divide the artery. The author places a pretied suture ligature on the artery for extra security.
4. Bluntly dissect the posterior pancreas from the retroperitoneal tissues at the site of the previously divided splenic artery. Elevate the gland medially (trocar #2) and laterally (trocar #4) with graspers to expose the area. The splenic vein should be on the posterior aspect of the gland. This is a delicate part of the operation and hemorrhage here must be avoided.
5. Once the posterior gland is fully mobilized, the dissector should be visible at the superior border of the pancreas at the previously divided splenic artery.

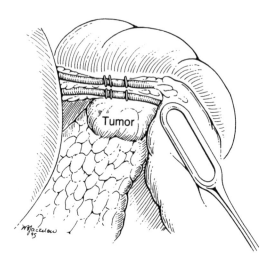

Figure 29.2. Once the lesser sac has been entered, lateral traction on the sple-nogastric attachments will allow exposure of the short gastric vessels. These can be clipped (as shown here) or divided with the LCS. Reprinted with permission from Salky BA and Edye M. Laparoscopic Pancreatectomy. Surg Clin N Am 1996; 76; 3: 539–45.

6. Pass the vascular endoscopic GIA stapler through trocar #3, and divide the gland and splenic vein as a unit (Fig. 29.3). Two applications of the stapler are usually necessary to completely transect the pancreas. The remainder of the dissection of the pancreatic tail, splenorenal ligament, and splenodiaphragmatic attachments is facilitated by the pancreatic division.
7. After the remaining attachments have been divided, remove trocar #3 and roll up a sturdy retrieval bag and insert it into the abdomen. The 5- × 7-cm Cook urological bag has worked well for the author.
8. Reinsert trocar #3 and regain pneumoperitoneum. The author prefers to insert another 5-mm trocar to hold the bag open with 3-point traction (graspers in trocars #2, 4, and 5).
9. Manipulate the specimen with a grasper inserted through trocar #3. Tilt the OR table to take advantage of gravity as the specimen is brought into the bag (see Chapter 8, Principles of Specimen Removal).
10. Thoroughly check hemostasis, irrigate, and place a closed suction drain via trocar #4. The operation is concluded in the usual fashion.

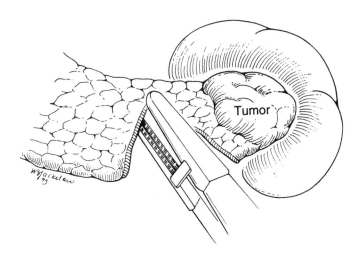

Figure 29.3. Distal pancreatectomy with splenectomy. The figure demonstrates the proper angle of approach when transecting the pancreatic body with the 30-mm GIA stapler. The posterior aspect of the pancreas must be dissected completely to allow free passage of the stapler. Include the splenic vein in the staple line, and transect pancreas and splenic vein at the site of the previously divided splenic artery. Reprinted with permission from Salky BA and Edye M. Laparoscopic Pancreatectomy. Surg Clin N Am 1996; 76; 3: 539–45.

F. Pancreatectomy with Splenic Salvage

Performing this procedure implies the benign pathology is not adherent to the splenic artery or vein. The size and location of the pathological process to the vessels determine the best approach. In general, there are multiple small vascular branches that have to be dissected. Traction and countertraction, meticulous avascular dissection, and fine working instruments are key here. Both sharp and blunt dissection techniques are employed, but sharp dissection tends to be more avascular.

1.   As the blood vessels are small, the LCS or 5-mm titanium clips are better choices for hemostasis. It is a good idea to limit the amount of electrocautery energy applied to the pancreatic tissue.
2.   Clip any identifiable pancreatic ductal branches to the main duct.
3.   As in pancreatectomy with splenectomy, trocars #2 and #3 are the operating ports with trocar #4 utilized for countertraction and suction.
4.   Hemostasis, irrigation, aspiration, and placement of a closed system suction drain via trocar #4 complete the procedure.

G. Complications

1. **Hemorrhage**
   a. **Cause and prevention:** The most common event leading to conversion to open procedure is inability to control hemorrhage. Both the splenic artery and vein are the main sources. Dissection in the proper adventitial plane and gentle laparoscopic techniques will limit this complication.
   b. **Recognition and management:** Rapid hemorrhage which cannot be controlled promptly requires laparotomy to treat. Temporary control may be obtained by exerting pressure with 10-mm instruments. This allows time to ascertain what exactly is the problem. Laparoscopic hemostatic techniques include vascular staples, titanium clips, electrocautery, LCS and suturing, and knot tying capability (Chapter 6, Principles of Laparoscopic Hemostasis).

2. **Pancreatic leak**
   a. **Cause and prevention:** Disruption of the pancreatic duct closure can lead to leakage of pancreatic juice. The enzymes in pancreatic fluid are caustic to surrounding tissue. Inspect the stump of the pancreatic remnant before closure. If necessary, suture-ligate the duct with a nonabsorbable suture.
   b. **Recognition and management:** A closed suction drain is routinely placed at the cut end of the pancreas. Check the drainage fluid for amylase on the second postoperative day, and remove the drain if the amylase level is normal. Elevation of amylase is consistent with a pancreatic leak. Management is dependent on amount of leakage and the clinical status of the patient. Barring a proximal obstruction of the pancreatic duct or a foreign body, the pancreatic leak should close. Adjunctive measures such as somatostatin analogues, total parenteral nutrition (TPN), and antibiotics may be required, depending upon the patient's clinical status.

3. **Infection**
   a. **Cause and prevention:** Pancreatic leak and hematoma formation at the surgical site in the left upper quadrant can lead to abscess formation. The incidence is around 5%. Meticulous hemostasis, closure of the pancreatic duct, gentle handling of the pancreatic gland, and minimal electrocautery usage will decrease, but not eliminate infection. There is no evidence that prophylactic antibiotics prevent infection in this setting. Most surgeons will place a closed-system suction drain at the time of surgery.
   b. **Recognition and management:** Respiratory difficulty, sepsis, pleural effusion, and left upper quadrant pain are all signs of a left subphrenic abscess, which is best confirmed by computed tomography (CT) scan. Antibiotics and percutaneous or opera-

tive drainage may be required. (See Chapter 31, Laparoscopic Splenectomy, for additional discussion of complications).

H. Suggested References

Gagner M, Ponp A. Laparoscopic pylorus-preserving pancreatoduodenectomy. Surg Endosc 1994;8:408–410.

Salky BA, Edye M. Laparoscopic pancreatectomy. Surg Clin North Am 1996;76:539–545.

30. Laparoscopic Cholecystojejunostomy and Gastrojejunostomy

Carol E.H. Scott-Conner, M.D., Ph.D.

A. Indications

1. **Laparoscopic cholecystojejunostomy** is indicated when bypass of the biliary tract is needed and the cystic duct is known to be patent. The procedure is most commonly used to palliate unresectable malignancies of the region of the ampulla of Vater. It may also be used in chronic pancreatitis. Internal stenting is an alternative procedure. Conditions in which this procedure is used include:
   a. Carcinoma of the head of the pancreas
   b. Chronic pancreatitis
   c. Other obstructive processes of the ampullary region for which no alternative treatment exists
2. **Laparoscopic gastrojejunostomy** is used alone or in conjunction with laparoscopic cholecystojejunostomy. Used alone, the procedure is indicated for bypass of distal gastric, pyloric, or duodenal obstruction, generally when the patient is not considered to be a candidate for a more definitive procedure. Such conditions include:
   a. Gastric carcinoma
   b. Severe peptic ulcer disease (often in conjunction with vagotomy)
   c. Carcinoma of the pancreas in the absence of jaundice
3. **Laparoscopic cholecystojejunostomy and gastrojejunostomy** are occasionally performed as a double-bypass procedure when both biliary and gastric diversion are indicated. This is occasionally needed in carcinoma of the ampullary region, particularly carcinoma of the pancreas.
4. These bypass procedures may be done at the time of laparoscopic exploration for resectability when unresectable gastric or pancreatic cancer is confirmed.

B. Patient Position and Room Setup

1. Position the patient supine on the operating table with arms extended.

2.   The surgeon stands at the right side of the patient. Some surgeons prefer to stand between the patient's legs, particularly if a sutured anastomosis is planned. This is a matter of individual preference.
3.   Place the monitors at the head, in positions similar to those used for laparoscopic cholecystectomy.

C. Trocar Position and Choice of Laparoscope (Fig. 30.1)

1.   Place the first trocar at or just below the umbilicus. Use an angled laparoscope (30 degree) to facilitate visualization of the anastomosis.
2.   Place a 5-mm trocar to the left of the midline, lateral to the rectus, at approximately the level of the umbilicus. Place a 10- or 12-mm trocar (use a 12-mm if a gastrojejunostomy is planned in addition to the cholecystojejunostomy) to the right of the midline, in the subcostal region but lateral to the gallbladder. The trocar on the right should be large enough (generally 10 mm, unless a smaller laparoscope is available) that the laparoscope can be passed through this port if needed. Use a long needle passed through the abdominal wall to test trocar locations and angles. These two trocars will be used for manipulation and suturing.
3.   The fourth trocar will be used for the endoscopic stapling device. It must be placed low on the right side (just above the iliac fossa). Placement of this trocar must be low enough to allow sufficient working space within the abdomen. If the trocar is placed too close to the gallbladder, it will be difficult to manipulate the stapling device (remember that the jaws must be completely out of the trocar in order to properly open the device). Take care to ensure that you are satisfied with the alignment and spatial relationships before you place this trocar. This trocar should be a 12-mm, to accommodate the stapler.

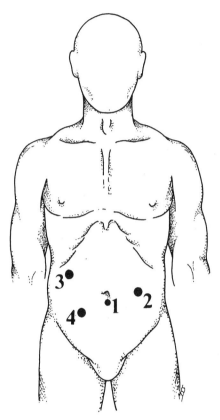

Figure 30.1. Trocar placement for cholecystojejunostomy. If you plan to do a gastrojejunostomy as well, modify the trocar placement as shown in Fig. 30.4. In each case, trocar placement must be individualized. A standard umbilical or subumbilical location for trocar #1 will place the laparoscope in a good position. Trocars #2 and #3 will be used to manipulate the bowel and gallbladder, and to place sutures. If you plan to use the endoscopic stapler to close the enterotomies, then trocar #2 must be sufficiently large (generally 12 mm) to accommodate this device. Otherwise a 5-mm trocar will suffice. Trocar #3 should be large enough to allow the laparoscope to be passed into this trocar should it become necessary to inspect the inside of the anastomosis. Trocar #4 will be used to pass the endoscopic stapling device. It must be placed low enough to allow sufficient working distance to open the jaws, and should also allow the stapler to line up with the long axis of the gallbladder, if possible. As with all advanced laparoscopic procedures, trocar placement is crucial and you should take time and explore your planned placement with a long needle, if necessary, to assure good alignment and positioning.

D. Performing the Cholecystojejunostomy

1. The simplest method is an **antecolic loop cholecystojejunostomy**, performed with the endoscopic linear stapling device. To perform this anastomosis,

    a. Identify the ligament of Treitz and run the bowel to a point at least 50 cm distal to the ligament of Treitz. The loop selected should reach comfortably to the gallbladder without tension, when passed in an antecolic fashion. Verify that the loop passes comfortably up into the right upper quadrant; if the loop does not pass easily, try selecting a more distal small bowel site (and hence farther from the ligament of Treitz).

    b. Place a stay suture on the loop of jejunum. With the same suture, take a bite of the fundus of the gallbladder. Use this stay suture to approximate the two hollow viscera in apposition. Tie the suture loosely and pass it out trocar #3. Place a second stay suture about 1 cm from the first, tie it loosely, and pass it out through trocar #2. The stab wounds will be placed between these two sutures. An alternative technique, without the use of stay sutures, may be used and is described below (see section D.2).

    c. Use electrocautery or endoscopic scissors to make two stab wounds, each large enough to accommodate one jaw of the endoscopic linear stapling device (approximately 8 mm long). Suction the bile from the gallbladder, note its color, and send for culture. The gallbladder bile should be golden. If the gallbladder bile is white (hydrops) the cystic duct is not patent and the procedure should not be performed (see Complications, below).

    d. Pass the endoscopic linear stapling device, with a 3.5-mm cartridge, from trocar #4. Place one jaw within each stab wound (Fig. 30.2). Take care to ensure that the jaws pass into the lumen of the two viscera rather than into a submucosal plane. When you are satisfied, close the stapler and fire it. Open the stapler and remove it from the region of the anastomosis. Some advocate keeping the stapler closed for 1 to 1½ minutes, feeling that this period of gentle compression facilitates hemostasis.

    e. Inspect the staple line for bleeding. Irrigate the staple line and check the color of the effluent (see Complications, below).

    f. Close the stab wounds by simple running suture (Fig. 30.3). An alternative method is to pass the endoscopic linear stapling device through the left lateral port and staple the closure.

    g. Inspect the completed anastomosis and place a closed suction drain in proximity. If there is omentum, place it in the right upper quadrant as well. Irrigate the abdomen and close in the usual fashion.

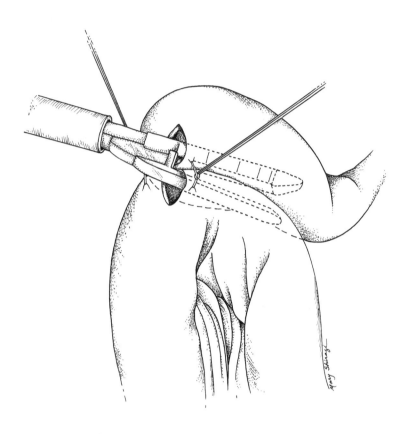

Figure 30.2. Stay sutures have been placed and tied. Two enterotomies have been made and the stapler is inserted into the two enterotomies. The bowel and gallbladder must be carefully positioned to fully utilize the entire length of the stapling device (by pulling the two viscera up into the "crotch" of the device) and to avoid catching other structures in the staple line. In this illustration the stapler is being passed through a trocar relatively high on the right side. This can only be done when the patient is large and the abdominal wall anatomy allows sufficient working distance. In smaller patients, the stapler will be passed from a trocar low in the right lower quadrant. (Reprinted with permission from Bogen GL, Mancino AT, Scott-Conner CE. Laparoscopy for staging and palliation of gastrointestinal malignancy. Surg Clin N Am 1996;76:557-69.)

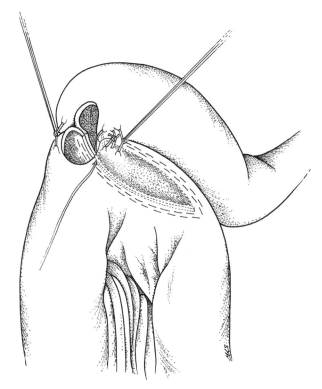

Figure 30.3. After inspecting the staple line for hemostasis, the enterotomies are closed with a running suture. (Reprinted with permission from Bogen et al. Surg Clin N Am 1996;76:557-69.)

2. **Alternate technique (no stay sutures):** Make the enterotomy in the jejunal loop first. Insert the narrow end of the linear stapler and gently close, but do not fire, the linear stapler. This will serve to hold the jejunal loop in position. Next, make an enterotomy on the gallbladder. Bring the stapler, carrying the jejunal loop, up into the right upper quadrant and open the jaws, taking care not to drop the jejunal loop. Pass the wide end of the stapler into the gallbladder. Use atraumatic graspers to position the bowel and gallbladder in the proper alignment. Close and fire the stapler.

E. Gastrojejunostomy

1. Trocar placements are similar (Fig. 30.4), with the exception that trocar #2 may be placed lower on the left side (to create sufficient working distance from the stomach).

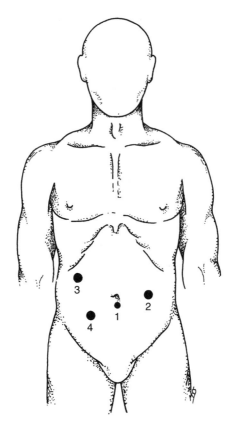

Figure 30.4. Trocar placement for gastrojejunostomy is slightly different, in that trocar #2 is placed lower, to allow adequate working distance from the stomach. If you plan to do both procedures, use this trocar arrangement (rather than that in Fig. 30.1).

2. Identify a loop of jejunum as previously described.
3. Choose a site low on the greater curvature of the stomach, but away from the tumor (if the bypass is performed for malignancy). Instillation of some air into the nasogastric (NG) tube will elevate the stomach, making it easier to identify the proper site.
4. Place two stay sutures to approximate the stomach and the jejunum. Pass these sutures out through trocars #2 and #3.
5. Make two enterotomies, pass and fire the stapling device with a 3.5 mm cartridge (Fig. 30.5). The 60-mm stapler provides an adequate lumen. If this is not available, perform a second firing of the 30-mm device, taking care to extend the stapling line directly back from the apex.

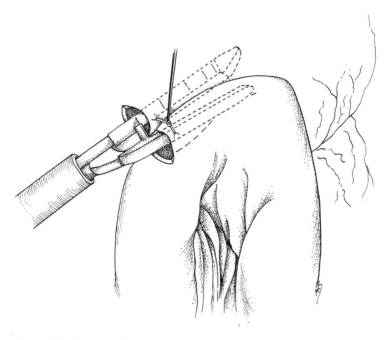

Figure 30.5. A loop of jejunum has been selected and affixed to the greater curvature of the stomach, above the gastroepiploic vessels, with two stay sutures. Two enterotomies have been made and the stapling device inserted.

6. Inspect the staple line for hemostasis. Close the enterotomies with a running suture or with the endoscopic stapler, passed through trocar #2 (Fig. 30.6). Check the anastomosis with air under saline, or by instillation of methylene blue into the NG tube.

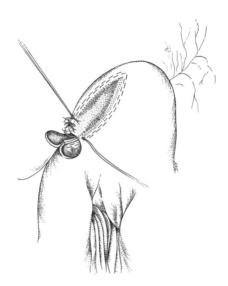

Figure 30.6. The stapler has been fired and removed. The staple line has been inspected for hemostasis and is being closed with a simple running suture.

F. Complications

1. **Leakage of the cholecystojejunostomy**
    a. **Cause and prevention:** Bile is a detergent and will go through a pinhole; hence, small leaks at biliary-enteric anastomotic sites are common. Many surgeons routinely place a closed suction drain in close proximity to a biliary-enteric anastomosis, so that any such leakage is easily recognized and controlled. The resulting bile leak usually subsides spontaneously in the absence of distal obstruction.
    b. **Recognition and management:** Bilious output from the closed suction drain should be monitored and outputs recorded. Excessive (more than 100–200 cc per day) or prolonged (more than one week) output may be a sign of distal obstruction. A radionuclide biliary scan is an easy, noninvasive way to confirm that the jejunal loop is patent. The scan will show passage of radionuclide into the distal small intestine if the loop is patent. Sequential scans over time will confirm rapid transit of bile through the gut. If the loop is obstructed or the leak is very large, the radionuclide will pass out through the drain or puddle in the right gutter and little or no activity will be seen to go into the gut.

Distal obstruction is generally mechanical in nature and requires operative correction.

If no drain has been placed, a subphrenic collection or generalized peritonitis may result. Generally this is signaled by fever or ileus, and diagnosed by CT or ultrasound. A localized collection may be amenable to percutaneous drainage. Generalized peritonitis will usually require exploration, with repair of the leak and establishment of adequate external drainage. Similar concerns about distal obstruction of the jejunal loop exist and should be kept in mind.

2. **Leakage of the gastrojejunostomy**
   a. **Cause and prevention:** To minimize the possibility of leakage, test the gastrojejunostomy by air under water, or by instillation of dilute methylene blue through the NG tube. Reinforce any areas that appear weak or are leaking.
   b. **Recognition and management:** A localized collection or generalized peritonitis may result. Fever, ileus, abdominal tenderness, and distention are symptoms. A Gastrografin upper gastrointestinal series may demonstrate the site of leakage. Revision of the anastomosis will generally be required.

3. **Bleeding from the staple line**
   a. **Cause and prevention:** All gastrointestinal stapling devices are designed to approximate tissues without strangulating or devascularizing them. The potential for bleeding always exists. The rich submucosal blood supply of the stomach makes it particularly prone to staple line bleeding. To avoid this complication, inspect the staple line carefully before closing the stab wounds. Use the suction irrigator to irrigate the staple line and carefully inspect the color and quantity of the effluent. The effluent should be clear or bilious in color.
   b. **Recognition and management:** If the effluent is persistently bloody, suspect a staple-line bleeder and place the laparoscope into the lateral port. You can then advance the laparoscope through the stab wounds to look inside. Cauterize or suture ligate any bleeding points under direct vision. Use cautery with caution to avoid thermal damage and delayed perforation.

4. **Failure of the cholecystojejunostomy to produce biliary diversion**
   a. **Cause and prevention:** Obstruction of the anastomosis by blood clot can cause recurrent jaundice. This can be avoided if hemostasis is carefully checked as noted above. An unrecognized blocked cystic duct will cause the anastomosis to fail. Avoid this complication by careful patient selection and knowledge of individual anatomy. The cystic duct enters the common duct at a variable distance from the duodenum. A cholecystojejunostomy uses the cystic duct as a conduit for bile from the common hepatic duct. If the cystic duct is not patent, or is blocked by tumor, the conduit will not function. At laparoscopy, the gallbladder should appear grossly distended (Courvoisier's sign). The cystic duct should be dilated and the gallbladder should contain bilious material. White bile (hydrops) indicates

the presence of cystic duct obstruction and is a contraindication to performing a biliary-enteric bypass.

Cholangiography is the best way to delineate biliary anatomy. If you are uncertain as to the anatomy, perform a transcystic cholangiogram by placing a needle in the gallbladder and injecting contrast. The cholangiogram should visualize the common duct.

b.   **Recognition and management:** If cholecystojejunostomy does not produce biliary diversion, or if the conduit fails as the tumor grows, stenting, transhepatic drainage, or conversion to choledochojejunostomy should be considered. Decision to employ one of these procedures should be based upon careful consideration of the anatomy and the patient's overall medical condition.

5.   **Obstruction of the jejunum at the anastomotic site**

a.   **Cause and prevention:** Problems during the construction of the anastomosis, particularly during closure of the enterotomies, can narrow the lumen of the jejunal loop or even totally obstruct it. This causes a high small bowel obstruction. Avoid this complication by taking care not to narrow the jejunal lumen, particularly if you use the stapler to close the enterotomies. Visually inspect the anastomosis after you construct it, and if it does not look right, consider revising it.

b.   **Recognition and management:** Signs of high small bowel obstruction (vomiting, inability to tolerate feeds) suggest the diagnosis, which may be confirmed by Gastrografin upper gastrointestinal series. The anastomosis must be revised or a jejunojejunostomy (to bypass the obstruction) constructed.

6.   **Distal mechanical obstruction of the jejunal loop**

a.   **Cause and prevention:** Avoid kinking by visually verifying that the chosen site allows the jejunum to lie in a comfortable and loose position as it passes over the transverse colon. Rarely, a trocar site hernia may present as small bowel obstruction.

b.   **Recognition and management:** Distal obstruction may cause the anastomosis to leak. If the anastomosis does not leak, obstructive symptoms of distention, inability to tolerate feedings, and vomiting suggest the diagnosis. The diagnosis may be confirmed by flat and upright abdominal films, HIDA scan (cholecystojejunostomy), or Gastrografin upper gastrointestinal series (gastrojejunostomy). Generally, revision of the anastomosis will be required.

G. Selected References

Bogen GL, Mancino AT. Scott-Conner CEH. Laparoscopy for staging and palliation of gastrointestinal malignancy. Surg Clin North Am 1996;76:557–569.

Cuschieri A. Laparoscopy for pancreatic cancer: Does it benefit the patient? Eur J Surg Oncol 1988;14:41–44.

Fletcher DR, Jones RM. Laparoscopic cholecystjejunostomy as palliation for obstructive jaundice in inoperable carcinoma of pancreas. Surg Endosc 1992;6:147–149.

Hawasli A. Laparoscopic cholecysto-jejunostomy for obstructive pancreatic cancer: technique and report of two cases. J Laparoendosc Surg 1992;2:351–355.

Nagy A, Brosseuk D, Hemming A, Scudamore C, Mamazza J. Laparoscopic gastroenterostomy for duodenal obstruction. Am J Surg 1995;169:539–542.

Nathanson LK. Laparoscopy and pancreatic cancer; Biopsy, staging, and bypass. Baillieres Clin Gastroenterol 1993;7:941–960.

Rangraj MS, Mehta M, Zale G, Maffucci L, Herz B. Laparoscopic gastrojejunostomy; a case presentation. J Laparoendosc Surg 1994;4:81–87.

Shimi S, Banting S, Cuschieri A. Laparoscopy in the management of pancreatic cancer: endoscopic cholecystojejunostomy for advanced disease. Br J Surg 1992;79:317–319.

Sosa JL, Zalewski M, Puente I. Laparoscopic gastrojejunostomy technique: case report. J Laparoendosc Surg 1994;4:215–220.

Targarona EM, Pera M, Martinez J, Balague C, Trias M. Laparoscopic treatment of pancreatic disorders: diagnosis and staging, palliation of cancer and treatment of pancreatic pseudocysts. Int surg 1996;81:1–5.

Wyman A, Stuart RC, Ng EK, Chung SC, Li AK. Laparoscopic truncal vagotomy and gastroenterostomy for pyloric stenosis. Am J Surg 1996;171:600–603.

31. Laparoscopic Splenectomy

Robert V. Rege, M.D.

A. Indications

1. **Laparoscopic splenectomy** is indicated in patients with hematological disorders that have not responded to medical therapy when removal of the spleen is expected to improve the patient's condition. Indications for laparoscopic splenectomy are essentially the same as for open splenectomy (Table 31.1).

Table 31.1. Disorders treated by splenectomy

Hematological disorders:
Idiopathic thrombocytopenic purpura (ITP)
AIDS-associated ITP
Hereditary spherocytosis
Idiopathic autoimmune hemolytic anemia
Felty's syndrome
Thalassemia
Sarcoidosis
Sickle cell disease
Gaucher's disease
Congenital and acquired hemolytic anemia
Thrombotic thrombocytopenic purpura
Miscellaneous diseases of the spleen:
Splenic artery aneurysm
Splenic cysts
Splenic abscesses*
Trauma*:
Acute rupture*
Delayed rupture*
Splenic tumors:
Hodgkin's lymphoma*
Non-Hodgkin's lymphoma*
Secondary hypersplenism

*Results of laparoscopic splenectomy not established.

2. Although laparoscopic splenectomy has been successfully performed for splenic artery aneurysms, ruptured spleens, tumors and tumor staging, and splenomegaly, **controversy exists about the use of the laparoscope for these disorders.** Results and safety compared to open splenectomy have not been clearly defined for these disorders and there is a possibility that otherwise curable tumors may be spread by laparoscopic techniques. Likewise, potential exists for spread of

a. Although short gastric vessels can be divided with cautery and clips, the author prefers the ultrasonically activated scissors since clips are sometimes accidentally dislodged and may interfere with placement of the vascular stapler later in the operation.

b. Reposition the Babcock clamp frequently to maintain visibility. This is especially important for the short gastric vessels to the upper pole of the spleen.

c. Gentle retraction of the upper pole of the spleen will aid in visualizing and dividing the highest short gastric vessel.

d. In some patients, division of the gastrosplenic ligament is best performed before posterior mobilization of the splenic attachments.

4. Identify the **hilum of the spleen.** Adipose tissue and/or remaining posterior attachments of the spleen often obscure the hilum and must be carefully dissected until the splenic vein is seen. Create a space in front of and behind the vein, and visualize the distal pancreas.

5. Divide **the splenic vein** with the vascular stapler, while avoiding injury to the pancreatic tail.

a. Pass an endoscopic lineal stapling device with a vascular cartridge through a left, posterior lateral port site. Pass the stapler cephalad along the left colic gutter so that it lies perpendicular to the vein.

b. Open the stapler, carefully place it across the entire vein, and close it. Ensure correct placement prior to closure. **Opening the device for repositioning without firing it is dangerous** and may tear the vein, causing bleeding.

c. Fire the stapling device, then open and remove it. Check the staple line for bleeding, which is unusual if the device is applied correctly. If bleeding occurs, control it with cautery, clips, sutures, or reapplication of the stapler.

6. Divide the **splenic artery** with the stapler (see above).

a. Depending on the splenic anatomy, 2 to 5 applications of the stapler may be required to divide all branches to the upper pole of the spleen.

b. Some surgeons prefer to ligate splenic hilar vessels with individual sutures. This can be difficult, time-consuming, and does not seem to have an advantage. Vascular staples are secure and bleeding from the staple line is rare.

7. A this point, **posterior attachments of the upper pole of the spleen** remain. Divide these attachments using the stapler, cautery, or the ultrasonically activated scissors.

a. Once the splenic blood supply is divided, the spleen can be safely retracted to visualize remaining attachments.

b. Posterior attachments may require retraction of the spleen anteriorly and to the right. This may be facilitated by rotating the table to the right.

8. When the spleen is free, place it in a **large plastic bag** and retrieve the bag through one of the large port sites (Fig. 31.4).

a. Morcellize the spleen using a Kocher clamp and/or ring forcep.

     b.   Remove the spleen in pieces, suctioning blood from the bag as needed. Place the bag on tension during morcellization, but take care to avoid damaging the bag.

9.   After removing the spleen, **reinsert the port** and examine the left upper quadrant to ensure that there is no hemorrhage. The operation is concluded in the usual fashion.

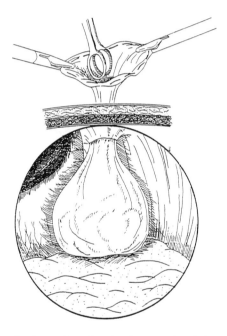

Figure 31.4. The plastic specimen bag has been retrieved through a large port site. A ring forceps is used to fragment the spleen and remove it piecemeal.

F. Complications

1.   Complications of laparoscopic splenectomy are the same as for the open operation. Although length of hospital stay and the time to full recovery is decreased, it is not clear that laparoscopic surgery is safer than open splenectomy. Laparoscopic splenectomy has the least benefit in patients with severe hematological disorders and/or medical comorbidities that necessitate prolonged hospitalization postoperatively in themselves. A potential exists for increased intraoperative bleeding and need for transfusion.

2. **Hemorrhage**
   a. **Cause and prevention:** The spleen is a pulpy organ that is easily injured during retraction. The hilar vessels are delicate and can be torn. Laparoscopic splenectomy requires excellent visualization of important structures, careful dissection, and rapid control of bleeding. Any coagulation deficits should be corrected before surgery. Patients with ITP should be treated medically to optimize platelet counts. Patients with refractory thrombocytopenia may require platelet transfusion, which should be delayed until after the splenic aretery and vein have been divided.
   b. **Recognition and management:** Monitor the operative field carefully during and after splenectomy for hemorrhage. Hemorrhage is the most common reason for conversion to open operation. Hemorrhage must be controlled rapidly with cautery, clips, or sutures, or the operation should be converted to an open procedure. It is prudent to set a limit for blood loss. If the limit is reached without end to the splenectomy in sight, conversion to open operation is justified.
3. **Postsplenectomy Sepsis**
   a. **Cause and prevention:** Warn all patients about this potential complication, and instruct them to contact their physician promptly if they develop febrile illnesses. Prompt treatment of bacterial illnesses with antibiotics is essential. Patients should receive preoperative vaccination against pneumococcal and hemophilus organisms.
   b. **Recognition and management:** Physicians should be aware of postsplenectomy sepsis. Prompt recognition and aggressive treatment of bacterial infections is required.
4. **Failure to control the primary disease:**
   a. **Cause and prevention:** Splenectomy will not improve every patient in which it is indicated. Careful selection of patients after assessment of all risks and benefits is important. Patients should be informed about expected results and the possibility of failure during discussions about the operation. Failure to recognize and remove an accessory spleen may result in persistent manifestation of the patients disease. Each operation should include a careful search for accessory spleens. They should be removed when found.
   b. **Recognition and management:** Patients with persistent disease require evaluation for accessory spleen. Accessory spleens can usually be visualized with a liver-spleen nucleotide scan. Removal of the accessory spleen is necessary, and may be performed laparoscopically. If no accessory spleen is found, treatment is medical and should involve a hematologist who is an expert with the disorder.
5. **Injury to adjacent organs (stomach, colon, or pancreas):**
   a. **Cause and prevention:** Injury to adjacent organs occurs during dissection of splenic attachments and division of vessels to the

spleen, or by tearing the organ during retraction. Careful dissection, exact application of instruments, staples, and clips, and gentle retraction are required to avoid these problems during laparoscopic splenectomy.

b. **Recognition and management**: Ideally, injury is recognized intraoperatively and can then be directly repaired (either laparoscopically or by conversion to open operation). Unrecognized injuries become manifest as prolonged postoperative ileus, intra-abdominal fluid collections, or postoperative abscess. Postoperative fluid collections and abscesses are often amenable to percutaneous drainage and antibiotic therapy. Measure the amylase concentration on any fluid drained from the abdomen to exclude pancreatic injury. If adequate drainage is obtained, infection can be controlled and fistulae will close. Failure of percutaneous drainage is an indication for reoperation.

6. **Subphrenic abscess**

a. **Cause and prevention:** Subphrenic abscess is a well-known complication of splenectomy. It may occur as an isolated complication or be caused by an injury to an adjacent organ (see above).

b. **Recognition and management:** Subphrenic abscess may causes persistent postoperative fever, elevated white blood count, and postoperative ileus. Subphrenic abscess can be diagnosed by computed tomography (CT) scan of the abdomen. Subphrenic abscess is treated with antibiotic therapy and percutaneous drainage of the abscess. If not amenable to or successfully treated by percutaneous drainage, operative drainage is indicated.

F. Selected References

Arregui M, Barteau J, Davis CJ. Laparoscopic splenectomy: techniques and indications. Int Surg 1994;79:335–341.

Cadiere GB, Verroken R, Himpens J, Bruyns J, Efira M, DeWit S. Operative strategy in laparoscopic splenectomy. J Am Coll Surg 1994;179:668–672.

Cushieri A, Shimi S, Banting S, Velpen GV. Technical aspects of laparoscopic splenectomy: hilar segmental devascularization and instrumentation. J R Coll Surg Edinb 1992;37(6):414–416.

Delaitre B. Laparoscopic splenectomy: the "hanged spleen" technique. Surg Endoscopy 1995;9:528–529.

Friedman RL, Fallas MJ, Carroll BJ, Hiatt JR, Pillips EH. Laparoscopic splenectomy for ITP: the gold standard. Surg Endosc 1996;10:991–995.

Gigot JF, Healy ML, Ferrant A, Michauz JL, Njinou B, Kestens PJ. Laparoscopic splenectomy for idiopathic thrombocytopenic purpura. Br J Surg 1994;81:1171–1172.

LeFor AT, Melvin S, Bailey RW, Flowers JL. Laparoscopic splenectomy in the management of immune thrombocytopenic purpura. Surgery 1993;114:613–618.

Phillips EH, Caroll BJ, Fallas MJ. Laparoscopic splenectomy. Surg Endosc 1994;8:931–933.

Poulin EC, Thibault C. Laparoscopic splenectomy for massive splenomegaly: operative technique and case report. Can J Surg 1995;38(1):69–72.

Rege RV, Merriam, LT, Joehl RJ. Laparoscopic splenectomy. Surg Clin of North America, 1996,76(3):459–468.

Robles AE, Andrews HG, Garberolgio C. Laparoscopic splenectomy: present status and future outlook. Int Surg 1994;79:332–334.

Schlinkert RT, Mann D. Laparoscopic splenectomy offers advantages in selected patients with immune thrombocytopenic purpura. Am J Surg 1995;170:624–627.

Yee JCK, Akpata MO. Laparoscopic splenectomy for congenital spherocytosis with splenomegaly: a case report. Can J Surg 1994;38(1):73–76.

Yee LF, Carvajal SH, de Lorimier AA, Mulvihill SJ. Laparoscopic splenectomy: the initial experience at University of California, San Francisco. Arch Surg 1995;130:874–879.

32. Lymph Node Biopsy, Dissection, and Staging Laparoscopy

Lee L. Swanstrom, M.D., F.A.C.S.

A. Indications

Laparotomy is commonly used to biopsy nodal tissue, to perform therapeutic lymphadenectomies, and to perform palliative gastrointestinal bypasses. Image-guided percutaneous biopsy is a less traumatic but significantly less accurate alterative. Most recently, laparoscopy has been advocated as an accurate, less invasive staging method and, in some cases, a procedure to allow extended lymphadenectomies for improved survival. Current **indications** for the use of laparoscopy for intra-abdominal node dissections or biopsies are listed in Table 32.1.

Table 32.1. Tumor sites for which laparoscopic lymph node biopsy or dissection has been reported, grouped by purpose of laparoscopic intervention

Purpose of Intervention	Tumor Site
Staging	Ovary Uterine Cervix Endometrium Prostate Bladder Testis (including germ cell) Hodgkin's lymphoma*
Determination of resectability for cure	Esophagus Stomach Pancreas Hepatobiliary Unknown retroperitoneal masses
Therapeutic lymph node dissection	Colon** Stomach** Nonseminomatous testicular Uterine cervix or endometrium

*Also see Chapter 12 for more details on staging laparoscopy for Hodgkin's lymphoma.
**As part of resection.

B. Patient Preparation, Positioning, and Setup

Informed consent for these procedures should include not only discussion of the procedure, risks, and alternatives, but also further treatment options for various scenarios. Patient and surgeon should reach consensus on how to proceed with surgical cancer treatment depending on the findings of the laparoscopic staging procedure. This allows the surgeon to proceed with an orderly plan of treatment that is consistent with the patient's wishes (e.g., to perform the formal resection under the same anesthesia, to attempt palliation, or to do nothing further) depending upon the intraoperative findings.

The details of preparation depend upon the anticipated site of dissection, duration of surgery, and associated pathology. Here are some general guidelines:

1. Place a **Foley catheter** for iliac node dissection, pelvic dissection, or long cases.
2. Retrogastric biopsy or other upper abdominal procedures require an orogastric tube.
3. Formal bowel preperation in advisable for para-aortic lymph node dissection as both the transabdominal and the retroperitoneal approaches involve extensive colon manipulation.
4. Patients with malignancy are at high risk for deep vein thrombosis (DVT), and the effects of position and pneumoperitoneum may contribute to intraoperative venous stasis. **Anti-DVT prophylaxis** is extremely important.
5. A single dose of **antibiotics** is given immediately preoperatively, usually a first-generation cephalosporin.
6. Patient position and OR monitor setup varies for these cases.
   a. Position the patient supine with the legs spread for **upper abdominal node biopsies, dissections, or Hodgkin's staging** (Fig. 32.1). Arms can be tucked or strapped onto arm boards at less than a 90-degree angle.
   b. **Para-aortic dissections** can also be done in this position (with the arms tucked), but are more commonly done through a retroperitoneal approach with the patient positioned in the lateral decubitus position (Fig. 32.2). This position requires a bean bag and attention to patient positioning, and padding of the axilla, arms, and legs. The monitors should be placed at the head and foot of the table.

338   Lee L Swanstrom

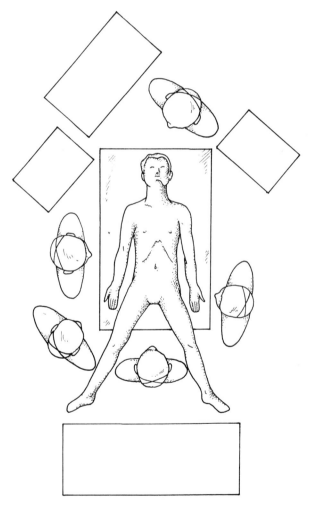

Figure 32.1. Room setup and patient position for upper abdominal node dissection.

C. Access Ports and Equipment for Laparoscopic Node Biopsy

Simple biopsy can often be performed with three ports (two 5 mm and one 10 mm), but more formal retroperitoneal node dissections may require up to six ports (three 10 mm and three 5 mm). Placement varies according to the area being biopsied.

Instruments that are typically needed are listed in Table 32.2.

Table 32.2. Instruments for laparoscopic node biopsy and dissection

Angled laparoscope	Large (10 mm) cup grasper
Atraumatic graspers (Glassman)	Specimen retrieval sac
Maryland dissector	Ultrasonic scissors*
Laparoscopic ultrasound probe	Dissecting balloons*
Endoscopic Metzenbaum scissor	Needle holders*

*Not needed in all cases.

D. Technique of Retrogastric Dissections

This procedure is approached much the same as for a laparoscopic antireflux procedure.

1. Position the patient on a split leg table with arms out on arm boards, as previously noted (Fig. 32.1) and in reverse Trendelenburg.
2. Place the initial trocar 3 cm above the umbilicus in the midline, the second (10 mm) trocar in the left mid-clavicular line, and the third (5 mm) in the right mid-clavicular line (Fig. 32.4).
3. Use a **25- or 30-degree angled laparoscope** to carefully perform a complete peritoneoscopy, which should include inspection of the pelvic cul-de-sac, Morrison's pouch, and the diaphragm. This is done to rule out any carcinomatosis that may obviate a more extended procedure.
4. Next use the **laparoscopic ultrasound** to assess the liver, portahepatic, celiac, and retrogastric nodes. Any nodes identified as enlarged should be targeted for biopsy.
5. If no adenopathy is noted, or the findings are equivocal, open the avascular portion of the gastrohepatic omentum and retract the lesser curvature of the stomach to the patient's left. This gives good access to the **celiac nodes** at the base of the patient's right crus. It also allows access to the head of the pancreas and the nodal tissue overlying this area as well as those immediately superior to the portal vein (Fig. 32.5).
6. Grasp the selected node(s) with an atraumatic grasper, and coagulate lymphatics and small feeding vessels with electrocautery or ultrasonic scissors.

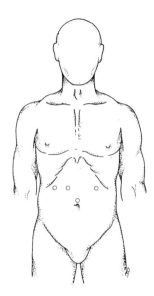

Figure 32.4. Trocar placement for upper abdominal dissection.

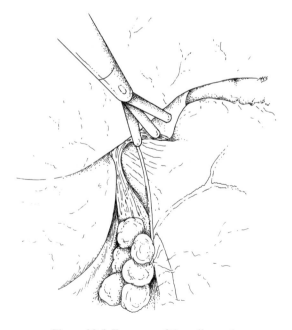

Figure 32.5. Exposure of the celiac nodes.

7. Access the **retrogastric nodes** by dividing the gastrocolic omentum and entering the lesser sac behind the stomach. Take care when dividing the gastrocolic omentum to avoid injury to the gastroepiploic vasculature (Fig. 32.6).
8. Inside the lesser sac, divide the avascular adhesions between stomach and pancreas and use an atraumatic fan retractor to elevate the stomach. This retractor is best held by a table mounted retractor holding system.
9. Node-bearing tissue also lies along the superior border of the splenic vein and pancreas and adjacent to the superior mesenteric vein and artery.
10. For simple staging, grasp and excise isolated nodes.
11. For more extended therapeutic dissections, the paraceliac and portahepatic nodes are usually dissected as one contiguous mass.
12. Node tissue between the superior mesenteric vein and splenic hilum is next removed in continuity.
13. The nodal tissue is placed in a specimen bag and removed through a trocar site (which may be enlarged if necessary).
14. Leave a closed suction drain in the field when an extensive node dissection is performed. This will control any postoperative lymphatic leakage. No drain is needed for simple biopsy.

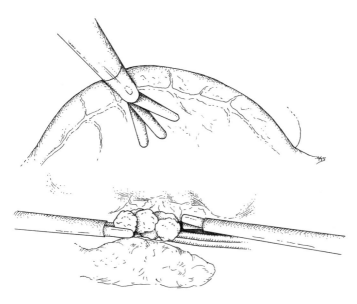

Figure 32.6. Retrogastric nodes exposed.

E. Staging for Hodgkin's Disease

Laparoscopic staging of Hodgkin's lymphoma typically involves biopsy of multiple node-bearing areas and solid organ tissue. This indication has enjoyed some renewed interest with the ability to do it laparoscopically because it yields a greater sensitivity and specificity than imaging techniques while minimizing patient morbidity and length of hospital stay. Chapter 12 contains some information about Hodgkin's staging. The discussion here will focus on the specific techniques of lymph node biopsy.

1. Position the patient supine with legs spread.
2. Five trocars are used (three 5-mm trocars and two 10-mm trocars).
3. Perform laparoscopic ultrasonography to identify any obvious retroperitoneal masses (Fig. 32.7).
4. Biopsy any visible nodes.
5. Obtain mesenteric nodes.
   a. Gently elevate the mid-jejunum with atraumatic graspers and dissect out several mesenteric nodes using sharp and blunt dissection.
   b. The ultrasonic coagulating shears are useful for control of lymphatics and vascular supply to the nodes.

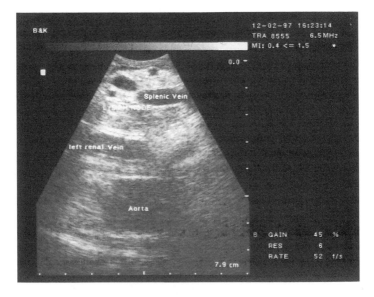

Figure 32.7. Ultrasonic image of retroperitoneal nodes.

    c.   Single nodes can be withdrawn through the 10-mm port, labeled, and fixed in formalin for pathologic assessment. One node from each area should also be sent fresh to allow touch prep slides to be made.

    d.   Obtain nodes from the transverse colon mesentery in the same way while the transverse colon is being elevated for mesenteric node sampling.

6.   Access para-aortic nodes by carrying the dissection down to the root of the mesentery adjacent to the ligament of Treitz.

7.   Liver biopsies are performed (see Chapter 12).

8.   Attention is then turned to the spleen. Laparoscopic splenectomy is performed (see Chapter 31, Laparoscopic Splenectomy).

F. Para-aortic Node Dissections

A formal para-aortic node dissection is usually indicated for staging or therapy of endometrial or cervical carcinomas, or as a treatment for early-stage germ cell tumors of the testicle. A formal dissection is best approached with retroperitonoscopy.

1.   Place the patient in the **lateral decubitus position** on a bean bag with the mid-abdomen positioned over the table break.

2.   **Flex the table** so that the abdominal musculature is stretched taut.

3.   **Take care to prevent nerve injury**: An axillary roll must be carefully positioned, the upper most arm supported, and abundant padding placed between the flexed leg.

4.   **Gain access** by a direct cut down to the preperitoneal plane in the mid-clavicular line 2 to 3 cm lateral to the umbilicus. Use blunt finger dissection to establish the working space. Introduce a dissecting balloon (Origin MedSystems, Menlo Park, California) and advance it posteriorly. Insufflate between 800 and 1600 ml into the balloon (with the scope in place to observe the resulting dissection). Stop the dissection when the aorta is visualized (Fig. 32.8).

5.   Use insufflation at 10 to 15 mm Hg to maintain the created space and insert **additional ports** (5 and 10 mm) under direct vision. Additional dissection can be done to allow full access to the aorta between the hypogastric takeoff and the renal artery.

6.   **Node sampling** is done throughout the entire area with the nodes removed either individually or by placing them in a tissue bag and removing the bag at the end of the procedure.

7.   Take care to **avoid injury** to the lumbar sympathetics, anterior spinal nerve roots, and ureters.

8.   While efforts are made to remove most of the nodes on the ipsilateral side of the tumor, it is also wise to **cross the midline** and sample nodes from the contralateral side.

9. For therapeutic dissections, take the nodes **in continuity** as much as possible. This may be combined with an ipsilateral iliac node dissection.

10. **No drains** are placed, and at the conclusion of the procedure the retroperitoneum is allowed to deinsufflate, the trocars withdrawn, and fascia closed.

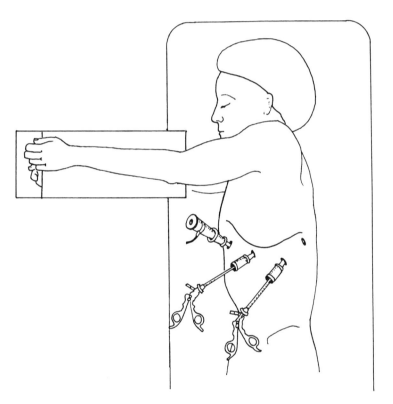

Figure 32.8. Trocar placement for retroperitoneal aortic node dissection.

G. Iliac Dissection

Iliac dissection can be performed either transabdominally or properitoneally. There is no clear-cut advantage of one approach over the other. Dissection is usually bilateral for prostate, cervical, or vulvar cancers, and unilateral (ipsilateral) for other malignancies confined to one side of the patient.

1. Room setup is the same for both approaches with a single monitor at the foot of the bed.
2. Place the patient supine with arms tucked at the side.
3. The surgeon stands on the side opposite the initial dissection (Fig. 32.3).
4. Three ports are used for both approaches; two 10 mm and one 5 mm.
5. Place the laparoscope through a trocar in the subumbilical site.
6. For the **transperitoneal approach**, the trocars are placed as shown in Fig. 32.9.
   a. Incise the peritoneum overlying the iliac artery in a longitudinal fashion and dissect the edges of the peritoneum back medial and lateral.
   b. The lymphatic tissue lies medial to the iliac artery and vein and within the obturator fossa (Fig. 32.10)
   c. Dissect out the nodal tissues in continuity, beginning at the femoral ring and working from top to bottom.
   d. Take care not to injure the obturator nerve, which marks the posterior boundary of the obturator fossa.

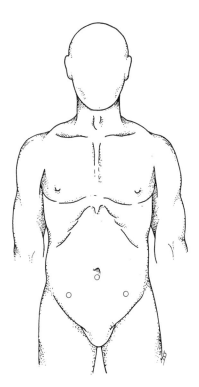

Figure 32.9. Trocar placement for transperitoneal iliac node dissection.

e.   Continue the dissection to the iliac bifurcation. Frozen section is usually obtained when doing nodes for prostate cancer, and if positive, there is no need to perform the contralateral node dissection.

f.   There is debate about closing the resulting peritoneal defect. If left open, there is a risk of bowel adhesions to this area. If closed, a lymphocele could form potentially compromising the iliac vein. If the peritoneum is closed, a closed suction drain may be advisable.

7.   The preperitoneal approach utilizes the same technique used for a TEP hernia repair (see Chapter 34, Laparoscopic Inguinal Hernia Repair).

a.   Enter the pre-peritoneal space via the infraumbilical port.

b.   Create the initial entry into the preperitoneal space by finger dissection.

c.   Pass a dissecting balloon or trocar into the space. If a dissecting balloon is not used the pressure of insufflation can be turned up (20 mm Hg) and the preperitoneum dissected bluntly using the laparoscope.

d.   Once this space is developed, additional trocars may be placed along the abdominal midline (Fig. 32.11). The same dissection as the transabdominal approach is then performed. A drain is not usually placed but the patient should be counseled to watch closely for extremity swelling.

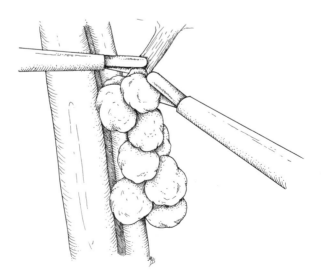

Figure 32.10. Exposure of iliac nodes.

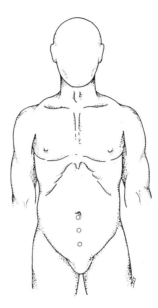

Figure 32.11. Trocar placement for properitoneal node biopsy.

H. Complications

1. **Diffuse bleeding from a peritoneal biopsy site**
   a. **Cause and prevention.** Cancer patients frequently bleed from simple biopsies because of hypocoagulability (from decreased platelet counts, antiinflammatory medications, clotting factor depletion, etc.) or portal hypertension secondary to hepatic or extrahepatic tumor involvement. Obtain a coagulation panel before surgery and correct any abnormalities. Look for clinical signs of portal hypertension (ascites, spider veins, history of variceal GI bleeds, etc.) during preoperative assessment; this may represent a relative contraindication for the surgery.
   b. **Recognition and treatment.** Bleeding from a biopsy site is usually recognized at the time of biopsy and should be treated by judicious electrocautery. If this fails a thrombogenic material can be inserted and 5 to 10 minutes of pressure applied. If bleeding continues, an endoscopically placed figure-of-eight suture tied intracorporally will almost always control the bleeding. Rarely an extended node dissection will result in diffuse

bleeding over a wide area. The laparoscopic argon beam coagulator can be useful in these circumstances.

Always check the security of hemostasis by lowering the insufflation pressure at the end of the procedure. In spite of this, delayed bleeding can occur and postoperative lymph node dissection patients should be carefully watched for the first 24 hours for signs of bleeding (tachycardia, increasing pain, dropping hematocrit (Hct), flank discoloration from a retroperitoneal bleed). Treatment of delayed bleed depends on the hemodynamic stability of the patient. Stable patients with mild symptoms may require fluids and/or blood, check of coagulation factors, and administration of appropriate factors if indicated. Unstable patients should be returned to the operating room without delay for a laparoscopic or open exploration.

2. **Bleeding from a liver biopsy**
   a. **Cause and prevention**. Cancer patients are at increased risk of bleeding. Patients with severe coagulopathy or known portal hypertension who have to have a liver biopsy should have blood products given before surgery to correct anemia and normalize coagulation indices. Maximal medical treatment should also be undertaken to control ascites (diuretics).
   b. **Recognition and treatment.** Bleeding from the site of a liver biopsy is hard to miss. Needle biopsy site bleeding is almost always controllable with cautery. Oozing is controlled with a monopolar device set on a high pure coagulating setting. This allows arcing of the current and prevents the resulting eschar from pulling away with the probe. High pressure bleeds require a lower setting and direct contact of the probe to apply pressure and heat simultaneously. Recalcitrant bleeding may require 15 to 20 minutes of direct pressure, argon beam coagulation or injection of fibrin glue into the needle tract.

   Bleeding from the exposed surface of a wedge resection should be controlled with a woven oxadized cellulose material and pressure. If this fails, the argon beam coagulator is useful.

3. **Chylous ascites**
   a. **Cause and prevention:** Rarely, disruption of major lymphatic chanels can lead to a massive lymphatic leak and chylous ascites. Clip or ligate large lymph ducts before division, and perform all extended dissections with ultrasonic coagulating shears or electrocautery.
   b. **Recognition and treatment:** Sometimes division of a major lymph channel is recognized at the time of the dissection when milky chyle appears. Identify the ends of the duct and ligate, cauterize, or clip it. Chylous ascites may present many weeks after the surgery with increasing abdominal distention and discomfort (rarely pain). Treatment almost always involves reexploration, identification of the severed duct, and ligation.

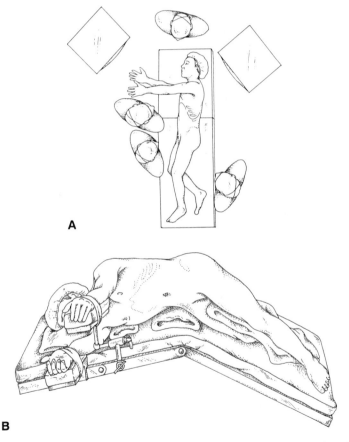

A

B

Figure 33.1. Patient position for laparoscopic transabdominal left adrenalectomy. A. Room setup for laparoscopic adrenalectomy. B. Placing the patient in the lateral decubitus position takes advantage of patient positioning to roll the viscera out of the operative field.

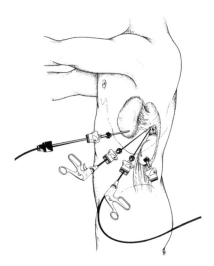

Figure 33.2. Placement of trocars in laparoscopic transabdominal left adrenalectomy. Three 10-mm trocars are usually placed initially; if a vascular stapler is needed, the middle trocar can be replaced to a 12-mm port.

3. **Performing the left adrenalectomy**

   a. Working with laparoscopic dissector and scissors, mobilize the splenic flexure medially to expose the lienorenal ligament (see Chapters 27, 28, and 31).

   b. Incise the lienorenal ligament inferosuperiorly approximately 1 cm from the spleen. Stop the dissection when the short gastric vessels are visualized posteriorly behind the stomach. This maneuver allows the spleen to fall medially, exposing the retroperitoneal space.

   c. If necessary, retract the spleen gently with an atraumatic retractor passed though the most posterior (fourth) trocar.

   d. **Laparoscopic ultrasound** may be used as an adjunct to identify the adrenal gland, the mass within the gland, and the adrenal vein (see Chapter 12).

   e. Grasping the perinephric fat, dissect the **lateral and anterior** part of the adrenal gland. Hook electrocautery or ultrasonic scalpel are useful instruments for this phase of the dissection.

   f. Avoid grasping the adrenal gland or tumor directly, as the fragile tissue is likely to tear. Sometimes it is possible to grasp the connective tissue around the tumor or adrenal gland. At certain points in the dissection, the shaft of an instrument may be used

to gently push the adrenal gland away from the region of interest, creating a space in which to work. The shaft of an instrument may also be used to elevate the adrenal gland.

g. Tilt the table to the **reverse Trendelenburg position**.

h. For **smaller adrenals (<5 cm)**, dissect the adrenal gland infe-
riomedially. The **adrenal vein** may be identified early in the
dissection, dissected using a right-angle instrument, and clipped
with medium to large titanium clips, using 3 clips proximally
and 2 clips distally. Continue the dissection superomedially,
clipping adrenal branches of the inferior phrenic vessels.

i. For **larger glands** (>5 cm), dissect the adrenal gland superiorly,
clipping the adrenal branches of the inferior phrenic vessels.
Clip and divide the adrenal vein last (Fig. 33.3).

j. Place the adrenal gland in an appropriately sized impermeable
nylon bag. Remove the bag through the original trocar site by
spreading the abdominal wall musculature using a Kelly clamp.
The abdominal incision may have to be enlarged to remove the
specimen (Chapter 8, Principles of Specimen Removal).

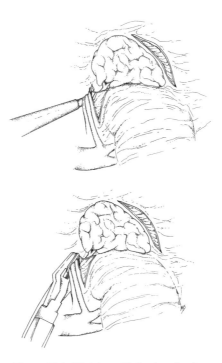

Figure 33.3. Division of left adrenal vein.

C. Transabdominal Laparoscopic Adrenalectomy—Right Adrenal

1. **Patient position and room setup** are the reverse of those described for the left adrenal.
2. **Trocar placement and choice of laparoscope**
    a. Insert a Veress needle at the right anterior axillary line, approximately 2 cm below and parallel to the costal margin. Palpate the liver carefully to avoid the edge of the liver. **Place a 10-mm trocar for the 30-degree angled laparoscope** at this site.
    b. Place three additional 10-mm trocars 2 cm below and parallel to the subcostal margin. Position one trocar in the right flank, inferior and posterior to the tip of the 11th rib, and the other two more anterior and medial. The most medial trocar should be lateral to the edge of the ipsilateral rectus muscle.
    c. The trocars should be at least 5 cm or, more optimally, 10 cm away from each other (Fig. 33.4).

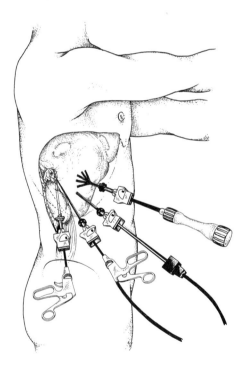

Figure 33.4. Trocar placement for transabdominal right adrenalectomy. Four 10-mm working trocars are used; if a vascular stapler is needed, one of these can be changed to a 12-mm port.

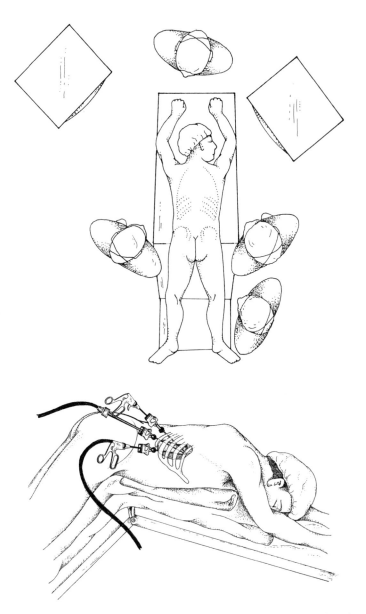

Figure 33.6. Placement of trocars in laparoscopic retroperitoneal adrenalectomy. Three 10-mm trocars are usually used. Bilateral adrenalectomies can be performed without repositioning the patient.

4. **Performance of right adrenalectomy**
   a. Identify the kidney and adrenal gland.
   b. Dissect the adrenal gland attachments to the vena cava infero-medially, clipping all vascular elements.
   c. Complete the dissection and remove the gland as described previously.

E. Complications

1. **Hemorrhage**
   a. **Cause and prevention:** Correct any preoperative coagulopathies. The dissection should consist of meticulous attention to hemostasis. Securely clip the proximal portion of the adrenal vein at least twice.
   b. **Recognition and management:** Intraoperative hemorrhage is easily identified and may require conversion to an open procedure if hemostasis cannot be achieved. (See Chapter 6, Principles of Laparoscopic Hemostasis.) Postoperative hemorrhage is best detected by carefully monitoring the patient's vital signs and urine output overnight.
2. **Damage to intraabdominal or retroperitoneal structures**
   a. **Cause and prevention:** Familiarity with intra-abdominal and retroperitoneal anatomy is an absolute must. Before clipping the adrenal vein, trace it back to the adrenal gland to avoid damaging an accessory renal vein. Take care along the superior aspect of a left adrenal dissection, as the tail of the pancreas may be injured. Retract liver and spleen gently to avoid injury and bleeding.
   b. **Recognition and management:** Damage to the liver or spleen will present as intraoperative or postoperative bleeding. Damage to the pancreas can present early as pancreatitis or later as pancreatic pseudocyst. These problems are usually self-limited, but may require medical or surgical management.

F. Selected References

Bax TW, Marcus DR, Galloway GQ, Swanstrom LL, Sheppard BC. Lapascopic bilateral adrenalectomy following failed hypophysectomy. Surg Endosc 1996;10:1150–1153.

Casaccia M, Toouli J, Fabiani P, Mouiel J. Initial experience of laparoscopic resection of adrenal tumors. Eur J Surg 1997;163:93–96.

Duh AY, Siperstein AE, Clark OH, et al. Laparoscopic adrenalectomy. Comparison of the lateral and posterior approaches. Arch Surg 1996;131:870–875.

Elashry OM, Clayman RV, Soble JJ, McDougall EM. Laparoscopic adrenalectomy for solitary metachronous contralateral adrenal metastasis from renal cell carcinoma. J Urol 1997;157:1217–1222.

Fernandez-Cruz L, Saenz A, Benarroch G, Astudillo E, Taura P, Sabater L. Laparoscopic unilateral and bilateral adrenalectomy for Cushing's syndrome. Transperitoneal and retroperitoneal approaches. Ann Surg 1996;224:727–736.

Ferrer FA, MacGillivray DC, Malchoff CD, Albala DM, Shichman SJ. Bilateral laparoscopic adrenalectomy for adrenocorticotropic dependent Cushing's syndrome. J Urol 1997;157:16–18.

Gagner M. Laparoscopic adrenalectomy. Surg Clin North Am 1996;76:523-537.

Gagner M, Breton G, Pharand D, Pomp A., Is laparoscopic adrenalectomy indicated for pheochromocytomas? Surgery 1996;120:1076–1080.

Gagner M, Lacroix A, Bolte E. Laparoscopic adrenal in Cushing's syndrome and pheochromocytomas. N Engl J Med 1992;327:1003–1006.

Gagner M, Lacroix A, Prinz R , et al. Early experience with laparoscopic approach for adrenalectomy. Surgery 1993;114:1120–1125.

Gagner M, Pomp A, Heniford BT, Pharand D, Lacroix A. Laparoscopic adrenalectomy: lessons learned from 100 consecutive cases. Ann Surg 1997;226:238–247.

Jacobs JK, Goldstein RE, Geer RJ. Laparoscopic adrenalectomy. A new standard of care. Ann Surg 1997;225:495–502.

Mugiya S, Suzuki K, Masuda H, Ushiyama T, Hata M, Fujita K. Laparoscopic adrenalectomy for nonfunctioning adrenal tumors. J Endourol 1996;10:539–541.

Prinz A. A comparison of laparoscopic and open adrenalectomies. Arch Surg 1995;130:489–494.

Rutherford JC, Gordon RD, Stowasser M, Tunny TJ, Klemm SA. Laparoscopic adrenalectomy for adrenal tumours causing hypertension and for "incidentalomas" of the adrenal on computerized tomography scanning. Clin Exp Pharmacol Physiol 1995;22:490–492.

Takeda M, Go H, Watanabe R, et al. Retroperitoneal laparoscopic adrenalectomy for functioning adrenal tumors; comnparison with conventional transperitoneal laparoscopic adrenalectomy. J Urol 1997;157:19–23.

Walz MK, Peitgren K, Hoermann R, Giebler RM, Mann K, Eigler FR. Posterior retroperitoneoscopy as a new minimally invasive approach for adrenalectomy: results of 30 adrenalectomies in 27 patients. World J Surg 1996;20:769–774.

Yamamoto H, Yoshida M, Sera Y. Laparoscopic surgery for neuroblastoma identified by mass screening. J Pediatr Surg 1996;31:385–388.

34. Laparoscopic Inguinal Hernia Repair: Transabdominal Preperitoneal (TAPP) and Totally Extraperitoneal (TEP)

Muhammed Ashraf Memon, M.B.B.S., D.C.H., F.R.C.S.I., F.R.C.S.Ed., F.R.C.S.Eng.
Robert J. Fitzgibbons, Jr., M.D., F.A.C.S.

A. Indications

Laparoscopic hernia repair may be performed for the same indications as conventional (anterior) repair. The role of laparoscopic inguinal hernia repair in treatment of an uncomplicated, unilateral hernia is **as yet unresolved**. Large, randomized, prospective trials will be needed to definitively settle the question of whether the added risks and costs are worth the benefits.

Transabdominal preperitoneal (TAPP) or totally extraperitoneal (TEP) laparoscopic inguinal herniorrhaphy may offer **specific benefit** in the following situations:

1. **Recurrent hernia:** Laparoscopic repair is a logical choice for patients with recurrent inguinal hernias. Conventional (anterior) repair for recurrent hernia is technically difficult because of scar tissue and distorted anatomy. It carries a failure rate as high as 30% in some series. The laparoscopic approach allows the repair to be performed through healthy tissue and may achieve a lower failure rate.

2. **Bilateral hernias:** Bilateral hernias can be repaired simultaneously without additional incisions or trocar sites.

3. **Patients undergoing another laparoscopic procedure:** A patient with an inguinal hernia can safely undergo laparoscopic herniorrhaphy following the completion of the primary laparoscopic procedure. For this to succeed:

   a. The primary procedure must not have created contamination by spillage of purulent material.

   b. Placement of additional trocars may be required. Hernia repair should not be performed using trocars in sub-optimal positions. Access and appropriate angles for dissection are critical for laparoscopic surgery.

B. Patient Position and Room Setup— TAPP or TEP

1. Position the patient supine with arms tucked at the side. Extending the arms on arm boards may not allow enough room for the surgeon to comfortably operate.
2. The Trendelenburg position allows the bowel to fall away from the pelvis, providing excellent access.
3. The surgeon stands on the opposite side of the table from the hernia.
4. Place a Foley catheter for continuous decompression of the bladder unless the patient voids immediately preoperatively.
5. Place a single video monitor at the foot of the operating table. Adjust the height of the monitor for comfortable viewing by both surgeon and assistants.

C. Transabdominal Preperitoneal (TAPP) Approach

1. Place the first trocar (10–12 mm) at the umbilicus.
2. Place two additional 10–12 mm trocars lateral to the rectus sheath on either side at the level of the umbilicus under direct vision (Fig. 34.1). Large trocars allow the laparoscope and stapler to be moved around for optimal dissection, depending upon anatomy. If 5-mm instruments are available, smaller trocars may be used. For a small, unilateral hernia, a 5-mm cannula may be substituted for the 10- to 12-mm cannula on the ipsilateral side of the hernia.
3. An angled laparoscope provides the best visualization of the inguinal region, which is somewhat anterior (Figs. 34.2 and 34.3).
4. Inspect both inguinal regions. Identify the median umbilical ligament (remnant of the urachus), the medial umbilical ligament (remnant of umbilical artery), and the lateral umbilical fold (peritoneal reflection over the inferior epigastric artery). If the median umbilical ligament appears to compromise exposure, divide it.
5. Use endoscopic scissors to incise the peritoneum along a line approximately 2 cm above the superior edge of the hernia defect, extending from the median umbilical ligament to the anterior superior iliac spine.
6. Mobilize the peritoneal flap inferiorly using blunt and sharp dissection.
   a. Expose the inferior epigastric vessels, and identify the pubic symphysis and lower portion of the rectus abdominis muscle.
   b. Dissect Cooper's ligament to its junction with the femoral vein.

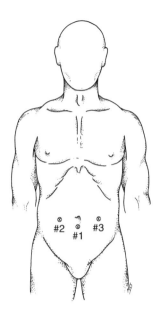

Figure 34.1. Trocar placement for TAPP.

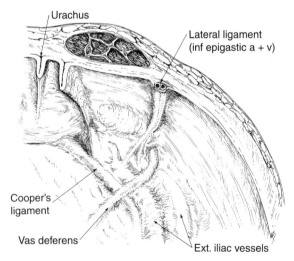

Figure 34.2. Male groin anatomy. In the female, the round ligament of the uterus leaves the pelvis at the internal ring.

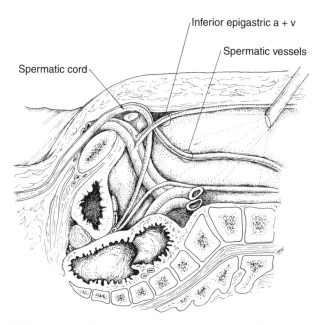

Figure 34.3. Anatomy of male pelvis as viewed by angled (30 degree) laparoscope.

    c.   Identify the iliopubic tract. Continue the dissection inferiorly, with care to avoid an injury to the femoral branch of the genitofemoral nerve and the lateral femoral cutaneous nerve which enter the lower extremity just below the iliopubic tract.

    d.   Complete the dissection by skeletonizing the cord structures.

7.   **Direct hernia**: Reduce the sac and preperitoneal fat from the hernia orifice by gentle traction.

8.   There are two options for **indirect hernias**:

    a.   A small sac is easily mobilized from the cord structures and reduced back into the peritoneal cavity (Fig. 34.4).

    b.   A large sac may be difficult to mobilize because of dense adhesions between the sac and the cord structures due to the chronicity of the hernia. Undue trauma to the cord may result if an attempt is made to remove the sac in its entirety. In this situation, divide the sac just distal to the internal ring leaving the distal sac *in situ*. This is most easily accomplished by opening the sac on the side opposite the cord structures and completing the division from the inside. Dissect the proximal sac away from the cord structures.

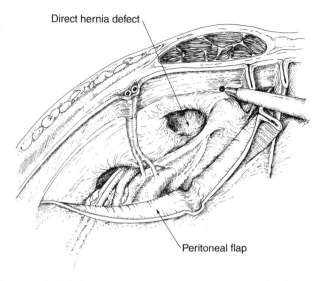

Direct hernia defect

Peritoneal flap

Figure 34.4. Mobilizing the peritoneal flap for a left direct inguinal hernia.

9. Next, place a large piece of mesh (at least 11 cm × 6 cm) over the myopectineal orifice so that it completely covers the direct, indirect and femoral spaces (Fig. 34.5).

    a. The mesh can either be simply laid over the cord structures or a slit can be made in the mesh to wrap around the cord structures. Most surgeons now avoid the slit in the prosthesis because recurrences have been noted through these slits (even when they have been closed around the cord).

    b. The large prosthesis allows the intra-abdominal pressure to act uniformly over a large area, thus preventing its herniation through the hernia defect in the abdominal wall.

10. Although not all surgeons think that **staple fixation** is necessary, most feel that migration or shrinkage may be prevented in some patients (Fig. 34.6).

    a. Begin stapling along the superior border of the prosthesis.

    b. Place the staples horizontally along the superior border to minimize the chance of injury to the deeper ilioinguinal or iliohypogastric nerves.

    c. Place these staples at least 2 cm above the hernia defect beginning medially above the *contralateral* pubic tubercle extending laterally to the anterior superior iliac spine.

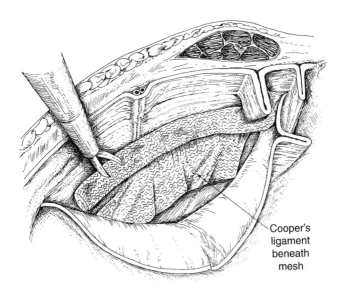

Figure 34.5. Placement of mesh. A large sheet of mesh is simply laid over the entire floor, covering the cord and all myopectineal orifices.

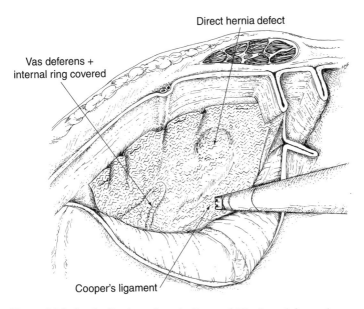

Figure 34.6. Staple fixation of mesh. **Beware!** The lateral femoral cutaneous nerve and the genital branch of the genitofemoral nerve cross under the iliopubic tract lateral to the cord structures.

    d.   Staple the inferior border to Cooper's ligament medially using either a horizontal or vertical orientation depending upon individual patient characteristics (i.e., how the staples best attach). Again the opposite pubic tubercle marks the area to begin placing staples for the inferior border and these are continued over the area of the ipsilateral pubic tubercle to the femoral vein. Do not place staples directly into either pubic tubercle because chronic postoperative pain (osteitis pubis) can result.

    e.   Affix the medial and lateral borders using vertically placed staples.This is the direction of the lateral cutaneous nerve of the thigh and the femoral branch of the genitofemoral nerve.

    f.   Lateral to the internal spermatic vessels, place all staples above the iliopubic tract. This avoids neuralgia from injury to the lateral cutaneous nerve of the thigh or the femoral branch of the genitofemoral nerve. It is useful to palpate the head of the stapler through the abdominal wall with the nondominant hand. This ensures that stapling is done above the iliopubic tract (Fig. 34.7).

11. After stapling is complete, excise any redundant mesh.

12. Close the peritoneal flap over the mesh with staples.

    a.   The goal should be to isolate the prosthesis from intra-abdominal viscera.

    b.   The authors do not feel that linear approximation of the peritoneum is necessary for all patients especially if this results in a tenting of the peritoneum because of excessive tension required to approximate the two edges. The tenting effect may leave a space between the peritoneal flap and the prosthesis. Bowel might migrate into this space resulting in bowel obstruction.

    c.   Occasionally, it is necessary to simply cover the mesh with the inferior flap leaving exposed transversalis fascia.

    d.   Avoid excess gaps between staples; bowel can herniate or adhere to the mesh through these defects.

    e.   It may be helpful to decrease the pneumoperitoneum prior to flap closure (Fig. 34.8).

13. Inject a long-acting local anesthetic such as bupivacaine into the preperitoneal space before closure, if desired, to decrease postoperative pain.

14. **Bilateral hernias** can be repaired using one long transverse peritoneal incision extending from one anterior superior iliac spine to the other.

    a.   Another option is to make two separate peritoneal incisions preserving the peritoneum between the medial umbilical ligaments but still dissecting the preperitoneal space over the symphysis pubis. This has the theoretical advantage of avoiding damage to a patent urachus.

    b.   A large single piece of mesh measuring 30 cm × 7.5 cm can be stapled from one anterior, superior iliac spine to the other anterior superior iliac spine.

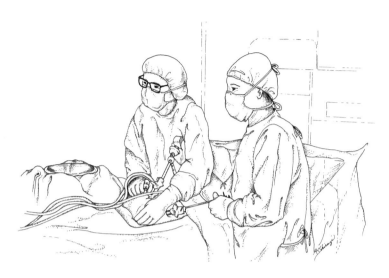

Figure 34.7. Surgeon using nondominant (left) hand to palpate the head of the stapler through the anterior abdominal wall, thus verifying stapler position relative to external landmarks and providing counterpressure.

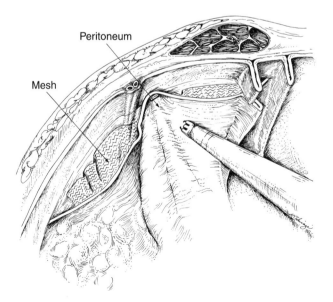

Figure 34.8. Closing peritoneal flap over the mesh with staples.

c.   Some surgeons prefer two separate pieces of mesh because of concern that placing the mesh across the bladder could interfere with bladder function. Also, it is technically easier to manipulate two pieces separately and tailor them more accurately to fit the preperitoneal space on either side.

D. Totally Extraperitoneal (TEP) Approach

1.   Make the skin incision for the first trocar (10–12 mm) at the umbilicus. Open the anterior rectus sheath on the ipsilateral side and retract the muscle laterally to expose the posterior rectus sheath.

   a.   Following the incision of the anterior rectus sheath and retraction of the muscle laterally, insert a finger over the posterior rectus sheath and gently develop this space.

   b.   Insert a transparent balloon tipped trocar into this space directed toward the pubic symphysis. Place the laparoscope in the trocar. Under direct vision, inflate the balloon to create the extraperitoneal tunnel or space.

2.   Place two additional trocars in the midline under direct vision: the second (5-mm) at the pubic symphysis and the third (10–12 mm) midway between the first and second (Figs. 34.9 and 34.10).

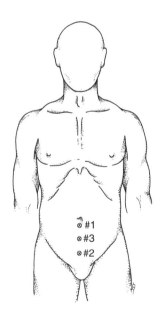

Figure 34.9. Trocar placement for TEP.

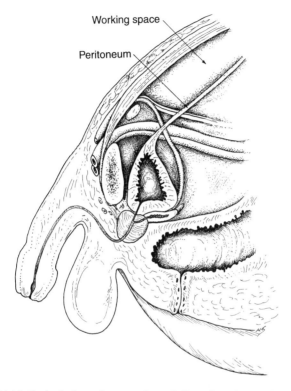

Figure 34.10. Sagittal view of extraperitoneal dissection. A space is developed between peritoneum and abdominal wall. Note that the bladder is mobilized downward.

    a.   Place these trocars by incising the skin with a scalpel, then blunt dissection with a hemostat under direct vision.

    b.   Avoid using a standard trocar, as inadvertent penetration through the narrow preperitoneal space into the peritoneal cavity may result.

3.   Use an angled laparoscope to provide the best visualization of the inguinal region (which is somewhat anterior).

4.   Complete the dissection of the preperitoneal space, placement of mesh and stapling in a similar manner to that described for TAPP procedure (Fig. 34.11).

5.   Bilateral hernias can be repaired with the use of either a single large prosthesis or two separate pieces.

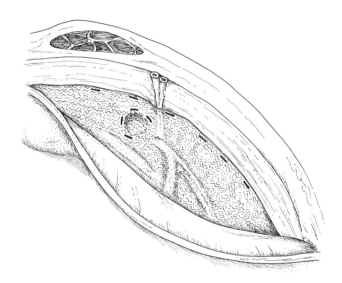

Figure 34.11. Mesh stapled in place using TEP approach.

F. Complications

As laparoscopic procedures, both TAPP and TEP may incur any of the complications of laparoscopy, including major vascular injury, injury to hollow viscera, complications of pneumoperitoneum, or complications associated with anesthesia. This section describes several specific complications related to the actual laparoscopic surgical procedures.

1. **Vascular injuries**

    a. **Cause and prevention:** Injuries to the inferior epigastric and spermatic vessels are the most common vascular injuries reported during laparoscopic inguinal herniorrhaphy in the literature. Other vessels at risk include the external iliac, circumflex iliac profunda, and obturator vessels. Of course, vascular injury can occur during the initial trocar or Veress needle insertion as with any laparoscopic procedure. Inexperience, anatomical variations, and confusion during dissection, especially if the patient has had previous lower abdominal surgery, predisposes patients to vascular injuries. Use of the open laparoscopic technique for insertion of the initial cannula, meticulous dissection, and absolute identification of important landmarks are essential in preventing these injuries.

    b. **Recognition and management:** Bleeding is easily recognized at the time of surgery. Delayed bleeding may present with signs and symptoms of hypovolemia. All vessels in the inguinal region except for the external iliacs can be safely ligated. Injury to the external iliac vessels requires immediate repair.

2. **Urinary tract complications**

   a. **Cause and Prevention:** Urinary retention, urinary infection and hematuria are the most common patient complications reported in the literature and are usually secondary to urinary catheterization, extensive preperitoneal dissection, general anesthesia, and/or administration of large volumes of intravenous fluids. Bladder injury is one of the more common complications of laparoscopic herniorrhaphy. It is most commonly seen in patients with previous "space of Retzius" surgery. **Previous surgery in this space (i.e., a prostate operation) should be considered a relative contraindication to laproscopic hernia repair.** Renal and ureteral injuries have been seen with off-center trocar insertion. Careful technique should prevent these injuries.

   b. **Recognition and management:** Transient urinary catheterization and a short course of antibiotics usually solves problems with retention or infection. If a bladder injury is recognized during hernia repair, it should be repaired immediately either laparoscopically or via conventional laparotomy if necessary. A conventional herniorrhaphy without a prosthesis should then be performed to avoid the need to place a foreign body next to the bladder repair. A high index of suspicion is the key to the diagnosis of a missed urinary tract injury. Lower abdominal pain, distended bladder, dysuria, and hematuria should be promptly investigated. Other signs may include azotemia, electrolyte abnormalities, and ascites. Indwelling catheter drainage alone may suffice for retroperitoneal bladder injuries, but intraperitoneal perforations are best closed either laparoscopically or by a laparotomy.

3. **Nerve injury**

   a. **Cause and prevention:** The femoral branch of the genitofemoral nerve, the lateral cutaneous nerve of the thigh, and the intermediate cutaneous branch of the anterior branch of the femoral nerve are at risk of damage during laparoscopic herniorrhaphy because of (a) failure to appreciate the anatomy from the posterior aspect; (b) difficulty in visualizing the nerves preperitoneally; (c) variable course of the nerves in this region; (d) improper staple placement; or (e) extensive preperitoneal dissection.

   b. **Recognition and management:** Symptoms of burning pain and numbness usually develop after a variable interval in the postoperative period. If the neuralgia is present in the recovery room, immediate reexploration is the best course of action. When the symptoms are delayed in onset, the condition is usually self-limiting. In the majority of cases nonsteroidal anti-inflammatory agents are sufficient. Reexploration and removal of the offending staple may occasionally be required.

4. **Vas deferens and testicular complications**

   a. **Cause and prevention:** The majority of these complications are transient and self-limiting including testicular pain, testicular swelling, orchitis, and epididymitis. Testicular pain may be the result of trauma to the genitofemoral nerve or to the sympathetic innervation of the testis during dissection around the cord structures or during separation of the peritoneum from the cord structures. Testicular swelling may be secondary to narrowing of the deep inguinal ring, ischemia, or from interruption of lymphatic or venous vessels resulting from attempts at complete removal of a large indirect inguinal hernia sac. Transection of the vas deferens or testicular atrophy are seen in about the same incidence as conventional surgery. Avoiding excessive tightening of the deep inguinal ring, gently dissecting around the cord structures, and avoiding complete removal of large indirect hernia sacs reduce vas deferens and testicular complications.

   b. **Recognition and management:** Most cord and testicular complications are treated by supportive care such as testicular support, limitation of activities, and analgesics. If the vas deferens is transected, the cut ends should be repaired with fine, interrupted sutures unless fertility is not a consideration. There is no treatment for unilateral testicular atrophy. The recommended treatment for bilateral testicular atrophy is the administration of parenteral testosterone usually by intramuscular injection.

5. **Complications related to the mesh**

   a. **Cause and prevention:** Migration of mesh, infection of mesh, mass lesions representing palpable mesh, adhesion formation, and erosion of the mesh into intra-abdominal organs have been reported following laparoscopic herniorrhaphy. Fixation of mesh prevents migration. The use of preoperative prophylactic antibiotics is recommended to prevent mesh infection. Adhesion formation is least likely to occur following the TEP procedure as the mesh is never in contact with intra-abdominal organs unless there are unrecognized perforations of the peritoneum. Following the TAPP procedure, adequate closure of the peritoneum over the mesh is the most important factor in preventing complications such as bowel herniating through large gaps and/or becoming adherent to exposed mesh. Minimizing trauma, avoiding infection, sparing the blood supply, and avoiding exposed mesh decreases the incidence of adhesion formation.

   b. **Recognition and management:** Mesh complications usually manifest themselves weeks to years following the repair in the form of small bowel obstruction, abscess or fistula. These may respond to conservative management or may require formal laparotomy.

6. **Recurrence of the hernia**
    a. **Cause and prevention:** Recurrence may be due to a variety of mechanisms (Table 34.1).

Table 34.1. Potential mechanisms for recurrence

Incomplete dissection
Missed hernias
Inadequate identification of landmarks
Prosthesis rolls up rather than lying flat
Mesh too small
Incomplete coverage of all defects
Migration of the mesh
Mesh slit and placed around cord
Slit may be site of recurrence
Folding or invagination of mesh into defect
Displacement of mesh by hematoma

The authors feel that a thorough dissection of the preperitoneal space with identification of all the landmarks followed by fixation of a large-size mesh that adequately covers and overlaps the entire myopectineal orifice without slitting or folding is the best way to avoid recurrence.

    b. **Recognition and management:** Recurrence is noted by the patient or physician as a lump or pain in the groin. Either a repeat laparoscopic repair or a conventional repair will be needed to correct the recurrence.

7. **Miscellaneous complications**
    a. **Cause and prevention:** Pubic and pelvic **osteitis** are usually caused by placing a staple into bone. Placing staples on the anterior and superior portion of Cooper's ligament or avoiding fixing mesh altogether prevents these complications. Groin **seroma** and **hematoma** usually occur due to extensive dissection or inadequate hemostasis. **Wound infection** may be prevented using meticulous sterile technique.
    b. **Recognition and management:** Pubic and pelvic osteitis are difficult to diagnose. The diagnosis is essentially one of exclusion. Simple measures such as anti-inflammatory agents and analgesia may be helpful. Groin hematoma or seroma may require evacuation or aspiration. Wound infection will require a course of antibiotics after drainage and may require removal of the mesh prosthesis if the infection extends to the groin.

G. Selected References

Arregui ME, Navarrete J, Davis CJ, Castro D, Nagan RF. Laparoscopic inguinal herniorrhaphy. Techniques and controversies. Surg Clin North Am 1993;73: 513–527.

Camps J, Nguyen N, Annibali R, Filipi CJ, FitzgibbonsRJ Jr. Laparoscopic inguinal herniorrhaphy: current techniques. In: Arregui ME, Fitzgibbons RJ, Jr, Katkhouda N, McKernan JB, Reich H, eds. Principles of Laparoscopic Surgery: Basic and Advanced Techniques. New York: Springer-Verlag, 1995;400–408.

Filipi CJ, Fitzgibbons RJ, Jr, Salerno GM. Laparoscopic herniorrhaphy. In: Hulka JF, Reich H, eds. Textbook of Laparoscopy 2nd ed. Philadelphia: WB Saunders, 1994;313–326.

Fitzgibbons RJ, Jr, Camps J, Cornet DA, et al. Laparoscopic inguinal herniorrhaphy. Results of a multicenter trial. Ann Surg 1995;1: 3–13.

Katkhouda N. Avoiding complications of laparoscopic hernia repair. Laparoscopic inguinal herniorrhaphy: current techniques. In: Arregui ME, Fitzgibbons RJ, Jr, Katkhouda N, McKernan JB, Reich H, eds. Principles of Laparoscopic Surgery: Basic and Advanced Techniques. New York: Springer-Verlag 1995;435–438.

Lowham AS, Filipi CJ, Fitzgibbons RJ Jr, et al. Mecahnisms of hernia recurrence after preperitoneal mesh repair. Traditional and laparoscopic. Ann Surg 1995;225:422–431.

Memon MA, Fitzgibbons RJ Jr. Assessing risks, costs and benefits of laparoscopic hernia repair. Annu Rev Med 1998;49:63–77.

Memon MA, Rice D, Donohue JH. Laparoscopic herniorrhaphy. J Am Coll Surg 1997;184: 325–335.

Tetik C, Arregui ME. Prevention of Complications of open and laparoscopic repair of groin hernias. In: Arregui ME, Fitzgibbons RJ, Jr, Katkhouda N, McKernan JB, Reich H, eds. Principles of Laparoscopic Surgery: Basic and Advanced Techniques. New York: Springer-Verlag, 1995;439–449.

35. Laparoscopic Repair of Ventral Hernia

Gerald M. Larson, M.D.

A. Indications and Contraindications

1. **The general indication** for a laparoscopic repair of a ventral hernia is the presence of a hernia with a fascial defect 3 cm or greater in patients who would otherwise meet the criteria for a traditional open surgical repair. Small hernia defects less than 3 cm in diameter are readily repaired by standard techniques, and the laparoscopic approach usually offers no advantage to the patient. Abdominal wall hernias in the midline or in the upper and lower quadrants are equally accessible by the laparoscopic approach. Special conditions include:
   a. **The incarcerated hernia** can be repaired laparoscopically if one can obtain a good laparoscopic view of the hernia and its contents, dissect the adhesions, and reduce the hernia.
   b. In the **multiply operated abdomen**, the extent and density of adhesions are the main determinants of length and difficulty of laparoscopic ventral hernia repair. Adhesion formation is unpredictable; therefore, multiple previous operations do not preclude the laparoscopic approach provided that an entry point for the first trocar can be obtained and a pneumoperitoneum safely established.
   c. **Swiss-cheese hernias** (multiple small defects) are actually a good indication for the laparoscopic approach because the number of fascial defects and extent of hernia formation are often greater than expected. The laparoscopic approach allows a clear delineation of all defects, so that the mesh prosthesis is tailored accordingly.
2. **Contraindications** to laparoscopic repair of ventral hernia include the densely scarred abdomen (in which it is impossible to safely introduce a trocar or establish pneumoperitoneum), and the acute abdomen with strangulated or infarcted bowel.

B. Patient Preparation and Room Setup

1. Place the patient supine on the operating table with arms extended.
2. For most midline hernias, the surgeon stands on either the patient's left or right with the video monitor positioned on the opposite side so

that the surgeon's view on the screen is parallel and in line with the laparoscopic repair of the hernia within the abdomen.

3. The assistant stands opposite the surgeon, and a second monitor is placed in a suitable position.

4. In addition to the standard preoperative preparation, consider bowel prep if an incarcerated hernia with colon involvement is suspected.

C. Trocar Position and Choice of Laparoscope (Fig. 35.1)

1. The author prefers open access with a Hasson cannula because of the likelihood of adhesions and bowel fixed to the abdominal wall. Place the cannula in the lower midline, 2 or 3 inches away from the lower extent of the hernia. Establish pneumoperitoneum and insert a direct view laparoscope (0 degree) to facilitate insertion of the other trocars.

2. Place two additional 10-mm trocars in the abdomen on the patient's left side as far lateral as possible. Specific port placement will depend on the size and location of the hernia. Establishing the pneumoperitoneum through a midline trocar facilitates safe placement of lateral trocars and minimizes the risk of injury to the colon. It is more difficult to place the initial trocar in a left lateral location because it is necessary to dissect through the three muscle layers rather than the linea alba only, the air seal is not always tight, and one is concerned about proximity to the colon.

3. Work with dissecting and grasping forceps and scissors to first take down the adhesions, reduce the hernia, and outline the defect in the fascia. The scope can be placed in any port so that the surgeon's view and the direction of the dissection are in the same direction.

4. For an optimal view and exposure it is best that the working ports be as far away from the hernia defect as possible. Since the mesh will overlap the defect by about 2 cm, a very lateral or inferior position of the trocar site maximizes the view and efficiency of the instruments when unrolling the mesh and placing the tacking sutures to hold the mesh in place. It may be necessary to place an additional trocar if none of the existing sites are optimal.

5. For most of the initial dissection, a straight (0 degree) laparoscope is preferred (some surgeons use it for the entire procedure). Once the hernia defect is exposed, an angled (30 degree) laparoscope provides a better view for proper placement of the mesh over the hernia defect and for suturing it in place.

6. An extra 5-mm port may be necessary in the opposite lower quadrant to assist with the dissection and then to position and suture the mesh to the muscle-fascia layer later in the procedure.

7. Trocar position is to some extent a matter of surgeon's choice and preference, and must be modified for hernias of various locations.

   a. Some surgeons may choose to stand on the patient's right but the same principles described above would apply.

b. For patients with subcostal hernias, the second and third trocar sites may move from the extreme lateral position to a more central inferior position in the abdomen, which will give good access to the length and breadth of the hernia defect.

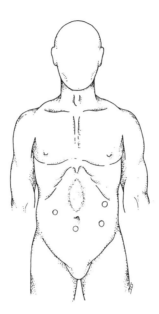

Figure 35.1. Demonstration of port placement for repair of a ventral hernia in the upper abdomen. Place the first trocar in the lower midline, 2 or 3 inches inferior to the ventral hernia. Ventral hernias in the lower abdomen require placement of the camera port in the upper abdomen.

D. The Technique of Laparoscopic Hernia Repair

This type of hernia repair is an intra-abdominal, intraperitoneal repair that uses a mesh prosthesis to close and cover the hernia defect. The hernia defect itself is not closed. The mesh is anchored and held in position with transfascial mattress sutures (2-0 or 0) at each corner of the repair; usually 4 mattress sutures, but for larger hernias 8 or more mattress sutures, are appropriate. The sutures are tied through a small stab incision in the skin and tied subcutaneously. In between the mattress sutures the mesh is tacked or stapled to the abdominal wall fascia at 1-cm intervals with special hernia staples or spiral tacks.

An important principle is that the mesh is tailored or trimmed so that it is 2 cm wider than the hernia defect on all four sides, thus permitting the prosthesis to be anchored and held in place to the solid musculofascial layer (Fig. 35.2). The mesh should be placed in some tension when it is sewn into place.

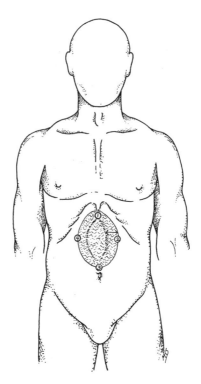

Figure 35.2. Cut the mesh prosthesis to the desired size and mark its intended location on the anterior abdominal wall. The shaded area indicates the approximate outline of the ventral hernia, and the mesh is indicated by crosshatches. The mesh should extend beyond the hernia defect by 2 cm or more on all sides. This 2 cm cuff will be used to anchor the mesh to the solid tissue surrounding the defect for the repair.

1. The first objective of the operation is to expose the hernia defect.
    a. Begin by dissecting the small bowel, omentum, and adhesions from the abdominal wall to expose the hernia defect (Fig. 35.3).
    b. External pressure applied to the abdominal wall and to the hernia assists in maintaining orientation and identifying the edge of the hernia. Frequently more than one defect is present.
    c. A variety of instruments aid in the dissection; standard grasping and dissecting forceps, a sharp scissor, bowel clamps, and Babcock forceps all may be useful. The ultrasonic scalpel can be invaluable for dividing tissue and avoiding bleeding. Dissecting forceps and scissors should have electrocautery attachments.
2. Identify the edge of the defect by one of several methods.

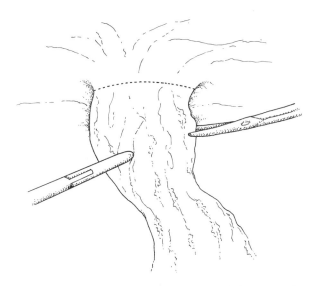

Figure 35.3. Laparoscopic view of a ventral hernia with incarcerated omentum. The hernia contents must be dissected free from the abdominal wall to expose the hernia defect.

    a.   Push an intra-abdominal instrument against a palpating finger on the abdomen and mark the position of the edge.

    b.   Pass needles through the abdominal wall, and confirm the position of the hernia defect relative to the needles by visual comparison.

3.   Mark the edges of the defect on the skin with a marking pen.

4.   Two types of mesh are currently available—a polypropylene mesh and an expanded polytetrafluoroethylene prosthesis. Choice is largely a matter of personal preference. Select a piece of appropriate size and tailor the mesh prosthesis in such a manner as to allow a 2-cm cuff or margin lateral to the fascial defect in all directions. Mark the mesh with a colored pen so that it is readily obvious which side faces the fascia and which side faces the viscera. It is also helpful to mark the corners of the mesh 1, 2, 3, and 4 (unless the defect is circular) to maintain the proper orientation when the mesh is being tacked in place (Fig. 35.4).

5.   Roll the mesh around a grasping forceps and insert it into the abdomen.

6.   Horizontal mattress sutures, passed through the mesh and all layers of the abdominal wall, anchor the four corners of the mesh to solid portions of the musculofascial layer.

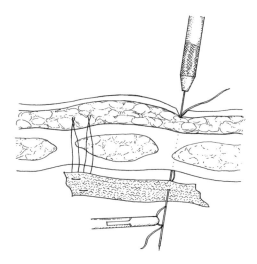

Figure 35.4. Method of mesh fixation with a suture passer. Use the suture passer to introduce the suture through the musculofascial layer, the mesh, and then back out through all layers as a mattress suture. Use four to eight mattress sutures to anchor the mesh, depending on the size of the hernia and the surgeon's preference. Knot the sutures subcutaneously. Use hernia tackers or staples to fix the mesh to the abdominal wall between the mattress sutures.

a. Either a short Keith needle or a specially designed suture passer may be used.

b. Use 2-0 braided or monofilament nonabsorbable suture for the suture passer. Heavier sutures do not pass easily.

c. Make a small incision in the skin. This will allow the suture to be tied subcutaneously.

d. Pass the suture through the abdominal wall (out to in), through and through the mesh (horizontal bite), and then back through the abdominal wall (in to out).

e. Tie the sutures subcutaneously.

f. The suture passer has a grasping jaw to carry a suture through a small skin incision through the abdominal wall (and solid fascia) into the abdomen and through the mesh. The suture is released, and the passer is removed and reinserted through the same skin site so that it will grasp the suture 1 cm away from the last entry point in the mesh and create a 1-cm mattress suture.

7. For hernias measuring 3 to 5 cm, four anchoring sutures located at 90-degree intervals around the defect are adequate. For hernias larger than 5 cm, the author prefers to place eight of these mattress sutures using the suture passer technique and then supplementing the fixation

of the mesh to the abdominal fascia with either a stapler or a spiral tacker in between at 1-cm intervals. The interval distance is important so that bowel has no entry point between the clips, which could cause an obstruction.

8. The horizontal bite through the mesh is important. This allows the mesh to act as a pledget, thus preventing the suture from cutting through the fascia.

9. Close the trocar sites and small skin incisions in the usual fashion.

E. Complications

Complications include trocar site and wound infection, urinary retention, and postoperative ileus. Dissection of adhesions and manipulation of bowel may result in injury (see Chapter 10.3, Previous Abdominal Surgery).

Recurrence is the complication unique to hernia repair. The risk can be minimized by adhering to sound surgical principles, clearly identifying all fascial defects, and placing the mesh properly with solid fixation to sound tissue. The mesh must be sufficiently large, and must be sutured under some (but not excessive) tension.

The **wound infection** rate should be no greater than for other laparoscopic procedures of similar magnitude. Infections can generally be treated by opening the wound. This must be done in a timely fashion so that the anchoring sutures are not jeopardized.

Mechanical bowel obstruction may result from internal herniation of bowel between anchoring sutures or clips. This may require laparotomy for repair.

F. Selected References

Felix EL, Michas C. Laparoscopic repair of spigelian hernias. Surg Laparosc & Endosc 1994;4(4): 308–310.

Holzman MD, Puret CM, Reintgen K. Laparoscopic ventral and incisional hernioplasty. Surg Endosc 1997;11 (1): 32–35.

Larson GM, Vandertoll DJ. Approach to repair of ventral hernia and full-thickness losses of abdominal wall. Surg Clin North Am 1984;64:335–349.

MacFadyen BV, Arregui ME, Corbitt JD. Complications of laparoscopic herniorrhaphy. Surg Endosc 1993;7:155–158.

Park A, Gagner M, Pomp A. Laparoscopic repair of large incisional hernias. Surg Laparosc Endosc 1996;6 (2):123–128.

Saiz AA, Willia IH, Paul DK. Laparoscopic ventral hernia repair: a community hospital experience. Am Surg 1996;62(5):336–338.

Temudom T, Siadati M, Sarr MG. Repair of complex giant or recurrent ventral hernias by using tension-free intraparietal prosthetic mest (Stoppa technique): Lessons learned from our initial experience (fifty patients). Surgery 1996;120(4):738–744.

36. Pediatric Laparoscopy: General Considerations

Thom E. Lobe, M.D.

A. Indications

Many common pediatric disorders can be treated using laparoscopy (Table 36.1). Just as with laparoscopic surgery in adult patients, the degree of benefit from the laparoscopic approach varies from procedure to procedure.

Table 36.1. Partial list of pediatric laparoscopic procedures

• Appendectomy
• Cholecystectomy
• Contralateral Exploration for Inguinal Hernias
• Pyloromyotomy
• Fundoplication for Gastroesophageal Reflux
• Splenectomy
• Staging for Cancer

B. Contraindications

Absolute **contraindications** to laparoscopy in children are similar to those in adult patients. These include:
1. Uncorrected coagulopathy
2. Hemodynamic instability or shock
3. Diffuse, dense abdominal adhesions that preclude safe access

C. Patient Position, Room Setup, and Preparation

The surgeon usually stands facing the structure to be operated on, and the video monitor should be in the line of sight of the operating surgeon. The general principles of room setup discussed in Chapters 1 and 2 apply to pediatric laparoscopy. Patient position is discussed with individual procedures in Chapter 37.

Specific considerations for preparing the pediatric patient include:

1. Credé's maneuver to empty the bladder for short or upper abdominal procedures.
2. Foley catheter for long procedures during which excessive blood loss is anticipated or for pelvic or lower abdominal procedures.
3. Naso- or orogastric suction to empty the stomach before beginning a laparoscopic procedure.
4. Consideration for prophylactic antibiotics to prevent trocar site infections.

D. Instruments and Choice of Laparoscope

Most pediatric procedures can be performed using 5-mm telescopes.
1. Zero-degree telescopes are suitable for many procedures.
2. Thirty-degree telescopes are useful for upper abdominal procedures and for laparoscopic suturing.
3. Smaller scopes, readily available in centers where pediatric cystoscopy or bronchoscopy are performed, are useful for some procedures, particularly in infants. These instruments vary from 1.7 to 4 mm in diameter and have viewing angles ranging from zero to 70 degrees.

Specially designed small-diameter pediatric laparoscopic instruments are available. These may be supplemented with arthroscopic knives and other specialized instruments as desired.

E. Access to the Abdomen

Infants and children have a "shallow abdominal cavity". The **first trocar** (usually at the umbilicus) is best inserted under direct visualization using an **open technique**:
1. Cleanse the umbilicus of the infant meticulously before the routine surgical prep since it is often full of debris.
2. Make a transverse incision in the inferior rim of the umbilical ring using a number 15 surgical blade.
3. Enlarge this incision by inserting the tips of a hemostat into the wound and spreading the jaws of the instrument perpendicular to the transverse incision. Perform this maneuver slowly and deliberately to allow the skin to separate along the direction of Langer's lines.
4. Grasp the midline fascia with two hemostats so that the wound can be opened in the midline, dividing the umbilical ring when appropriate.
5. Open the peritoneum and insert the trocar under direct vision.
6. Insert the laparoscope to assure that the trocar is in the proper position and that there is a free space in the peritoneal cavity.
7. Secure the trocar in place with sutures or other securing mechanisms to prevent its dislodgment.
8. Begin insufflation with CO_2 to 8-12 mm Hg as tolerated.
9. Insert **secondary trocars** sharply.

a. Make a small skin incision at the trocar insertion site.
b. Insert the trocar while observing the procedure with the laparoscope in place.
c. As the trocar is inserted with a steady downward pressure, elevate the abdominal wall medial to the point of insertion to flatten the abdominal wall.
d. As soon as the tip of the trocar can be seen entering the peritoneal cavity (and thus "snagging" the peritoneum), aim the trocar directly for the camera, which is withdrawn into its cannula. (In this way, with the trocar aimed at the camera, the tip of the trocar is always in site and cannot cause visceral or vascular injury).

10. Trocar sites can be infiltrated with a **long-lasting local anesthetic** (at the time of trocar insertion for short procedures and at the end of the procedure for long procedures), keeping in mind appropriate dose limitations to avoid drug toxicity.

F. Selected References

Blucher D, Lobe TE. Minimal access surgery in children: The state of the art. Internat Surg 79:317-321, 1994.

Lobe TE. Laparoscopy in infants and children. In Spitz L, Coran AG (eds) Rob and Smith's Operative Surgery, Chapman and Hall Medical, London UK, pp 308-319, 1995.

Lobe TE, Schropp KP, eds. Pediatric Laparoscopy and Thoracoscopy. Philadelphia, WB Saunders, 1994.

Lobe TE. Evolving Laparoscopic and Thoracoscopic Procedures in Infants and Children in Gadacz TR, Howell CG Jr (eds) Laparoscopic Surgery, Decker Periodicals, Hamilton, Ontario, Canada, pp 184-204, 1993.

Rogers Da, Lobe TE, Schropp KP. Evolving uses of laparoscopy in children. Surg Clin N Amer 72:1299-1313, 1992.

37.1. Pediatric Laparoscopy: Specific Surgical Procedures I

Anthony Sandler, M.D.

A. Appendectomy

Laparoscopic **appendectomy** may be a beneficial procedure for the obese patient, a teenage female patient, and for the patient with chronic abdominal pain in whom the diagnosis of appendicitis is in question. For the thin, small child, this approach is not beneficial. The potential advantages of the laparoscopic approach should be weighed individually and this technique should be used selectively in children.

1. Place a 12-mm cannula through the umbilical "cut-down" site, and two 5-mm ports in the left lower quadrant and suprapubic region, respectively.
2. Pass a grasper (held in the left hand) through the suprapubic port and grasp the appendix. Elevate the appendix toward the anterior abdominal wall.
3. Use a dissector (held in the right hand) to create a window in the mesoappendix.
4. Once exploration, dissection, and mobilization are complete, place a 5-mm laparoscope through the left lower quadrant port.
5. Pass an endoscopic linear stapling device (vascular load) through the umbilical port.
6. Ligate and divide the mesoappendix and appendix with the endoscopic stapler.
7. An alternate technique similar to that of adults can be used in larger children. This technique utilizes a 5-mm umbilical port for the camera, a 5-mm right upper quadrant port for instrumentation, and a 10- to 12-mm port in the right lower quadrant for clips and stapling instruments.

B. Cholecystectomy

Laparoscopic cholecystectomy is preferred to an open technique and is indicated in children with cholelithiasis. Causes of cholelithiasis in children include chronic hemolysis, total parenteral nutrition, and cystic fibrosis.

1. Use a four-cannula technique similar to that for adults with some modifications.
   a. Consider placing the epigastric port more to the patients left.

    b.   In infants and small children, the liver can extend well below the costal margin; thus, the subcostal ports should be placed with this in mind.

    c.   The right-sided lowest port can be placed closer to the inguinal crease and a 5-mm telescope is satisfactory for use in smaller children.

    d.   A 10- or 5-mm port is required for insertion of the endoscopic clip applier.

2.   The technique of laparoscopic cholecystectomy is similar to that for adults.

3.   If cholelithiasis is present in a child with hereditary spherocytosis undergoing laproscopic splenectomy, the gallbladder is removed prior to splenectomy at the same laparoscopic operative setting.

C. Splenectomy

Laparoscopic Splenectomy may be the procedure of choice for removal of the normal or near-normal-sized spleen.

1.   Position the patient in the right lateral decubitus position (Fig. 37.1.1). Utilize a four-port technique.

2.   The operating table can be **flexed at the flank position** to widen the distance between the rib edge and the superior iliac crest. This will improve the work space of the left lateral port.

3.   A 30-degree laparoscope will improve exposure of the left upper quadrant.

4.   Divide the inferior attachments of the spleen, including the splenocolic and peritoneal attachments, with cautery or the ultrasonic scalpel.

5.   Make a window in the gastrosplenic ligament and individually divide the short gastric vessels with the ultrasonic scalpel or hemoclips.

6.   Control the splenic hilar blood supply with an endoscopic vascular loaded linear stapler (author's preference), or individually ligate the artery and vein with hemoclips.

7.   Use a large, spring-loaded, sturdy laparoscopic bag for splenic retrieval and morcellation.

8.   Morcellate the spleen by passing a ring forceps into the mid-subcostal port site and crushing and extracting the spleen.

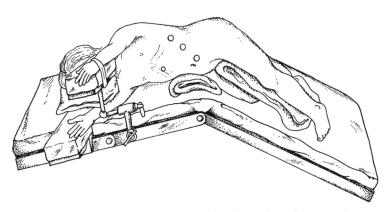

Figure 37.1.1. Patient position and trocar sites for pediatric laparoscopic splenectomy. Note that the patient is in the lateral position, and the operating table has been flexed to increase the distance between costal margin and superior ilac crest.

D. Fundoplication

Avoiding a large upper abdominal incision is of special benefit to neurologically impaired children in need of an antireflux procedure. Due to the high incidence of postoperative pulmonary complications, this group of patients can benefit immensely from a laparoscopic approach.

1. Position the patient supine.
2. Use a four-cannula technique. A fifth cannula may be needed for retraction of the left hepatic lobe (Fig. 37.1.2).
3. Port positioning and technique is similar to that for adults (see Chapter 16).
4. Complete and partial (posterior or anterior) fundoplication can be satisfactorily performed in children.
5. The short gastric vessels may be divided with the ultrasonic scalpel or hemoclips, but this step is not always necessary if a loose and tension free wrap is easily achieved.
6. An endostitch suturing device is useful for creating the fundic wrap of choice.

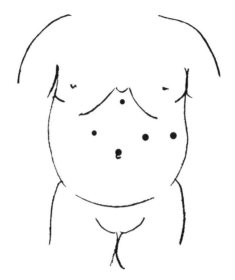

Figure 37.1.2. Port site placement for pediatric laparoscopic fundoplication. The right upper quadrant port is optional and used for retracting the left hepatic lobe.

7. Judge the correct size of bougie to use while constructing the wrap by the size of the esophagus. Generally a 26- to 28-French bougie is used in small infants, a 40-French bougie in young children, and a 50-to 60-French bougie in adolescents.
8. Several techniques for placing a gastrostomy tube following fundoplication have been described, but placement of a percutaneous endoscopic gastrostomy (PEG) tube under direct vision with the laparoscope is safe and efficient.

E. Gastrostomy

The laparoscopically guided technique is especially useful in children needing a gastrostomy tube who have marked spinal deformities. PEG placement is often difficult and hazardous in these patients due to the abnormal anatomic position of the stomach. The technique is essentially a laparoscopically guided PEG technique (see Chapter 43.2.6, Percutaneous Endoscopic Feeding Tube Placement).

1. This technique is useful when the "light reflex" reflected from the endoscope through the anterior abdominal wall is unsatisfactory.
2. Place a 5-mm laparoscope through an umbilical port and use minimal insufflation—just sufficient to obtain a clear view of the stomach during PEG placement.
3. The PEG is performed in the usual fashion, with laparoscopic confirmation.

F. Laparoscopy for Undescended Testis

The benefits of an initial laparoscopic approach in the management of a nonpalpable testis include the ability to explore for an intraabdominal testis, and the opportunity to ligate vessels for the first stage of a Fowler-Stevens orchiopexy. Laparoscopic orchiectomy is also advocated in teenagers and younger children with an atrophic testis or ambiguous external genitalia. In approximately 15 to 20% of patients with an empty scrotum, the testis is not palpated and laparoscopic exploration via an umbilical port is then performed:

1. If an **intraabdominal testis** is found, the vascular pedicle is ligated approximately 1 cm from the testis using a 2 or 3 port technique. Six to nine months later, the patient returns for the second stage of the Fowler-Stevens orchiopexy at which time the testis is nourished by vasal collateral supply.
2. If an **atrophic residual intraabdominal testis** is noted, a laparoscopic orchiectomy can be performed.
3. If **no testis** is detected on laparoscopic exploration and a blind ending cord is noted, the procedure is concluded.
4. If **the cord passes into the internal inguinal ring**, the laparoscope is removed and an inguinal exploration is done in standard fashion.

G. Ovarian Pathology

Ovarian pathology can cause abdominal pain in adolescents as the result of rupture of a cyst, hemorrhage, or torsion.

1. Laparoscopic exploration is carried out through an umbilical port.
2. Insert an additional 5 mm trocar either suprapubically or on the ipsilateral side to aide in detorsion of the ovary.
3. Identify a torsed ovary by the congested appearance of the adnexa. If no permanent injury is observed, untwist the lesion.
4. If the ovary is not viable, or if a neoplastic lesion is suspected, then the ovary may be removed laparoscopically or the procedure converted to an open laparotomy.
5. Ovarian cystectomy can also be performed laparoscopically if a simple cyst is noted.

H. Pull-Through Operation for Hirschsprung's Disease

Hirschsprung's disease is characterized by bowel obstruction secondary to congenital absence of ganglia in both the myenteric and submucosal plexus of the distal colon. The extent of the diseased colon is variable, but always involves the rectum and extends proximally. Absence of ganglia in the enteric plexuses results in failure of relaxation and peristalsis of the involved bowel. Long-term follow-up is needed for validation of laparoscopic techniques in the management of this disease, but the Duhamel, Swenson, and Soave type colo-anal pull-through procedures have all been performed by a laparoscopic approach.

1. Three 5 mm ports and one 10 mm port are used with the patient placed horizontally across the table (Figure 37.1.3).
2. A one or two stage procedure protected with a colostomy may be used.
3. In both a "Swenson and Soave type" laparoscopic approach, the extramuscular dissection is done laparoscopically from above, while the mucosectomy and anastomosis are performed from below.
4. The "Duhamel type" procedure is performed by mobilizing colon from above and then pulling it through retrorectally from below.
5. The "Duhamel" is completed with the endo GIA stapler which is used to fashion the common channel between the aganglionic rectum and ganglionic retrorectal colon by transecting and stapling the common spur from below.

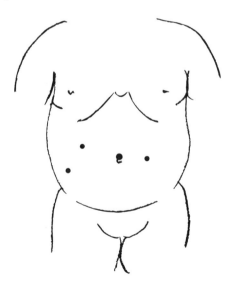

Figure 37.1.3. Port site placement for the laparoscopic approach to colo-anal pull-through in Hirschsprung's disease.

I. Meckel's Diverticulectomy

A Meckel's diverticulum usually presents with massive, painless, lower gastrointestinal bleeding in children. More rarely, intussusception and/or abdominal pain can be the presenting scenario. The diagnosis is often made preoperatively with a technetium Meckel's scan (99^m Tc).

1. Explore the abdomen through a 5 or 10 mm umbilical port.
2. Place a 5 mm port on the right side and another 10 or 5 mm port is placed on the left. (Lower quadrants in larger children).
3. Identify the ileocecal junction then follow the small bowel retrograde using blunt grasping forceps.
4. The vascular supply of the diverticulum can either be dissected separately or included in the resection of the diverticulum.
5. Place a stapling device across the base of the diverticulum transversely to avoid narrowing the lumen with transection.
6. Remove the diverticulum through the 10 mm port.
7. Check the staple line for both hemostatis and leakage.
8. Open the resected specimen on the back table to confirm complete resection of aberrant ectopic mucosa.
9. If inadequate resection is noted, the bowel can be exteriorized or a laparotomy should be performed using a right lower quadrant transverse incision to complete the resection.

J. Selected References

Collins JB 3rd, Georgeson KE, Vicente Y, Hardin Jr WD. Comparison of open and laparoscopic gastrostomy and fundoplication in 120 patients. J Pediatr Surg 1995;30(7):1065–1071.

Fitzgerald PG, Langer JC, Cameron BH, et al. Pediatric laparoscopic splenectomy using the lateral approach. Surg Endosc 1996;10:859–861.

Kim PC, Wesson D, Superina R, Filler R. Laparoscopic cholecystectomy versus open cholecystectomy in children: Which is better? J Pediatr Surg 1995;30(7):971–973.

Georgeson KE, Fuenfer MM, Hardin WD. Primary laparoscopic pull-through for Hirschsprung disease in infants and children. J Pediatr Surg 1995;30(7):1017-1022.

Curran TJ, Raffensperger JG. Laparoscopic Swenson pull-through: A comparison with the open procedure. J Pediatr Surg 1996;31(8):1155-1157.

Brock JW 3rd, Holcomb GW 3rd, Morgan WM 3rd. The use of laparoscopy in the management of the nonpalpable testis. J Laparoendosc Surg 1996;6(1):S35-39.

Teitelbaum DH, Polly TZ, Obeid F. Laparoscopic diagnosis and excision of Meckel's diverticulum. J Pediatr Surg 1994;29(4):495-497.

37.2. Pediatric Laparoscopy: Specific Surgical Procedures II

Thom E. Lobe, M.D.

A. Diagnostic Laparoscopy and Cancer Staging

This topic is also discussed in Chapter 12, Elective Diagnostic Laparoscopy and Cancer Staging.

1. **Formal abdominal staging** procedures in children are rarely performed today. Lymphomas, germ cell tumors, rhadbomyosrcomas, liver tumors, neuroblastoma, and Wilm's tumor are among the malignancies for which staging may be appropriate. Splenectomy, lymph node sampling, liver, and other biopsies can all be done laparoscopically.
   a. Start with the splenectomy.
   b. Extend the dissection down to the pelvis for the retroperitoneal node sampling.
   c. Perform liver biopsies as the last procedure.
2. **Liver biopsies** can be accomplished by any one of several techniques.
   a. Superficial biopsies can be carried out using a cup biopsy forceps.
   b. Percutaneous Tru-Cut needle biopsies under direct laparoscopic control.
   c. The endoscopic stapler can be used for an excisional biopsy.
   d. Endoscopic sutures can be placed for a standard wedge biopsy.
3. **Retroperitoneal node sampling.**
   a. Position the patient in the lateral position for the para-aortic node dissection, and in reverse Trendelenburg position for pelvic nodes.
   b. Divide the peritoneum in an avascular plane.
   c. Sample individual nodes according to the specific disease protocol.
   d. If biopsies are being performed based upon lymphangiograms, x-rays can be taken in the operating room to confirm excision of the proper nodes.

B. Pyloromyotomy

1. Position the patient supine.
2. The surgeon stands on the patient's right side with the assistant on the patient's left.
3. Two video monitors are used, one on either side, at the head of the table in the line of sight of the surgeon and surgical assistant. It is easiest for the camera operator to stand immediately to the left of the assistant.
4. Insert a 5-mm or smaller cannula into the infraumbilical site for the laparoscope.
5. With the laparoscope in place, use a #11 blade to make a stab wound just above the level of the umbilicus, lateral to the rectus muscle. A retractable, round-ended, disposable arthroscopy blade is inserted via this stab wound.
6. Make a mirror image stab wound for the direct insertion of a 2.7-mm grasper to grasp the stomach proximal to the pyloric tumor.
7. Make a shallow incision in the pyloric muscle, beginning on the distal antrum and extending it distally to a point just shy of the pyloric vein.
8. Retract the blade and use its protective sheath to deepen the incision by inserting the sheath into the incision and turning the instrument perpendicular to the axis of the incision.
9. Replace the arthroscopy blade with a 2.7-mm pyloric spreader and use it to gently spread the muscle.
10. Grasp the edges of the muscle and confirm that they move independently of each other, indicating that the pyloric ring has been suitably divided.
11. Inflate the stomach via a naso- or orogastric tube to check for leaks.
12. Close the umbilical incision with sutures. Simply Steri-strip the stab wounds.

C. Contralateral Groin Exploration During Herniorraphy

1. Position the patient supine on the operating table.
2. The surgeon stands on the side of the symptomatic hernia.
3. Place the video monitor at the foot of the table or directly across from the surgeon.
4. Open the hernia sac on the symptomatic side.
5. Insert a 4-mm cannula into the peritoneal cavity.
6. Use a suture to secure the hernia sac and prevent leakage of CO_2.
7. Pass an angled 70° laparoscope into the cannula to inspect the contralateral side.

D. Selected References

Bufo AJ, Merry C, Shah R, Cyr N, Schropp KP, Lobe TE. Laparoscopic pyloromyotomy: A safer technique. Pediatr Surg Int, (in press).

Lobe TE, Rao BN: Laparoscopy for paediatric oncology patient. Gaslini 27:119-129, 1995.

Lobe TE, Schropp KP, Joyner R, Lasater O, Jenkins J. The suitability of automatic tissue morcellation for the endoscopic removal of large specimens in pediatric surgery. J Pediatr Surg 29:232-234, 1994.

Lobe TE, Schropp KP. Inguinal hernias in pediatrics: Initial experience with laparoscopic inguinal exploration of the asymptomatic contralateral side. Laparoendosc Surg 2:135-140, 1992.

38. Pediatric Laparoscopy: Complications

Thom E. Lobe, M.D.

A. General Laparoscopic Complications

1. **Veress–needle associated visceral and vascular injuries**
    a. **Cause and prevention:** The Veress needle does not offer any particular advantage in pediatric cases, except perhaps in the obese child. An open technique is preferred.
    b. **Recognition and management:** These injuries are usually recognized upon introduction of the telescope for initial inspection and should be treated according to the nature of the injury (see Section 4, Access to Abdomen).
2. **Trocar site hernias**
    a. **Cause and prevention:** Close the fascia for all trocar sites greater than 3 mm.
    b. **Recognition and management:** A bulge is usually noted at the site of a trocar insertion. Operative repair is usually required.
3. **Abdominal wall hemorrhage**
    a. **Cause and prevention:** This occurs when abdominal wall vessels are injured at the time of trocar insertion. Care should be taken to avoid abdominal wall vessels during trocar insertion.
    b. **Recognition and management:** This is usually a self-limiting problem in children and rarely requires suture repair.
4. **Abdominal wall crepitus**
    a. **Cause and prevention:** This is caused by dissection of CO_2 gas into tissue planes and is often seen after extensive laparoscopic surgery in children.
    b. **Recognition and management:** This is usually self-limiting and disappears in 24 to 36 hours. If the problem persists and is accompanied by high fever with erythema and tenderness of the abdominal wall, infection with a gas-producing organism should be suspected and aggressive antibiotic coverage with or without operative debridement should be considered.
5. **Remote bowel injury**
    a. **Cause and prevention:** Monopolar electrocautery has been implicated in bowel injuries to segments of intestine that were not visible to the telescope during the procedure. The use of alternative energy sources such as bipolar devices or the ultrasonically activated scissors should minimize the risk of these injuries.

b. **Recognition and management:** Such injuries should be searched for carefully. If they are recognized at the time of laparoscopy, antibiotics should be started or continued and the area of injury should be repaired. Unrecognized injuries present late, with signs and symptoms of peritonitis. Abdominal exploration with repair or ostomy should be undertaken.

B. Complications of Specific Surgical Procedures

1. **Laparoscopic appendectomy**
   a. **Wound infection**
      i. **Cause and prevention:** Contamination of wound during procedure. Can be prevented by extracting appendix using tissue pouches or by extracting the appendix through the cannula without allowing it to touch the abdominal wall tissue directly. Prophylactic antibiotic use with a broad-spectrum cephalosporin may prevent wound infections in trocar sites.
      ii. **Recognition and management:** Red erythematous wound, or purulent drainage. Incision and drainage of wound and appropriate antibiotic coverage if significant cellulitis exists should be sufficient to treat most infections.
   b. **Postoperative pelvic fluid collections and abscesses**
      i. **Cause and prevention:** These conditions may be seen after laparoscopic appendectomy for ruptured appendicitis, but are no greater in their frequency than similar complications after open appendectomy for ruptured appendicitis. They may be related to inadequate evacuation of irrigation fluid. Meticulous evacuation of all irrigant should be the rule as should evacuation of all pus.
      ii. **Recognition and management:** Patients may do well initially, but later have increasing symptoms of abdominal pain, fever, and possibly bowel obstruction. These fluid collections should be drained by percutaneous methods under diagnostic imaging if possible or by surgery.
   c. **A lost fecalith**
      i. **Cause and prevention:** Disruption of the appendix during its removal may cause this problem. Careful attention should be paid to location of the fecalith and removing it if one is present.
      ii. **Recognition and management:** Being aware of this possibility is half the battle. If the fecalith is lost, most likely it will form the nidus for an infection or abscess that will require drainage.

2. **Cholecystectomy**
   a. The complications of cholecystectomy in children are the same as in adults.
   b. **Bile duct injury at the time of cholangiography and/or common duct exploration**
      i. **Cause and prevention:** The bile duct in infants and children is much smaller than it is in adults. Great care should be taken if these procedures are performed.
      ii. **Recognition and management:** Injury to the bile ducts should be foremost on the mind of the surgeon carrying out these maneuvers. If the injury is minimal, a simple suture repair may be sufficient. A T-tube may be difficult to place in these small ducts using laparoscopic technique. An open repair, with or without a choledochojejunostomy, should be considered.

3. **Hernia exploration**
   a. **Tear of the hernia sac on the symptomatic side**
      i. **Cause and prevention:** Rough handling of the thin hernia sac in small infants can result in a tear of the sac.
      ii. **Recognition and management:** This problem is recognized immediately. The torn sac can be repaired using a purse-string suture at the internal inguinal ring to close the defect.
   b. **Missed hernia or patent processus vaginalis**
      i. **Cause and prevention:** Any abnormality may represent a hernia. If exploration is not performed, then there remains the risk of the development of a symptomatic hernia.
      ii. **Recognition and management:** Inspection of the inguinal canal from inside the abdomen should demonstrate a flat or concave surface with no opening. The slightest pin hole can represent a hernia as can a veil covering the opening to the inguinal canal. If the anatomy is not perfectly normal, the open exploration of the contralateral groin should be undertaken.

4. **Pyloromyotomy**
   a. **A mucosal tear**
      i. **Cause and prevention:** The pyloric mucosa is close to the pyloroduodenal junction. Care should be taken not to extend the pyloromyotomy too far distally.
      ii. **Recognition and management:** Insufflation of air into the stomach by the anesthesiologist while the surgeon watches the pyloromyotomy site for leaks should be routine. If a leak is noted, a simple suture repair with 6-0 or 7-0 suture should be done and the omentum, if sufficient, should be tacked over the repair.

b. **An inadequate pyloromyotomy**

   i. **Cause and prevention:** The pyloromyotomy should extend from the distal antrum of the stomach to just short of the pyloric vein.

   ii. **Recognition and management:** The upper and lower margin of the pyloromyotomy should be grasped and moved from side to side to assure that the two margins move independently and that the muscular pyloric ring is disrupted. If this is not the case, the pyloromyotomy should be extended by additional spreading of the muscle with the pyloric spreader. Occasionally, an additional cut toward the duodenum will be necessary. Great care should be taken in this case to avoid a mucosal injury. If persistent vomiting exists postoperatively, an upper gastrointestinal contrast study should be carried out to confirm that the pylorus is still causing an obstruction. If this is the case, a redo pyloromyotomy must be performed.

5. **Fundoplication**

a. The complications of fundoplication are essentially the same in children and adults.

b. **Gastric volvulus**

   i. **Cause and prevention:** This can result from placing the gastrostomy too close to the pylorus.

   ii. **Recognition and management:** Acute gastric distention and shock may result. A plain abdominal radiograph will demonstrate a hugely dilated stomach. Immediate laparotomy after fluid resuscitation and antibiotic administration should be performed to detorsion the stomach and to replace the gastrostomy in a better location.

c. **Esophageal tear**

   i. **Cause and prevention:** The esophagus can be injured during its dissection mobilization. Placing a bougie in the esophagus as large as the esophagus can accommodate during the initial dissection will aide in identification of the structure and help to prevent dissection through its wall into the lumen.

   ii. **Recognition and management:** During dissection of the esophagus, careful inspection for mucosa or luminal contents should be routine. If the esophagus is injured, a simple suture repair that is covered by the wrap should be sufficient.

d. Hourglass stomach

   i. **Cause and prevention:** In severe stricture disease, the esophagus may be shorted and thus difficult to mobilize into the abdomen. Caution must be taken in these cases to assure that the wrap is not misplaced onto the cardia of the stomach to form an hourglass stomach.

    ii. **Recognition and management:** Careful inspection of the gastroesophageal junction should be the rule. The wrap should sit at this level and not at the junction of the cardia and body of the stomach. If the esophagus is too short for a proper wrap, consideration should be given to a Collis-Nissen procedure.

  e. **Liver hemorrhage**

    i. **Cause and prevention:** The liver in the child is often floppy and difficult to retract. Sharp instruments and needles can easily injure the liver and cause hemorrhage.

    ii. **Recognition and management:** The problem can be prevented by using blunt instruments for liver retraction. A ratcheting grasper, grasping the diaphragm above the esophageal hiatus, makes a useful retractor in some cases. Placement of an additional grasper from the left lateral costal margin to grasp the falciform ligament may help to elevate a floppy left lobe of the liver. Deflation of the abdomen with gentle pressure on the area of injury should be sufficient to stop most hemorrhage as long as no coagulopathy exists. Major hemorrhage warrants laparotomy and resection or repair of the injured segment of liver or repair of any injured vessels.

  f. **Hemorrhage from short gastric vessels**

    i. **Cause and prevention:** Short gastric vessels that are divided before adequate hemostasis is achieved will retract and can be difficult to control. Meticulous hemostasis should be established before division of these vessels.

    ii. **Recognition and management:** Hemorrhage and the inability to stop it is obvious. It may be difficult to see the vessels that are the source of the hemorrhage in the left upper quadrant. Additional instruments may need to be inserted for retraction and exposure. If hemodynamic instability develops, conversion to laparotomy should be considered.

6. **Splenectomy**

  a. **Missed accessory spleen**

    i. **Cause and prevention:** Accessory spleen should be searched for and removed.

    ii. **Recognition and management:** In cases of ITP or hereditary spherocytosis that remain symptomatic after laparoscopic splenectomy, and in which a radionuclide spleen scan shows residual splenic tissue, reexploration with removal of the retained accessory spleen should be performed.

  b. **Hemorrhage from short gastric vessels**

    i. **Cause and prevention:** Short gastric vessels that are divided before adequate hemostasis is achieved will retract and can be difficult to control. Meticulous hemostasis should be established before division of these vessels.

ii. **Recognition and management:** Hemorrhage and the inability to stop it is obvious. It may be difficult to see the vessels that are the source of the hemorrhage in the left upper quadrant. Additional instruments may need to be inserted for retraction and exposure. If hemodynamic instability develops, conversion to laparotomy should be considered.

c. **Hilar vessel hemorrhage**

i. **Cause and prevention:** Hilar vessels can be a source of hemorrhage if they are not properly ligated. Mass ligature is effective and has not caused any arteriovenous fistulae or other problems.

ii. **Recognition and management:** Hemorrhage is immediately apparent. If hemorrhage is severe enough to cause hemodynamic instability, immediate conversion to laparotomy should be performed. If hemorrhage is minor, the placement of additional clips, staples or sutures, or the use of an energy source to stop the hemorrhage may be sufficient.

d. **Pancreatic injury**

i. **Cause and Prevention:** The pancreas can be injured in the course of dissection if care is not taken to differentiate fat from pancreas.

ii. **Recognition and management:** Stapling across the tail of the pancreas if the injury is distal will usually treat the injury.

e. **Colon injury**

i. **Cause and prevention:** The colon can be injured in the course of dissection if care is not taken.

ii. **Recognition and management:** Suture repair may be possible. If the injury or fecal contamination is severe, particularly in immune-suppressed patients, then colostomy should be considered.

f. **Gastric injury**

i. **Cause and prevention:** Care should be taken not to injure the stomach when dividing the short gastric vessels. The use of energy devices to cauterize and divide these vessels is the usual cause.

ii. **Recognition and management:** If a gastric injury is suspected because the short gastric vessels were particularly short, then suture reinforcement of the stomach should be performed. Postoperative peritonitis or massive free air should raise suspicion of a gastric injury. The injury can be confirmed with an upper gastrointestinal contrast study, and laparotomy should be performed for repair.

g. **Splenic disruption during attempted retrieval**

   i. **Cause and prevention:** Large spleen may be too big for the tissue retrieval sac.

   ii. **Recognition and management:** That the spleen is too large for the retrieval sac should be obvious, especially if repeated attempts to place the spleen in the bag fail. After being freed, the large spleen can be divided in the left upper quadrant in a controlled fashion and removed in segments. The right upper quadrant should then be copiously irrigated to remove any splenic remains. This approach has not resulted in any splenosis such as may be seen after traumatic splenic injury.

h. **Postsplenectomy sepsis**

   i. **Cause and prevention:** Postsplenectomy sepsis can occur and thus patients should receive the appropriate vaccines against pneumococcus and *Haemophilus influenzae*, and should take prophylactic penicillin daily.

   ii. **Recognition and management:** Postsplenectomy sepsis can occur at any time after splenectomy and is usually recognized by the rapid onset and progression of a febrile illness to a picture of full-blown sepsis and shock in a matter of hours. Aggressive broad-spectrum antibiotics and hemodynamic and respiratory support should be taken as appropriate.

i. **Shoulder pain**

   i. **Cause and prevention:** While the precise cause is unknown, diaphragmatic irritation during dissection is probably causative.

   ii. **Recognition and management:** This is usually rare in children and is self-limited. If it persists and is accompanied by fever, a left subphrenic abscess should be searched for.

7. **Staging for cancer**

a. **Vascular injury**

   i. **Cause and prevention:** Vascular injury can be avoided be careful dissection.

   ii. **Recognition and management:** Major injuries may require conversion to laparotomy and vascular repair.

b. **Ureteral injury**

   i. **Cause and prevention:** Care should be taken during dissection in the retroperitoneum and pelvis to identify the ureter in order to prevent its injury.

   ii. **Recognition and management:** Immediate injury, recognized by urine leak, should be repaired. Delayed injury, recognized by the development of a urinoma with or without associated signs of sepsis or obstructive uropathy should be treated by drainage and repair.

c. **Liver hemorrhage**
   i. **Cause and prevention:** Care should be taken at the time of liver biopsy.
   ii. **Recognition and management:** Simple deflation of the abdomen with gentle pressure for 5 or 10 minutes will stop most hemorrhage unless a coagulopathy is present. Microfibrillar collagen or fibrin glue application may be useful. Brisk live hemorrhage that is uncontrolled by simple pressure maneuvers or suturing may require conversion to laparotomy for control with suture ligation or segmental resection as necessary.

39. Characteristics of Flexible Endoscopes, Troubleshooting, and Equipment Care

Jeffrey L. Ponsky, M.D., F.A.C.S.
Carol E.H. Scott-Conner, M.D., F.A.C.S.

A. Characteristics of Flexible Endoscopes

Flexible endoscopy provided a quantum leap in the area of diagnosis and therapy of the aerodigestive tract.

1. **Optical properties** of flexible endoscopes. Two types of flexible endoscopes are currently in use: flexible fiberoptic endoscopes and video endoscopic systems. Each will be considered briefly here.

    a. **Fiberoptic endoscopes** are based upon fiberoptic light transmission technology. Light is conveyed through a bundle of fine glass fibers, each smaller than a human hair (8 to 10 Mm in diameter), packed tightly together.

        i. Each individual fiber is clad in a wrapping of greater optical density, creating a reflective layer that causes light to bounce back and forth within the fiber with little loss of light. This cladding does not transmit light itself, creating a dark rim around the portion of the image produced by each fiber and accounting for the characteristic newsprint-like image produced by fiberoptic endoscopes (Fig. 39.1).

        ii. Thousands of fibers are packed tightly together in a bundle, each carrying a small parcel of light to or from a portion of the viewing area.

        iii. One bundle of fibers carries light into the examined organ, and a second bundle transmits the image from the organ interior to the viewing optic.

        iv. The latter bundle must have all the fibers arranged in a "coherent bundle" (that is, in the same spatial arrangement at both ends of the fiber so that the portion of the total image that each carried would be in its proper position).

        v. Major disadvantages with flexible fiberoptic endoscopes include fragility. When individual fibers break, light transmission is decreased and the visual image develops dark spots (corresponding to the broken fibers).

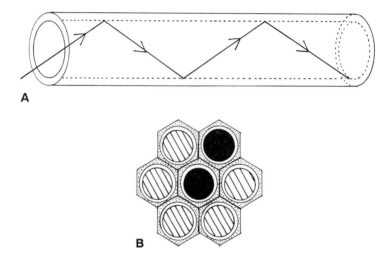

Figure 39.1. A. Internal reflection is assured by cladding each fiber with a coating of high refractive index. Virtually all light is reflected back and forth within the fiber with little loss. B. The image produced by a fiberoptic endoscope is composed of a multitude of images transmitted by each individual fiber. Broken fibers do not transmit light, resulting in black dropouts in the image.

      vi. These endoscopes are generally direct-viewing endoscopes. The endoscopist looks directly into an eyepiece. An optical beam splitter allows a second observer to view the image. Alternatively, a small video camera may be placed on the end of the endoscope and the image viewed on a video screen.

  b. **Video-endoscopy** applies video technology to endoscopy, with significant improvements in image quality and endoscope durability. An increasing number of the endoscopes in use today are video-endoscopes.

      i. Light is transmitted to the tip of the endoscope through a fiberoptic bundle, as in the endoscopes described above.

      ii. The viewing fiberoptic bundle is replaced with a charge-coupled device (CCD) chip camera placed at the tip of the endoscope. This chip carries a digital image back to a video processor, which displays an image on a color monitor.

      iii. The CCD chip camera uses a dense grid of photocell receptors, each of which generates a single pixel on the monitor. Resolution depends on the density of receptor packing on the chip camera.

      iv. Some video-endoscopes use a single color (e.g., black-white) CCD chip and create color images by rapidly cycling through a color wheel. Newer video-endoscopes use three-color CCD chips and provide the most accurate color resolution.

      v. Most video-endoscopes incorporate an automatic iris in the system to decrease the problem of glare due to tissue reflection.

2. Flexible endoscopes provide one or more **channels** for passage of diagnostic and therapeutic instruments as well as for suctioning. Air and water insufflation channels permit distention of the bowel and cleaning of the lens.

3. **Tip deflection** is controlled by rotating wheels on the headpiece. Locks are provided. For most purposes, the wheels should be allowed to move freely (Fig. 39.2).

4. Modern endoscopes also include electronic systems to capture still images and record video footage.

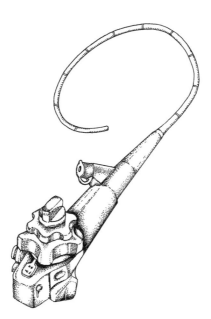

Figure 39.2. Rotating wheels on the headpiece of the endoscope control tip deflection. Instruments may be passed through an access port, which is kept capped when not in use (to prevent loss of insufflation and splashing with fluids).

B. Equipment Setup

The equipment for flexible endoscopy is generally arranged on a multiple level cart, which allows access to all the equipment and easy mobility. The cart generally includes a monitor, video processor, light source, water bottle, and an image printer (Fig. 39.3).

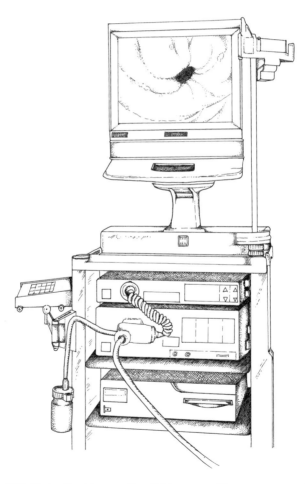

Figure 39.3. Cart with video monitor, light source, video processor, water bottle, and image printer. A keyboard allows entry of patient and physician name, patient number, date, and any additional documentation desired.

1. A fiberoptic cable connects the endoscope to the light source. This umbilical cable also contains connectors for suction, water, and insufflation.
2. Air (for insufflation) and water are introduced through a common channel by depression of a trumpet-like valve on the control head of the scope.
    a. Partial depression of the valve insufflates air.
    b. Complete depression of the valve forces the air backward, causing increased pressure in the attached water bottle and forcing a stream of water to the tip of the instrument where it serves to wash the lens.
    c. Depression of an adjacent trumpet valve enables the suction function of the instrument.
    d. Insufflation, irrigation, and suction should be tested each time the endoscope is used.
3. Common problems include sticky valves, lack of water in the water bottle, failure to secure all connections, or leaks in the valve apparatus.
4. Become well versed in the construction and function of the particular endoscopic system in use. Accurate assessment of problems arising during a procedure often allows rapid resolution.
5. Adopt a standard approach to equipment setup. Problems commonly arise when one or another step is forgotten.
    a. Choose the appropriate size (length and diameter) and type of endoscope for the intended purpose. Both pediatric and adult upper gastrointestinal endoscopes are available, for example.
    b. Connect the umbilical cable of the endoscope to the light source.
    c. Turn on all electronic equipment on the cart, even if use of a particular item (for example, a VCR) is not planned. The connections of the various pieces of equipment may require that all be on for any to work properly.
    d. Ensure that the water bottle is filled with clean water.
    e. Connect the hose from the water bottle to the side of the umbilical cable, near where it enters the light box. Generally the fittings are arranged with a Luer-lock or other mating set of connectors, so that the hose can only connect to one place.
    f. Connect suction to the remaining site on the umbilical cord.
    g. Obtain a cup or basin of water and test insufflation (by insufflation air under water and observing bubbles), water irrigation (with the tip of the endoscope out of the water), and suction (by aspirating the water from the cup). If any of these functions are sluggish or nonfunctional, first check the connections. (See Troubleshooting, below, for additional tips.)
    h. Take the light source off standby and aim the tip of the endoscope into the cupped fingers of one hand. A sharp image of the fingers should be seen on the monitor.
    i. Check the tip deflection controls and verify that any locking devices are "off" so that the tip is free to move.

j. Verify that any additional items that may be required (such as biopsy forceps, polypectomy snares) are available, of appropriate size, and in good working order.

C. Troubleshooting

A systematic approach to identifying the problem, followed by creative measures to circumvent or repair the difficulty, will usually permit satisfactory completion of the examination. As mentioned previously, attention to detail during the setup phase can help minimize problems during the examination. Common problems and solutions are listed in Table 39.1.

Table 39.1. Common problems with flexible endoscopes and suggested solutions.

Problem	Check the Following
No light at distal end	1. Light source plugged in and turned on 2. Light source ignited 3. Not in "standby" mode 4. Lense at distal tip is dirty 5. Bulb burned out
Out of focus	1. Adjust focus ring 2. Fiberoptic scope—clean lens
No irrigation	1. Water bottle contains water 2. Water bottle connected to umbilical cord 3. Connection tight 4. Lid of water bottle screwed on tightly 5. Power turned on 6. Valve stuck or occluded
No insufflation	1. Umbilical cord firmly seated into light source and screwed in if necessary 2. Power turned on 3. Valve stuck or occluded
Clogged valve or nozzle	1. Take valve apart and clean 2. Flush channel of endoscope with cleaning solution, followed by clean water

Table 39.1. continued

Problem	Check the Following
Difficulty passing instrument	1. Check tip angulation; decrease angulation and try again 2. Ensure that the instrument is fully closed 3. Check size of instrument relative to instrument channel; try smaller diameter instrument.

D. Equipment Care

Flexible endoscopes are expensive and relatively fragile. Attention to care is important.

1. The light fibers are fragile and easily broken. Coil the endoscope into gentle curves, rather than folding it in acute angles. Do not drop the endoscope, allow a wheeled cart to roll over it, or allow the patient to bite down on the endoscope.

2. Avoid extreme angulation of the tip wherever possible. Do not force biopsy forceps or other instruments down the channel when the tip is sharply angulated, as damage to the biopsy channel may result.

3. Ensure that polypectomy snares and sclerosing needles are fully withdrawn into the sheath before passing through the channel. Lubricate instruments with a suitable lubricant to facilitate passage.

4. The outer coating of the endoscope is delicate, particularly in the region near the tip. A rubber sheath, designed to flex as the tip bends, covers this region of the endoscope.

5. After each use, wash off any gross contamination and suction water through the endoscope. Do not allow blood, mucus, stool, or other foreign matter to dry on the endoscope or in the channels or valves.

6. Endoscopes are rarely actually sterilized. Generally high-level disinfection with a chemical agent (such as gluteraldehyde) is used. Disinfection does not work well when foreign matter (mucus, blood, enteric contents) are present. Therefore, the endoscope must be mechanically cleaned before disinfection. Many endoscopy suites use automated cleaners that rapidly wash, disinfect, and rinse the endoscope. Ultrasonic cleaners are available in some units.

7. Ethylene oxide gas sterilization is an option, but requires an overnight cycle. Newer methods of sterilization and newer endoscopes that are more tolerant of sterilizing conditions are being developed. Be careful to follow the manufacturer's instructions for sterilization to avoid potentially severe damage to the endoscope.

E. Selected References

Bordelon BM, Hunter JG. Endoscopic technology. In: Endoscopic Surgery. Greene FL, Ponsky JL (eds.). Philadelphia: WB Saunders, 1994, pp. 6–18.

Kawahara I, Ichikawa H. Fiberoptic instrument technology. In: Gastroenterologic Endoscopy. Sivak MV (ed.). Philadelphia: WB Saunders, 1987, pp. 20–41.

40. Endoscope Handling

Jeffrey L. Ponsky, M.D., F.A.C.S.

A. Room Setup

The room should have oxygen, suction, and monitoring devices. It should be sufficiently large to allow free movement around the gurney. Most endoscopic examinations are performed in rooms or suites specially designed for the purpose. Occasional endoscopy is done at the bedside in the intensive care unit, in the operating room, or in some other location.

Take a few minutes to consider the room layout and the proposed endoscopic examination before bringing the patient into the room or setting up the equipment.

1. The nature of the examination influences patient position and room setup.
   a. For **upper gastrointestinal endoscopy**, the patient will be positioned with the left side slightly down. The endoscopist faces the patient, standing at the patient's left side near the head of the bed. This provides easy access to the mouth and oropharynx.
   b. For **colonoscopy or flexible sigmoidoscopy**, the patient is usually positioned in the left lateral decubitus position and the endoscopist stands facing the back of the patient, just below the patient's buttocks. This generally puts the endoscopist on the opposite side of the gurney and requires an inverse room setup.
   c. If **both an upper gastrointestinal endoscopy and a colonoscopy** or flexible sigmoidoscopy are to be done on the same patient, it is often worthwhile to take the time to reverse the position of the patient (head to foot) on the gurney, or turn the gurney around, rather than deal with a less-than-optimal room setup for one of the two examinations.
2. The primary video monitor should be placed across from the endoscopist, in a direct line of sight. The endoscopy cart must be close to the intended working area.

B. Manipulation of the Endoscope

Some endoscopists use both hands to manipulate the controls of the endoscope, and ask an assistant to advance and withdraw the endoscope. Significantly greater control is attained if the endoscopist manipulates the controls with the left hand, and advances and withdraws the endoscope with the right hand. This is the method described here. There are no left-handed endoscopes, and this method is used by both right- and left-handed endoscopists. Specific techniques useful for performing various endoscopic examinations are given in the sections that follow.

1. Stand in a comfortable position, facing the patient and the video monitor (Fig. 40.1).

2. If the endoscope is a direct-viewing fiberoptic endoscope, hold it comfortably up to your eye. Avoid a hunched-over posture, which contributes to back and neck strain.

3. Cradle the endoscope in the upper palm of the left hand. Rest the controls between the thumb and forefinger. Endoscopists with small hands will need to experiment to find a comfortable position that will allow access to all controls. The key is to keep the hand rotated so that the thumb can manipulate the control wheel.

4. The index and long finger work the two trumpet valves and thus control suction and insufflation. The ring and little finger hold the control handle firmly against the palm.

5. The thumb of the left hand manipulates the large control wheel on the right side of the scope. This wheel angulates the scope tip in an up or down direction.

6. The endoscopist's right hand works the small outer wheel, which controls right and left motion of the instrument tip. There are locking brakes associated with each control knob so that a postion may be held while the hand is removed to perform another function.

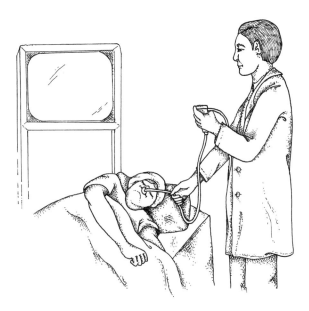

Figure 40.1. Stand comfortably, facing the patient and the video monitor. Generally the video monitor will be across the gurney from the endoscopist, directly in the endoscopist's line of sight.

7.   While the control knobs provide motion at the tip of the endoscope, experienced endoscopists know that equal if not more vital directional control is provided by rotation and elevation of the scope's control head in concert with gentle torsion of the scope shaft. These often imperceptible maneuvers of the endoscopist occur throughout the procedure, and in combination with tip control allow for complex manipulations to be performed. An accomplished endoscopist is rarely motionless during a procedure, but continually makes a complex "endoscopic dance."

8.   Try to maintain the endoscope in a relatively straight or only slightly curved path. Minor deflections of the tip combined with gentle torsion and gentle advancing motions will allow the endoscope to traverse bends (Fig. 40.2). In contrast, sharply angulating the tip may prevent advancement and promote paradoxic tip motion (where the target actually gets farther away). Never use force to advance the endoscope.

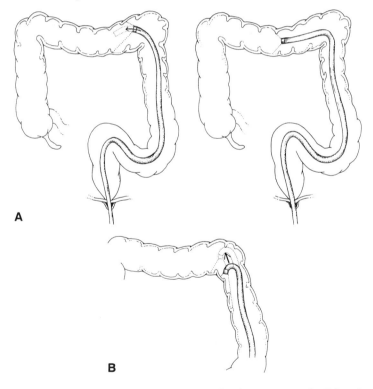

A

B

Figure 40.2. A. Minor tip deflection with gentle advancement and mild torsion allows the endoscope to traverse bends while maintaining a gentle curve. B. Sharp angulation of the tip (like a candy cane) hinders advancement and may result in paradox motion, where the target gets farther away rather than closer, or contribute to perforation.

C. Documentation of Findings

Early endoscopes provided visualization of the gastrointestinal tract but lacked the ability to record images for documentation or discussion. Cameras soon were developed that utilized film to record endoscopic images. Some models, such as the "gastrocamera," were designed specifically for this purpose and sacrificed visualization for the ability to record. These are primarily of historic interest.

Modern endoscopes enjoy the ability to record and document findings in a variety of formats. While cameras are still available for fixation to the viewing optic of fiberoptic systems, newer video endoscopes produce a digital signal that can be recorded on film, video tape, or computer disk. The images can then be incorporated into reports or teaching programs. With the digital format large numbers of images can be stored in a small environment. Some problems have developed as individuals have attempted to transmit images across different systems. The electronic formats of all systems are not the same and communication can be difficult. International standards for digital transmission of images are currently in development.

It is important that the practicing endoscopist record important findings in order to allow the entire health care team to appreciate the patient's pathology and to permit comparison with subsequent (or previous) examinations. The simplest way to do this is to print an image for inclusion in the patient's medical record. Some endoscopy units keep separate files for teaching or research purposes. Many use specialized forms designed for each examination. Whatever system is employed, the record should be clear and easily interpretable.

41. Monitoring, Sedation, and Recovery

Jeffrey L. Ponsky, M.D., F.A.C.S.

A. Monitoring

Continuous patient assessment by a second trained individual is crucial and allows the endoscopist to concentrate on the examination. Level of consciousness, responsiveness, and pain should all be watched closely. Most endoscopy units use a special form on which pulse, blood pressure, medications, and other measures can be recorded. Continuous monitoring of the following parameters is commonly used and generally recommended:

1. Pulse (usually by electrocardiograph)—rate and rhythm
2. Blood pressure (usually with periodic recordings)
3. Pulse oximetry

Even when conscious sedation is not used, bowel distention from insufflation may decrease ventilation. It is important to remember that oxygen saturation is not always an accurate reflection of ventilation, and depression of respiration with hypercapnea may occur despite adequate oxygen levels. Capnography is cumbersome and not readily available; hence, it is not currently the standard. All monitoring devices must be supplemented by constant nursing observation of the patient's ventilation, discomfort, and state of consciousness.

Because hypoxemia is common, many endoscopists routinely administer supplemental oxygen during endoscopy and recovery. Care must be taken not to depress respiration if the patient suffers from chronic obstructive pulmonary disease.

Suction must be available, and resuscitation equipment should be conveniently located.

Monitoring must continue into the recovery phase (see below).

B. Conscious Sedation

Safe and effective administration of conscious sedation is as important as the endoscopy itself. While some endoscopic procedures can be performed without any sedation, most patients prefer to have intravenous sedation in order to facilitate the intervention. The characteristics of conscious sedation are enumerated in Table 40.1. Most agents used for conscious sedation also produce amnesia. This is regarded as desirable and facilitates patient acceptance of repeat examinations if necessary. The Joint Commission on Accreditation of

Healthcare Organizations (JCAHO) regards sedation with certain medications, such as midazolam, to be anesthesia.

Table 41.1. Characteristics of conscious sedation

Conscious sedation is a state of minimally depressed consciousness in which the patient:
- Retains protective airway reflexes
- Responds appropriately to physical stimuli and verbal commands
- Maintains continuous communication with caregivers

An intravenous line must be maintained during endoscopy. The line is used for administration of agents used for conscious sedation, and is crucial if resuscitation is required. Agents commonly used for conscious during endoscopy are listed in Table 41.2. Most are benzodiazepines, and provide both sedation and amnesia.

Table 41.2. Agents commonly used for conscious sedation during endoscopy

Name of Drug	Advantages	Disadvantages
Diazepam	1. Reduces anxiety 2. Causes amnesia 3. Minimal cardio-vascular effects 4. Relatively flat dose-response curve	1. Pain on injection 2. High incidence of chemical phlebitis
Midazolam	1. More rapid onset 2. Less pain on injection 3. More amnesia	1. Significantly more potent, requiring dose adjustment 2. Avoid combination with narcotic agents
Demerol	1. Analgesic effect	1. Minimal amnesia 2. Cardiopulmonary depression

C. Recovery

Continue monitoring (and recording information) until the patient has fully recovered from the procedure and any sedation. The benzodiazepine antagonist flumazenil has been used after endoscopy in an attempt to shorten recovery time. Flumazenil rapidly reverses the central effects of diazepam or midazolam but may not completely reverse the respiratory depression. Resedation may occur after 1 to 2 hours. Patients should be cautioned against driving and released into the care of a responsible accompanying person.

D. Selected References

Andrus CH, Dean PA, Ponsky JL. Evaluation of safe, effective intravenous sedation for utilization in endoscopic procedures. Surg Endosc 1990;4:179–183.

Arrowsmith JB, Gerstman BB, Fleischer DE, Benjamin SB. Results from the American Society for Gastrointestinal Endoscopy/US Food and Drug Administration collaborative study on complication rates and drug use during gastrointestinal endoscopy. Gastrointest Endosc 1991;37:421–427.

Bartelsman JFWM, Sars PRA, Tytgat GNJ. Flumazenil used for reversal of midazolam-induced sedation in endoscopy outpatients. Gastrointest Endosc 1990;36:S9–S12.

Council on Scientific Affairs, American Medical Association. The use of pulse oximetry during conscious sedation. JAMA 1993;270:1463-1468.

Holzman RS, Cullen DJ, Eichhorn JH, Philip JH. Guidelines for sedation by nonanesthesiologists during diagnostic and therapeutic procedures. J Clin Anesth 1994;6:265–276.

Keeffe EB, O'Connor KW. 1989 A/S/G/E survey of endoscopic sedation and monitoring practices. Gastrointest Endosc 1990;36:S13–18.

Lewis BS, Shlien RD, Wayne JD, Knight RJ, Aldoroty RA. Diazepam versus midaxolam (versed) in outpatient colonoscopy: a double-blind randomized study. Gastrointest Endosc 1989;35:33–36.

McCloy RF, Pearson RC. Which agent and how to deliver it? A review of benzodiazepine sedation and its reversal in endoscopy. Scand J Gastroenterol Suppl 1990;179:7–11.

42. Diagnostic Upper Gastrointestinal Endoscopy

John D. Mellinger, M.D., F.A.C.S.

A. Indications

1. Diagnostic upper gastrointestinal endoscopy, or esophagogastroduo-denoscopy (EGD), may be indicated for symptom evaluation, malignancy surveillance, and in several special circumstances (Table 42.1).

Table 42.1. Indications for EGD

Indication	Specific examples
Symptoms	• Dyspepsia* • Dysphagia • Odynophagia • Pyrosis* • Nausea and vomiting *If persistent, recurrent despite medical management, or associated with other gastrointestinal symptoms or signs such as weight loss
Malignancy surveillance	• Barrett's epithelium • Gastric polyps • Familiar polyposis syndromes • Gastric ulcer • Esophageal ulcer • Marginal (postgastrectomy) ulcer
Other circumstances	• Occult gastrointestinal bleeding • Cirrhosis (to evaluate varices) • Malabsorption (for small intestine biopsy)

2. Therapeutic EGD is appropriate for acute upper gastrointestinal bleeding, foreign body ingestion, polyp removal, dilation of stenoses, placement of feeding or drainage catheters, eradication of esophageal varices, and palliative therapy of obstructing neoplasms (see Chapters 43.1.1-43.2.6).

B. Patient Preparation

1. Keep the patient NPO for 6 to 8 hours before routine elective EGD. This minimizes aspiration risks associated with a sedated procedure, and facilitates a complete and unhampered examination.
2. Consider a **longer period of preparation** (NPO, and/or liquid diet) if gastric outlet obstruction or impaired gastric motility is anticipated.
3. If retained ingested material, secretions, or blood are likely, consider **preprocedural gastric aspiration or lavage**.
4. **Obtain informed consent** for the procedure. This includes a discussion of specific complications as well as anticipated outcomes and their general frequency. Review alternative therapies, the information to be gained from the proposed study, and anticipated practical impact on the patient's care. If a new technique is likely to be employed, frank discussion of experience with the new method is in order.
5. Apply monitoring devices (see Chapter 41) and ensure that a secure intravenous line is in place.
6. Have the patient **remove dentures.**
7. **Topical anesthesia** is usually employed prior to EGD. Effective topical anesthesia facilitates intubation and comfort of the otherwise neurologically intact patient (especially when sedation is not employed), and may allow a smaller amount of sedation to be used.
    a. Deliver the topical agents to the posterior pharynx by spray or gargle, rather than to the oral cavity and tongue only.
    b. Topical anesthetics take a few minutes to work. Use this time to check the endoscope (see Chapter 39) and verify that all items that might be needed (such as biopsy forceps) are available.
    c. Test the patient's gag response before attempting endoscopy. This is a good indicator of patient tolerance.
    d. Several applications may be required.
    e. Topical agents are probably of marginal importance when deeper conscious sedation is required.

C. Performance of Diagnostic Upper Gastrointestinal Endoscopy—Normal Anatomy

1. Place the patient in the left lateral decubitus position with a pillow under the head.
2. Place a bite block between the teeth.
3. Lubricate the endoscope with water-soluble lubricant and hold it in front of the patient's mouth. The initial insertion is best done under visual guidance:
    a. Hold the endoscope in the right hand, approximately 20 to 30 cm from the tip.

b. This facilitates passage through the upper esophageal sphincter without releasing and regrasping the instrument. If the endoscope is held farther back, it may buckle.

c. Position the endoscope in front of the mouth in such a way that a simple deflection of the large (up/down) control wheel with the thumb of the left hand moves the tip to the desired curve (inferiorly in the axis of the patient's midline).

d. Rotate the instrument with the right hand to orient this downward deflection in the appropriate axis.

e. Next, straighten the instrument, pass it through the bite block, and insert it to the level of the posterior pharynx.

f. Maintain the endoscope in the midline of the pharynx, and deflect the tip inferiorly by repeating the maneuver as rehearsed above. Attention should now shift to the video monitor. The base of the tongue and epiglottis will be seen anteriorly.

g. Advance the endoscope slowly and smoothly to minimize gagging, using torque with the right hand to accomplish right/left movements and left thumb deflections to make anterior/posterior adjustments. Visualize the laryngeal cartilages and vocal cords, and advance the scope in the midline immediately posterior to the arytenoid cartilages (Fig. 42.1).

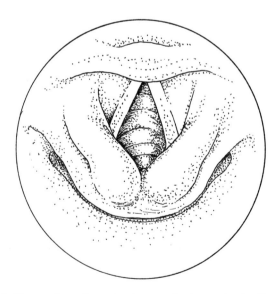

Figure 42.1. The esophageal opening is recognized as a simple slit at the base of the triangle formed by the glottis, just behind the arytenoid cartileges. The two pyriform sinuses lie on each side of the esophageal opening.

    h.   Passage through the upper esophageal sphincter is facilitated by having the patient swallow, which relaxes the sphincter.

        i.   Often the simple presence of the instrument in this area will initiate a swallow and allow passage through the upper esophageal sphincter.

        ii.   If the patient is not too deeply sedated, asking him or her to perform a swallow may achieve the same.

        iii.   If gentle pressure in the appropriate midline position does not achieve the above, withdraw the scope and repeat the maneuver; lateral deflection into the pyriform sinus area can easily occur and lead to injury if increasing pressure is applied.

    i.   Alternative techniques, such as placing two fingers in the patient's mouth to guide the endoscope and keep it in the midline, are especially useful for patients who are under anesthesia.

    j.   If an endotracheal tube is in place, it is crucial that someone hold the endotracheal tube to prevent accidental dislodgment. It may be necessary to deflate the balloon to allow the endoscope to pass.

4.   Advance the endoscope slowly down the length of the esophagus, again using torque and limited deflection of the up/down control wheel to allow preservation of a luminal view at all times. Never advance the endoscope without a visible lumen (Fig. 42.2).

5.   Watch for peristaltic activity, distensibility, and mucosal appearance. Measure the distance from the incisors to the squamocolumnar junction (where the white esophageal epithelium abruptly gives way to pink gastric mucosa). Identify the location of the diaphragm by asking the patient to sniff. Visible contraction of the diaphragm will produce extrinsic compression of the esophagus.

6.   As soon as the endoscope enters the stomach, step back from the table and allow the instrument to assume an unrestrained, straightened posture. This is often best accomplished by completely letting go of the scope with the right hand as one steps back.

7.   With the patient on the left side, this will typically orient the instrument in the stomach such that the greater curve will be at the 6 o'clock position, the lesser curve at 12 o'clock, and the anterior and posterior walls to the left and right, respectively (Fig. 42.3). Insufflate sufficient air to obtain a good view, and note rugal folds, peristaltic activity, and distensibility. Avoid overdistention, as this may trigger pylorospasm.

8.   Continue to advance the endoscope down the length of the stomach, maintaining upward deflection of the tip in a gentle curve to preserve an antegrade view and hug the lesser curvature (Fig. 42.4).

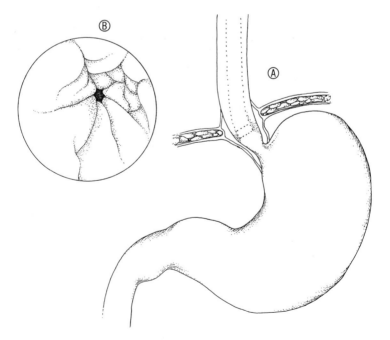

Figure 42.2. A. The endoscope is advanced down the relatively straight esophagus until the lower esophageal sphincter is identified. B. The lower esophageal sphincter often coincides with the transition from squamous epithelium (white) of the esophagus to mucosa (pink) of the stomach.

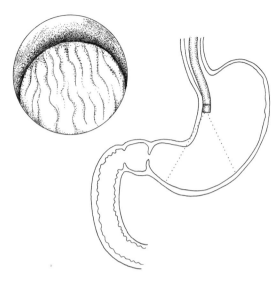

Figure 42.3. With the patient in the left lateral decubitus position, the endoscopist facing the patient, and the scope relaxed as described in the text, entry into the stomach will generally give a view oriented with the lesser curvature at 12 o'clock, the greater curvature at 6 o'clock, anterior at 9 o'clock, and posterior at 3 o'clock.

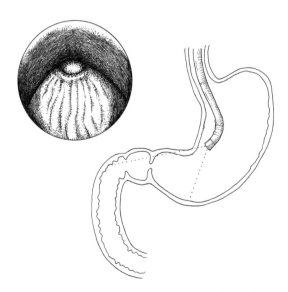

Figure 42.4. As the endoscope is advanced, the lumen is kept in view. A gentle upward deflection of the tip helps the endoscope hug the lesser curvature.

9. Advance the endoscope to the pylorus and carefully note the pyloric channel and duodenal bulb. Often some of the best views of the bulb are achieved prior to pyloric intubation via such an antegrade view. Make very fine maneuvers of the deflection wheels to hold the pylorus in the center of the visual field as gentle continued advancement of the scope allows it to pass into the proximal duodenum (Fig. 42.5).

10. Rarely, application of a brief period of suction will allow the pylorus to be drawn over the scope if it seems unwilling to otherwise admit the same, provided the suction is applied as the tip of the scope sits immediately in front of the opening of the pyloric channel.

11. Carefully visualize the duodenal bulb before advancing the instrument further. The posterior bulb is often the most challenging area to visualize well. Inspection of this area can be achieved by withdrawing the endoscope and using torque and fine deflections of the tip to achieve an adequate view (Fig. 42.6).

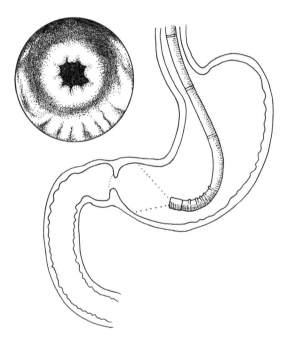

Figure 42.5. The pylorus is viewed from the gastric antrum. The endoscope is gently advanced while keeping the pylorus directly in the center of the visual field. Sometimes the pylorus will be observed to open and close. Position the endoscope ready to pass through the pylorus when it opens.

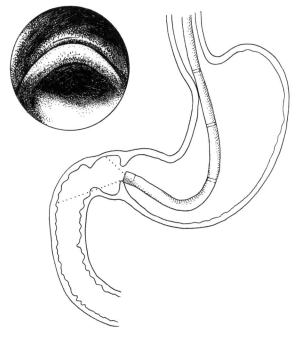

Figure 42.6. The duodenal bulb lacks folds. At the distal and superior aspect is the superior duodenal fold, which marks the entrance to the second portion of the duodenum.

12. Advance the endoscope as far into the second portion of the duodenum as luminal visualization permits (Fig. 42.7).
     a. In some cases, full introduction into the second and third portion of the duodenum is easily achieved in this fashion.
     b. More commonly, the posterior sweep of the duodenum requires some further maneuvering. In such settings, the luminal view is lost as the duodenum turns posteriorly near the junction of its first and second portions.
     c. Deflect the tip of the instrument slightly upward with the left thumb on the larger control wheel and simultaneously rotate the left wrist 90 degrees clockwise. This is best accomplished with the right hand completely off the endoscope.

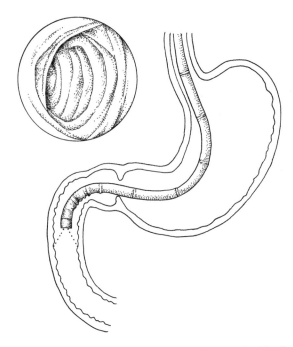

Figure 42.7. The second portion of the duodenum is recognized by its concentric semicircular folds.

    d.   Next, pull back on the endoscope to straighten it and achieve further advancement of the tip. This "paradoxic motion" occurs as the instrument moves from the looped, greater curvature position in the stomach (which usually follows initial antegrade intubation), to a lesser curve or "short stick" position.

    e.   Further antegrade intubation can also be accomplished after this maneuver, if deeper duodenal entry is desired.

13. As the endoscope is withdrawn, carefully inspect all areas.

14. Position the endoscope with its tip in the gastric antrum and retroflex it.

    a.   Deflect the tip of the instrument upward, using the left thumb on the larger control wheel, while simultaneously rotating the left wrist 90 degrees counterclockwise. Frequently an "owl's eye" view of both pylorus and cardia may be seen as the tip crosses the incisura to look directly back at the cardia (Fig. 42.8).

    b.   This maneuver is easily accomplished with the right hand off the endoscope.

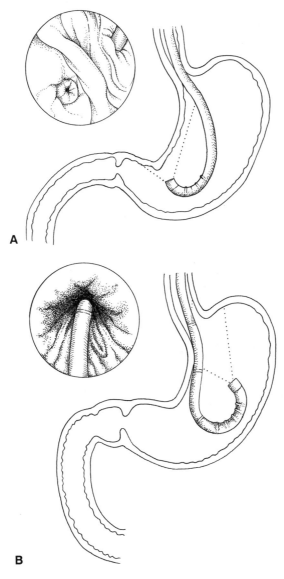

Figure 42.8. Retroflex the endoscope to visualize the cardia. A. Perform this maneuver by deflecting the tip sharply back. An owl's eye view of both pylorus and cardia may be seen as the tip crosses over the incisura. B. As the cardia is identified, move the tip in a circular manner to inspect the entire cardia. Pull the endoscope back to bring the tip (now sharply retroflexed) closer to the area of interest.

    c. Manipulate the endoscope with the right hand (torque, advancement, withdrawal) to obtain optimal visualization of the incisura, cardia, fundus, and remaining proximal stomach. Grasp the endoscope 10 to 20 cm from the patient's mouth to allow a wide range of movements to be done with fluid motions.

    d. Often the "gastric lake" of dependent fundic fluid is seen from this vantage point, and should be suctioned to allow complete inspection. Suction of fluid is most efficient when the meniscus of the fluid surface is oriented transversely across the endoscopic field of visualization. In this position, the suction port (at 6 o'clock in the visual field) is located completely under the fluid, while a luminal view is preserved above the same. Short bursts of suction at a lower setting minimize capturing of the gastric mucosa in the port, which requires repositioning before continuing the suction process. By proceeding in this fashion, fluid evacuation can be accomplished efficiently while continuing dynamic inspection of the lumen.

15. Return the endoscope to its normal (straight, antegrade) position and gradually remove it, reinspecting all areas as the instrument is removed.

16. Suction excess air after the stomach is reinspected during withdrawal. Carefully inspect the esophagus, hypopharynx, and larynx during removal.

D. The Postoperative Stomach

The postoperative stomach offers some special challenges worthy of brief mention. Foregut disease states, which may prompt surgical intervention and the associated anatomic changes, are listed in Table 42.2. As a general rule, the endoscopist does not need to change the technique of the examination because of these alterations, other than being sensitive to, capable of recognition of, and able to identify specific problems related to, their presence. Preendoscopic review of prior operative reports or contrast studies can be invaluable, particularly in patients with multiple previous operations.

A few additional techniques assist the endoscopist in these special situations. These techniques, in conjunction with a sound understanding of anatomy and the basic maneuvers described in section C, will enable the endoscopist to conduct the postoperative exam with the same facility as in the normal anatomic setting. When difficulty is encountered or anticipated, consider one or more of these special techniques:

Table 42.2. Anatomic alterations associated with specific surgical interventions.

Disease Category	Anatomic Changes	Surgical Procedures
Gastroesophageal reflux	• Augmentation of the cardia	• Fundoplication
Peptic ulcer disease	• Gastric outlet alteration • Partial absence of stomach	• Pyloroplasty • Gastroduodenostomy • Gastrojejunostomy • Antrectomy with Billroth I, II, or Roux-en-Y reconstruction
Neoplasia	• Partial or complete absence of stomach	• Subtotal or total gastrectomy, varying reconstructions
Morbid obesity	• Gastric partitioning • Gastric bypass	• Vertical banded gastroplasty • Gastric bypass

1. **Longer but small caliber instruments**, such as a pediatric colonoscope, are useful for accessing the jejunal limbs after gastrojejunostomy (Fig. 42.9).

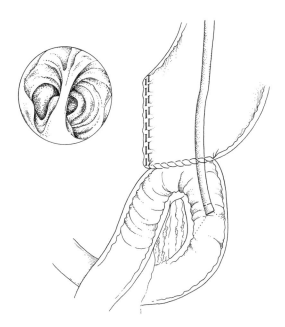

Figure 42.9. A pediatric colonoscope facilitates intubation of the jejunal limbs, particularly the afferent limb, after gastrojejunostomy.

2. A **side-viewing duodenoscope** may facilitate visualization of the proximal stomach when a small, surgically reduced pouch precludes normal retroflexion.

3. **Vital staining** or other special tests are used to visualize subtle mucosal changes (Lugol's solution, methylene blue), or to monitor postvagotomy parietal cell function (pH indicators).

4. Change the **position of the patient** to avoid retained material (bezoars), or to place the area being intubated in a more dependent location.

E. Tissue Sampling Techniques

Biopsy and brushing techniques are an important adjunct to endoscopic visualization in the conduct of upper gastrointestinal endoscopy. Brush cytology, forceps biopsy, large particle biopsy, and chromoscopic techniques enhance the diagnostic yield beyond that provided by endoscopic inspection alone.

Cytology is particularly useful in the evaluation of fungal and viral infections of the foregut, and is also an acceptable way to evaluate for *Helicobacter pylori* infection. It can add 10% to the diagnostic yield of biopsy alone in the evaluation of upper gastrointestinal malignancy. Brush cytology for malignancy is 85% to 90% sensitive and close to 100% specific in the foregut setting. Touch cytology is a technique where a standard biopsy is processed by rolling it on a slide and then fixing and staining the same for cytologic review. This technique has been shown to be a useful adjunct to biopsy alone when evaluating for infectious organisms including *Candida*, *Helicobacter*, and *Giardia*.

Standard biopsy techniques offer high diagnostic yields for a number of foregut pathologies, provided the disease is manifested at the mucosal level. Appropriate targeting of the tissue being sampled can be important in optimizing diagnostic yield. In the setting of evaluation for *H. pylori*, it has been shown that diagnostic yields are comparable from all areas of the stomach, and virtually all infected patients can be identified by a combination of three biopsies obtained from the prepyloric antrum, lesser curve near the incisura, and greater curve body. With malignant ulcers, yields are highest with multiple biopsies (7 to 10), obtained from the rim of the ulcer as well as its base. Such approaches, particularly when combined with brush cytology and salvage cytology of material retained in the endoscope biopsy channel following forceps biopsy, allow documented diagnostic accuracies of 100% with malignant gastric ulcers.

1. Perform **brush cytology** by passing a sheathed brush through the endoscope biopsy channel.
   a. Position the sheath adjacent to the area to be sampled and extend the brush.
   b. Vigorously move the sheath-brush complex to and fro across the area being evaluated. This dislodges cells onto the brush.

    c.   Retract the brush back into the sheath to prevent sample loss while the sheath is being withdrawn through the endoscope biopsy channel.

    d.   The material obtained is then processed onto slides for cytologic evaluation.

    e.   Washing the brush itself in balanced salt solution may allow recovery of additional material for pathology review.

2.   **Forceps biopsy** provides sufficient tissue (generally limited to the mucosa) for histologic examination. Several kinds of biopsy forceps are available, and it is important to choose the proper type for the intended purpose.

    a.   **Spiked forceps** have a tiny needle-like projection between the jaws of the forceps. These facilitate obtaining multiple biopsies on a single pass of the forceps, and may enhance the endoscopist's ability to grasp tissue that is oriented tangentially to the endoscope by helping the forceps to firmly engage the tissue to be sampled.

    b.   **Large cupped forceps**, or jumbo forceps as they are often called, require a therapeutic size endoscope with a 3.7-mm biopsy channel. They typically provide a larger mucosal specimen, but do not usually allow submucosal sampling.

3.   **Endoscopic mucosal resection** is sometimes useful when larger areas of mucosa are to be biopsied or excised. This allows more complete removal of areas of suspicious mucosal pathology. It is particularly applicable in the setting of early gastric cancer, where it is used in concert with endoscopic ultrasound evaluation.

    a.   **Inject saline** underneath the target lesion to elevate the mucosa and produce an easier target to snare. Hypertonic saline prolongs the effect.

    b.   Resect the target lesion with a **standard snare technique**.

    c.   The technique may be modified by using two small-caliber endoscopes simultaneously. This allows the first endoscope to provide forceps traction after injection, while the second endoscope applies the snare around the base of the lesion.

    d.   Another modification utilizes a single cap-fitted endoscope capable of applying suction to the tissue, which is snared after being drawn into the cap.

4.   **Large particle biopsy** allows submucosal tissue sampling in the setting of infiltrative submucosal pathology not amenable to standard mucosal biopsy techniques. The risk of perforation is higher with such techniques, and other alternatives for submucosal evaluation and sampling are becoming available via endoscopic ultrasound (see below).

    a.   Use a **therapeutic, two-channel endoscope**. Pass a snare down one channel and a biopsy forceps down the second.

    b.   **Open the snare** and place it over the area to be sampled.

      c. **Pass the biopsy forceps** through the snare. Pick up and elevate both mucosa and submucosa, thus allowing the snare to incorporate a deeper level of tissue than would otherwise be possible.

   5. **Chromoscopic techniques** are briefly mentioned above because of their particular utility in the postoperative setting. Chromoscopy is probably underutilized in the United States, and can be employed along with magnification video-endoscopy to enhance detection of neoplastic and preneoplastic mucosal abnormalities.

      a. **Lugol's solution** (typically 20 cc or more of a 1% to 2% solution applied directly via an endoscopic catheter) stains glycogen containing tissue, which is present in normal esophageal squamous mucosa. Areas of intestinal metaplasia, carcinoma, and inflammation stain negatively with this agent, and may thus be more apparent for biopsy sampling after its application.

      b. **Methylene blue** is usually applied as a 0.5% to 1% solution in similar volume following application of a mucolytic agent, and is taken up selectively by absorptive epithelium, such as intestinal metaplasia.

F. Endoscopic Ultrasound

Endoscopic ultrasound (EUS) is an area of expanding significance in diagnostic upper gastrointestinal endoscopy. Current **areas of application** include the diagnosis and staging of upper aerodigestive tract neoplasia, diagnosis of submucosal pathology, and diagnosis of choledocholithiasis. A specially designed endoscope is required.

EUS-guided **fine-needle aspiration cytology** offers great promise in adding to the diagnostic potential of this modality, and may make it a diagnostic procedure of choice in the setting of esophageal, gastric, pancreatic, and even pulmonary neoplasia. Its staging potential in these settings, particularly in view of this tissue sampling capability, is increasingly being shown to be superior to radiologic methods such as computed tomography. EUS is also showing promise in the diagnosis and monitoring of submucosal pathology such as stromal and neuroendocrine lesions, and varices.

With continuing technologic improvements, including the availability of instruments capable of combined luminal visualization and EUS, through the scope high-frequency/high-resolution probes, Doppler capability, therapeutic echoendoscopes with elevator-equipped biopsy channels, and improved tissue sampling instrumentation, EUS is poised for increasing importance and utilization in the years ahead. Factors which may limit its application include instrument cost, a steep learning curve required for meaningful interpretation (50-100 cases), low reimbursement, and dearth of studies documenting significant and cost-effective changes in patient management based on its use. References at the end of this section give further information on this emerging diagnostic tool.

G. Selected References

Botet JF, Lightdale C. Endoscopic ultrasonography of the gastrointestinal tract. Gastrointest Endosc Clin North Am 1995;24:385–412.

Cooper GS. Indications and contraindications for upper gastrointestinal endoscopy. Gastrointest Endosc Clin North Am 1994;4:439–454.

Jaffe PK. The use of endoscopic ultrasonagraphy in the evaluation and diagnosis of gastric lesions. Gastrointest Endosc Clin North Am 1996;6:566–584.

Jane PK. Technique of upper gastrointestinal endoscopy. Gastrointest Endosc Clin North Am 1994;4:501–521.

Mellinger JD, Ponsky JL. Endoscopic evaluation of the postoperative stomach. Gastrointest Endosc Clin North Am 1996;6:621–639.

Misumi A, Murakami A, Harada K, Donahue PK. Endoscopic dye techniques in the upper gastrointestinal tract: evaluation of esophageal and gastric pathology. Prob Gastrointest Endosc 990;7:75–86.

Sivak MV. Technique of upper gastrointestinal endoscopy. In Gastroenterologic Endoscopy. Sivak MV (ed.). Philadelphia: WB Saunders, 1987, pp. 272–295.

43.1.1. Variceal Banding

Gregory Van Stiegmann, M.D., F.A.C.S.

A. Indications

Documented hemorrhage from esophageal varices is the indication for endoscopic treatment of bleeding esophageal varices.

1. Perform **diagnostic upper gastrointestinal endoscopy** as soon as possible after the patient who presents with an upper gastrointestinal hemorrhage has been resuscitated and is hemodynamically stable.
2. Confirm hemorrhage from varices by observing:
   a. Actively bleeding varices,
   b. A varix with a fibrin plug ("cherry red spot" or pigmented pro-tuberance), or
   c. The presence of varices with no other identifiable source of up-per gastrointestinal bleeding.

B. Patient Positioning, Room Setup, and Special Considerations in the Bleeding Patient

1. Place the awake sedated patient in the left lateral decubitus position.
2. Adequate monitoring, suctioning and resuscitation apparatus must be readily available, particularly in patients who are actively bleeding.
3. Patients who are combative, encephalopathic, or are bleeding briskly may require **endotracheal intubation**. This protects the airway, and allows sufficient sedation for the procedure to be performed. Intu-bated patients may be treated in the left lateral or supine position (see Chapter 41, Monitoring, Sedation, and Recovery).

C. Technique of Endoscopic Variceal Band Ligation

Both endoscopic band ligation and sclerotherapy (see Chapter 43.1.2) are effective techniques for management of bleeding varices. This section describes endoscopic ligation performed with a "single shot" device.

1. Insert an endoscope overtube, using the endoscope itself or an eso-phageal dilator as an obturator. Newer ligators allow multiple liga-tions without an overtube.
2. Attach the ligating device to the endoscope and insert it through the overtube. The overtube facilitates removal and reloading for multiple ligations.
3. A multifire ligator eliminates need for the overtube, but care must be exercised when introducing the multifire devices to avoid damage to the hypopharynx.
4. Ligate the most distal esophageal varices first, usually beginning at or just caudad to the gastroesophageal junction.
    a. Perform subsequent ligations at the same level or more cepha-lad.
    b. Treat actively bleeding patients in the same manner, unless a bleeding site is identified. In this case, it is ligated first, either by placing the band on the rent in the varix or by ligating proximal and distal to the rent. Subsequent ligations are performed as above until all varices in the distal esophagus are ligated at least once.
5. Identify the target lesion and advance the endoscope under direct vi-sion until the banding cylinder is in full 360-degree contact with the target.
6. Activate endoscopic suction, drawing the lesion into the banding chamber (Fig. 43.1.1.1). When the target has filled the chamber, as witnessed by a complete redout, pull the trip wire to securely fix the latex "0" ring around the base of the target.
7. Repeat ligation treatments aimed at eradication of varices are con-ducted at 1 to 3 week intervals until varices in the distal esophagus are obliterated. Elective repeat treatments are performed on an outpa-tient basis.

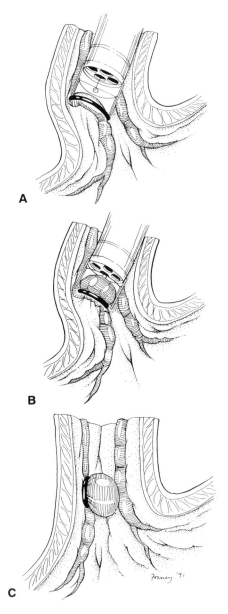

Figure 43.1.1.1. A. The endoscopist makes contact with the varix to be ligated. B. The varix is aspirated into the ligating device using endoscopic suction and the elastic band is ejected from the ligator to ensnare the varix. C. The ligated varix. (Reprinted with permission from Springer-Verlag; World J Surg 1992;16:1034–1041.)

D. Complications of Endoscopic Band Ligation

1. **Overtube complications**
   a. **Cause and prevention:** Mechanical complications caused by introduction of the overtube consist of partial or complete cervical esophageal perforations or mucosal trauma causing bleeding. The cause is usually "pinching" of the esophageal wall in the gap between the overtube and the endoscope when the latter was used as an obturator for introduction. Using an esophageal dilator (which completely fills the lumen of the overtube) as an obturator should prevent this problem.
   b. **Recognition and management:** Bleeding from overtube trauma to the mucosa is usually self-limited. Esophageal perforation should be suspected when intense cervical pain or crepitance is observed. Perforation should be confirmed with water soluble x-ray contrast studies. Antibiotic administration, primary repair of the perforation, and drainage is usually indicated. When perforation is suspected clinically (e.g., cervical crepitance) but no leak is seen on x-ray contrast studies, a 5-day course of antibiotics effective against oral flora may be indicated.

2. **Other complications** directly related to endoscopic ligation are infrequent. Bleeding from ligation site ulcers occurs in up to 8% of patients. Shallow ulcers occur at each treated site when the ligated tissue bolus sloughs (usually 3 to 6 days following ligation) and are not preventable. There is no evidence that sucralfate or acid blocking agents decrease this risk. Diagnosis and treatment is usually by repeat endoscopy and repeat ligation or sclerotherapy. Many such bleeding episodes are self-limited.

E. Selected References

Conn HO, Lebrec D, Terblanche J. The treatment of oesophageal varices: a debate and a discussion. J Intern Med 1997,241:103-108.

Grace ND. Diagnosis and treatment of gastrointestinal bleeding secondary to portal hypertension. American College of Gastroenterology Practice Parameters Committee. Am J Gastroenterol 1997;92:1081-1091.

Van Stiegmann G, Isshi K. Elastic band ligation for bleeding esophagogastric varices. Hepatogastroenterology 1997;44:620-624.

43.1.2. Sclerotherapy of Variceal Bleeding

Choichi Sugawa, M.D.

A. Indications and Results

Endoscopic sclerotherapy (ES) and variceal banding (Chapter 43.1.1) are currently accepted as primary treatment modalities for bleeding esophageal varices. When variceal hemorrhage is found to be the cause of bleeding by initial diagnostic endoscopy, the patient is best served if the endoscopist proceeds to definitive control of bleeding with ES or variceal banding.

Indications for ES are similar to those for banding and (1) actively bleeding varices; (2) nonbleeding varices with stigmata of bleeding (an erosion, clot, or red or brown elevations on the surface of the varix); and (3) nonbleeding varices without any other lesion or source of bleeding. Prophylactic ES in patients who have not yet experienced variceal hemorrhage is controversial. There are both positive and negative reports on this. In Japan, prophylactic ES or variceal banding is standard procedure. Currently, we do not perform prophylactic ES.

Sclerotherapy controls acute variceal bleeding in 75% to 95% of patients. Most clinical reports show that ES reduces recurrent bleeding from esophageal varices. Hospital mortality rates of 25% to 30% have been reported. There have been a few controlled studies indicating that ES of esophageal varices, compared with medical therapy, improves overall survival.

B. Contraindications

There are no contraindications to the use of ES in the acute phase of hemorrhage. Endoscopy should be performed after adequate resuscitation. In case of massive bleeding, we usually intubate the patient to prevent aspiration, which is relatively common in massively bleeding patients. With torrential bleeding, a Blakemore or Minnesota tube may be necessary for 12 to 24 hours before attempting sclerotherapy.

C. Technical Considerations

1. **Timing and preparation:** Perform ES at the earliest possible time in a patient's hospital course. ES can be done in the endoscopy examination room, or in the intensive care unit. An expert endoscopist and

a skilled assistant should be available since emergency endoscopy requires the utmost skill and clinical judgment. Carefully monitor the bleeding patient during the procedure.

2. **Endoscopy:** Video endoscopes are preferred for ES. The author uses a double-channel or large, single-channel video endoscope for acute upper gastrointestinal bleeding, but switches to a single-channel endoscope for elective sclerotherapy or band ligation. The author does not use an overtube or balloon cuff to tamponade the injection site.

3. **Needle (injector):** Single-use disposable sclerotherapy injectors are available from several manufacturers. These provide a catheter or sheath with a 23- or 25-gauge needle capable of advancing 5 mm beyond the end of the catheter.

4. **Sclerosant:** Geography and operator preference determine the choice of sclerosant. In the United States, three effective sclerosing agents are available (Table 43.1.2.1).

Table 43.1.2.1. Sclerosing Agents Available in the United States

Sodium morrhuate	
Sodium tetradecyl sulfate	0.75–1.5% solution, or 1% in combination with 33% ethanol and 0.3% normal saline
Ethanolamine oleate	Used extensively in Europe and Japan Most expensive agent Author's sclerosant of choice

5. **Volume of sclerosant:** The volume of sclerosant varies according to the type of sclerosant used, number, size and length of varices, and the presence of active bleeding. The average volume injected per puncture is 1 to 3 ml, although larger varices will require more volume. The total volume of solution injected during the first procedure varies from 10 to 20 ml, depending on the size and number of varices.

6. **Injection site:** The sclerosant may be injected into the varix (intravariceal) or in the tissue adjacent to the varix (paravariceal) (Fig. 43.1.2.1).

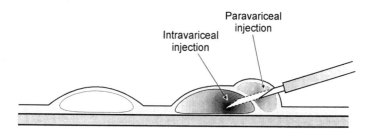

Figure 43.1.2.1. In intravariceal injection, the sclerosant is injected directly into the varix. In paravariceal injection, sclerosant is injected in the surrounding tissues.

D. Technique of Variceal Injection

This section describes the technique of intravariceal injection. This is the method most commonly used.

1. **Pass the injection needle** through the biopsy channel of the endoscope and advance it into view.

   a. **Choose a target** for injection. Begin the injections at two or three points in each line of varices at 2- to 3-cm intervals, from just above the gastroesophageal junction up to the proximal esophagus. Successful obliteration of varices in the distal esophagus usually eliminates the proximal varices or at least decreases their size.

   b. **Advance the needle** out of the sheath and pass it directly into the lumen of the varix.

   c. In most cases, the injections are made in a direction tangential to the varix (Fig. 43.1.2.2).

   d. An assistant performs the injection while the endoscopist controls the position of the needle within the varix.

   e. The goal of the **intravariceal injection** is to introduce the sclerosant directly into the lumen of the varix, resulting in acute variceal thrombosis.

2. If a site of active variceal bleeding is seen, begin injections distally, continue proximally, and finally into and around the site until bleeding is controlled.

   a. Usually 6 to 9 ml of sclerosant are injected (2 to 3 ml for three or four injections).

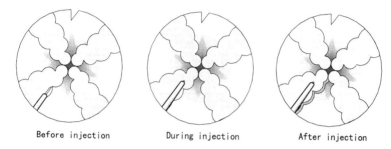

Before injection   During injection   After injection

Figure 43.1.2.2. The injections begin just above the gastroesophageal junction and progress up into the proximal esophagus.

    b.   Then inject other varices.

    c.   The author injects sclerosant directly into the varices, and removes the needle slowly while injecting to tamponade the injection site (Fig. 43.1.2.1).

3.   **Bleeding gastric varices** are difficult to treat endoscopically and results are not as good as ES of esophageal varices. Injection of a large volume of sclerosant or bucrylate into gastric varices has been described. There are two types of gastric varices: junctional varices and fundic varices.

    a.   **Junctional varices** are gastric varices seen as an extension of esophageal varices and without extension into the fundus. These are treated with standard intravariceal sclerotherapy from the proximal, connecting, esophageal varices.

    b.   **Fundic varices** are gastric varices confined to the fundus, with channels extending distally to the gastroesophageal junction.

        i.   In patients with fundic varices, the author performs sclerotherapy only on varices that are bleeding or have stigmata of bleeding, using the retroflexed view. The author's preference is to inject 2 ml into the varices, with a total of 6 to 9 ml of 5% **ethanolamine oleate.**

       ii.   **Cyanoacrylate** has been used for the control of gastric variceal hemorrhage. Either isobutyl-2 or N-butyl-cyanoacrylate is mixed with Lipiodol and injected directly into the varices, producing a virtual acrylic cast of the varices. It appears to be quite effective, but major concerns include the lack of a licensed, deliverable agent and the potential for endoscopic damage.

c. **Control of gastric pH** with high-volume continuous intravenous infusion of H_2 blockers or oral omeprazole (20 to 40 mg every 12 hours) has been recommended to decrease the risk of bleeding from injection site erosions.

E. Injection Schedule and Timing of Therapy

After successful initial hemostasis by ES, ES is repeated during hospitalization. The number and intervals of injections for obliteration of varices differ according to the sclerosant and injection methods. The authors inject two to four times electively, in 2- to 3-day intervals during hospitalization, and repeat at 6- to 8-week intervals until the varices are believed to be obliterated.

Repeat outpatient sclerotherapy is necessary every 2 to 6 months to prevent rebleeding from residual or new varices. If bleeding vessels or varices are still apparent during follow-up examination, they should be injected. For the most part, recurrent bleeding is not as severe as the initial episode and can be controlled by repeat ES. Compliance with follow-up sclerotherapy and abstinence from alcohol abuse improve the prognosis. Patients who adhere to these recommendations but still have progressive liver failure may benefit from liver transplantation.

F. Complications

The complication rate is reported to be from 12% to 50%. Complications may be divided into major and minor ones. **Major complications** are severe bleeding, perforations, mediastinitis, adult respiratory distress syndrome, sepsis, and stricture formation. Major complications occur in about 2% to 3% of patients. Among the minor complications are fever, transient chest pain, odynophagia, and pleural effusion, which are usually transient and inconsequential. Esophageal ulcers are commonly seen a few days after injection and usually heal spontaneously.

G. Selected References

Fardy JM, Laupacis A. A meta-analysis of prophylactic endoscopic sclerotherapy for esophageal varices. Am J Gastroenterol 1994;89:1938–1948.

Goff JS. Esophageal varices. Gastro Endosc Clin North Am 1994;4:747–771.

Infante-Rivard C, Esnaola S, Villeneuve J-P. Role of endoscopic variceal sclerotherapy in the long-term management of variceal bleeding: a meta-analysis. Gastroenterology 1989;96:1087–1092.

Kitano S, Iso Y, Koyanagi N, et al. Ethanolamine oleate is superior to polidocanol (Athoxysklerol) for endoscopic injection sclerotherapy of esophageal varices: a prospective randomized trial. Hepatogastroenterology 1987;34:19–23.

Laine L, El-Newihi HM, Migikovsky B, et al. Endoscopic ligation compared with sclerotherapy for treatment of bleeding esophageal varices. Ann Intern Med 1993;119:1–7.

Lyons SD, Sugawa C, Geller EF, Vandenberg DM. Comparison of 1% sodium tetradecyl sulfate to a thrombogenic sclerosant cocktail for endoscopic sclerotherapy. Am Surg 1988;54:81–84.

McKee RE, Garden OJ, Anderson JR, Carter DC. A trial of elective versus on demand sclerotherapy in "poor risk" patients with variceal hemorrhage. Endoscopy 1994;26:474–477.

Nakamura R, Bucci LA, Sugawa C, et al. Sclerotherapy of bleeding esophageal varices using a thrombogenic cocktail. Am Surg 1991;57:226–230.

Stiegmann GV, Goff JS, Michaletz-Onody PA, et al. Endoscopic sclerotherapy as compared with endoscopic variceal ligation for bleeding esophageal varices. N Engl J Med 1992;326:1527–1532.

Sugawa C. Endoscopic diagnosis and treatment of upper gastrointestinal bleeding. Surg Clin North Am 1989;69:1167–1183.

Sugawa C, Okumura Y, Lucas CE, Walt AJ. Endoscopic sclerosis of experimental eosophageal varices in dogs. Gastrointest Endosc 1978;24:114–116.

Sugawa C, Steffes CP, Nakamura R, et al. Upper GI bleeding in an urban hospital. Ann Surg 1990;212:521–527.

The Veterans Affairs Cooperative Variceal Sclerotherapy Group. Sclerotherapy for male alcoholic cirrhotic patients who have bled from esophageal varices: results of a randomized, multicenter trial. Hepatology 1994;20:618–625.

43.2.1. Control of Nonvariceal Upper GI Bleeding

Choichi Sugawa, M.D.

A. Introduction

Early endoscopy has an important role in the evaluation and treatment of the patient with upper gastrointestinal bleeding. Definition of the precise appearance of the lesions by endoscopy gives important information about the prognosis, risk of rebleeding, and indications for surgery. There are several effective endoscopic modalities for the control of bleeding. This section describes several techniques currently used for endoscopic management of nonvariceal upper gastrointestinal bleeding.

B. Diagnosis

Although individual series vary, peptic ulceration generally is the most common cause of upper gastrointestinal bleeding, followed by acute erosive gastritis, esophageal varices, and Mallory-Weiss tears. Other sources include esophagitis, tumors, vascular malformations, and gastric varices. Before endoscopic hemostasis can be achieved, the exact sites of bleeding must be accurately identified and the visual field must be clear. Endoscopic hemostasis should be attempted only under the following circumstances: the precise bleeding site can be visualized, hemostatic devices can be accurately placed near the bleeding vessels, and hemorrhage is not torrential.

C. Indications

The strongest endoscopic predictor of persistent or recurrent bleeding is ongoing active bleeding at the time of endoscopy. The presence of a discrete protuberance within the ulcer crater is important. This is referred to as a "visible vessel" or "sentinel clot" (Fig. 43.2.1.1). Some pigmented protuberances (e.g., red, blue, purple) imply a high risk of rebleeding.

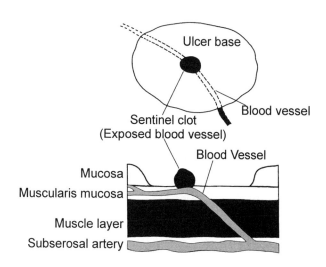

Figure 43.2.1.1. A visible vessel or sentinel clot on the base of the ulcer.

Indications for hemostasis include active bleeding from a peptic ulcer or ulcers with a sentinel clot. Mallory-Weiss tears, acute gastric mucosal lesions, and esophagitis usually cause only minor bleeding. If severe bleeding does occur in these lesions, there will be a discrete ulcer with either an arterial bleeder or a sentinel clot. Multiple clinical and endoscopic risk factors can be used to predict the occurrence of continued or recurrent bleeding (Table 43.2.1.1).

Table 43.2.1.1. Clinical and endoscopic risk factors for continued or recurrent bleeding

Clinical risk factors
Patient history
Age >60 years
Coexistent major organ system disease
In-hospital onset
Admission hemoglobin <8.0
Other clinical criteria
Shock (systolic blood pressure <90)
Transfusion requirements > 5 U packed erythrocytes
Coagulopathy

Table 43.2.1.1. continued

Endoscopic risk factors
Endoscopic appearance
Torrential hemorrhage
Ulcer location in posterior bulb or high on lesser curvature
Active spurting or oozing from base
Pigmented protuberance (visible vessel)
Adherent clot
Doppler-positive lesion

Many terms have been used to describe mucosal and submucosal vascular lesions: telangiectasia, arteriovenous malformation, and angiodysplasia. Endoscopic distinction of these three lesions is seldom possible. Endoscopic treatment should aim at the submucosal level and avoid full-thickness burn. A small lesion can be easily treated directly by endoscopic hemostasis. With a larger lesion, treatment proceeds from the periphery to the center of the lesion.

D. Methods and Results

Several modalities are available for endoscopic control of hemorrhage. These include thermal devices (including electrocautery), injection therapy, clips, and other methods. Each will be described here. The author has employed a variety of methods, but, because of laboratory and clinical experience, currently favors the use of epinephrine injection, heater probe, and multiple coagulation, sometimes in combination with epinephrine and a thermal modality.

1. **Thermal therapy**. Thermal devices are among the most commonly employed and effective. Localized heating causes tissue edema, shrinkage, protein denaturation, contraction of blood vessels, and tissue desiccation to achieve hemostasis.

    a. **Heater probe:** This device is preferable because of cost and portability, in addition to effectiveness. Probes are available in diameters of 3.2 and 2.4 mm. They are designed to allow the simultaneous application of heat and pressure (coaptive coagulation) (Fig. 43.2.1.2).

        i.   Apply the heater probe to the bleeding vessel with firm pressure. The objective is to coapt the vessel walls (Fig. 43.2.1.3). The large-diameter probe (3.2 mm) is more effective.

        ii. When the vessel is occluded by pressure, apply three to four sequential pulses of 30 joules each in tandem for a total of 120 joules, with no cooling period between pulses.

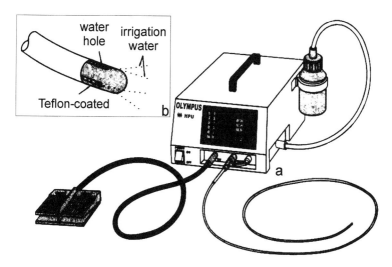

Figure 43.2.1.2. Heater probe power unit with foot pedal and large probe (Olympus Corp. Ltd., Tokyo, Japan). Irrigation from the tip of the heater probe. Simultaneous tamponade and washing of a bleeding arterial lesion are feasible with the heater probe.

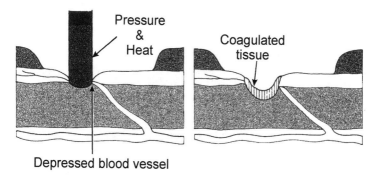

Figure 43.2.1.3. Simultaneous application of heat and pressure (coaptive coagulation).

iii. Recommended techniques for heater probe hemostasis for different types of bleeding lesions are shown in Table 43.2.1.2. Fewer joules and total pulses are recommended for Dieulafoy's disease, Mallory-Weiss tears, and gastrointestinal angiomas.

Table 43.2.1.2. Techniques for heater probe hemostasis

Lesion	Tamponade pressure	Setting (joules)	Pulses/ tamponade station	Site of hemostasis
Chronic peptic ulcer*	Very firm	30	4	Only on visible vessel
Acute ulcer or Dieulafoy's disease**	Firm	25	3	Only on bleeding point
Mallory-Weiss tear**	Moderate	20	2–3	Only on bleeding point
GI angiomas***	Gentle	10	1–2	Entire angioma

*Treatment of visible vessel (either actively bleeding or nonbleeding) only is recommended.
**Treatment of actively bleeding lesions only.
***For treatment of all angiomas in the bowel segment causing GI bleeding.
Source: Jensen DM.

b. **BICAP (multipolar) endoscopic probe**. New types of the bipolar electrode, called the bipolar circumactive probe (BICAP), and the Gold probe have been developed. These have equally spaced microelectrodes along the side and over the tip, and can contact the bleeding lesion from any direction. The power unit incorporates a water pump, allowing water irrigation of the target area intermittently or constantly. Bipolar probes produce less damage compared with monopolar electrocoagulation or YAG lasers.

i. Press the probe against the bleeding site in order to find the precise point that tamponades bleeding.

ii. When the exposed bleeding artery (sentinel clot with bleeding) is demonstrably occluded by pressure, apply heat to seal the vessel (Fig. 43.2.1.3).

iii. The optimal technique for bipolar electrocoagulation should include the use of the large (3.2 mm) probe, positioning of the tip of the endoscope *en face* as close as possible to the bleeding lesion, lower watt settings of 3 to 5 (i.e., 15–25 W), and prolonged periods of coagulation.

iv. Multiple 2-second pulses given in rapid succession appear to be as effective as a single, long pulse of identical duration.

c. **Laser photocoagulation.** The intense monochrome light energy produced by a laser can be directed through safe flexible light guides and effectively coagulate tissue. Currently there are two lasers suitable for endoscopic therapy: the neodymium yttrium-aluminum-garnet (Nd:YAG) laser and the argon laser.

    i. The standard recommendation for use of the Nd:YAG laser is 80 watts of energy over 0.5-second pulses from a distance of 1 cm.

    ii. Begin laser therapy at least 2 to 3 mm away from the visible arterial segment.

    iii. Depending on the distance (0.5 cm, for example), a lower and shorter setting may be required.

    iv. The control trials of ulcer hemostasis generally suggest that laser photocoagulation is effective treatment for both actively bleeding and nonbleeding visible vessels. The lasers are not portable, are extremely costly, and require a high level of training for both the laser endoscopist and technician.

2. **Injection therapy.** Injection sclerotherapy of esophageal varices has been shown to be relatively safe and effective in the control of bleeding esophageal varices (see Chapter 43.1.2). This technique has been expanded to include nonvariceal bleeding lesions. Injection therapy is simple, inexpensive, readily available, and can be performed at the time of diagnostic endoscopy. Injection therapy with saline or water provides effective hemostasis mainly by tamponade. Several other agents have been used.

a. **Epinephrine (1:10,000).** Epinephrine injection is more effective for immediate hemostasis and preferable to ethanol injection because of greater overall effectiveness, ease, and lessened tissue damage.

    i. This solution is made by mixing 1 ml of epinephrine (1:1,000) with 9 ml of normal saline (0.9%).

    ii. The total volume used ranges from 5 to 10 ml, with a larger volume used to stop spurting vessels.

    iii. Inject this solution directly around the blood vessel in 3 to 4 increments (Figs. 43.2.1.4, 43.2.1.5).

    iv. Recent controlled studies concluded that endoscopic epinephrine injection was effective in stopping bleeding, and decreased the transfusion requirement and the need for emergency surgery. No complications were reported.

b. **Absolute ethanol**

    i. The total dose of 0.6 to 1.2 ml of 98% dehydrated ethanol (Abbott Laboratories) is injected through a 1 ml disposable plastic tuberculin syringe in amounts of 0.1 to 0.2 ml per injection.

    ii. Inject this solution at three or four sites surrounding the bleeding vessel, and 1 or 2 mm from the vessel, causing thrombosis, to dehydrate and fix the blood vessel (Figs. 43.2.1.4, 43.2.1.5).

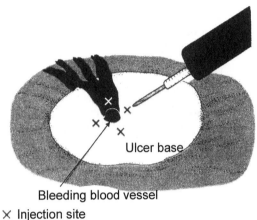

× Injection site

Figure 43.2.1.4. Epinephrine or ethanol is injected around and into the bleeding point at the base of the ulcer.

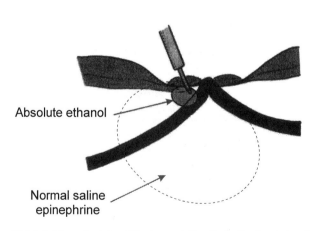

Figure 43.2.1.5. The principle of the hemostatic effect of epinephrine (tamponade) and ethanol (dehydration and fixation of tissue).

    iii. Permanent hemostasis with absolute ethanol injection re-
      portedly has a success rate of greater than 90%. Ethanol
      injection is technically more difficult, as it is injected pre-
      cisely in small volumes.

   c. **Epinephrine followed by other sclerosing agents** or thermal
    therapy.

    i. Epinephrine (1:10,000, 5 to 10 ml) is injected submucosally
     directly around the blood vessel to obtain initial hemostasis
     by compression and vasoconstriction.

    ii. To achieve definitive hemostasis by obliterating the vessel,
     5 ml of 1% polidocanol or multipolar electrocoagulation or
     heater probe is applied into the blood vessel after initial in-
     jection of the epinephrine solution.

    iii. Research shows that application of further therapy after
     initial injection therapy improves the hemostatic results.

 3. **Other therapies.** Many other forms of endoscopic therapies have
  been assessed for the treatment of bleeding ulcers.

   a. **Metallic clip** (hemoclip). Hemoclips (miniature metal clips) can
    be applied to bleeding vessels by a special flexible slip applica-
    tor through the biopsy channel of an endoscope. With recent im-
    provements in the clip and applicator, this technique is easier to
    perform. It is very popular in Japan, where good results are re-
    ported. Recently, this clip has become available in the United
    States.

   b. **Argon plasma coagulator.** Activated argon gas is currently
    used by surgeons to promote hemostasis on the surface of the
    diaphragm or the liver. Inert argon gas is delivered into the in-
    testinal lumen through a small catheter in the biopsy channel of
    the endoscope. Once the wire at the tip of the catheter is acti-
    vated, the argon gas becomes electrically energized, and an
    electric spark is formed from the tip of the sheath to the intesti-
    nal wall. This is a noncontact thermal modality. The argon
    plasma coagulator is an excellent modality to stop bleeding from
    superficial lesions such as radiation proctitis, vascular malfor-
    mations, and polypectomy-induced bleeding.

E. Complications

Complications include perforation, induced acute hemorrhage, and delayed
hemorrhage. The incidence of perforation from endoscopic hemostasis has been
low, with rates of 1% to 2% commonly quoted. Induced bleeding can occur
more commonly during thermal therapy than injection therapy. It is desirable to
limit the area and depth of treatment as much as possible in clinical applications in order to prevent ulceration caused by endoscopic therapy itself. (See
Chapter 44, Complications of Upper Gastrointestinal Endoscopy.)

F. Selected References

Chung SCS, Lau JYW, Sung JJY, et al. A randomized comparison between adrenaline injection alone and adrenaline injection plus heat probe treatment for actively bleeding ulcers. BMJ 1997;314:1307–1311.

Haber G, Dorais J, DuVall A, et al. Argon plasma coagulation: a new effective technique of noncontact thermal coagulation. Experience in 44 cases of GI angiomata. Gastrointest Endosc 1996;43:293.

Jensen DM. Endoscopic coagulation therapy. Part A: Heater Probe. In: Gastroinstestinal Bleeding. Sugawa C, Schuman BM, Lucas CE (eds.). New York: Igaku-Shoin, 1992, pp. 298–313.

Jensen DM, Kovacs TOG, Freeman M, et al. A multicenter randomized prospective study of gold probe versus heater probe for hemostasis of very severe ulcer or Mallory-Weiss bleeding. Gastroenterology 1991;100:1492.

NIH Consensus Conference. Therapeutic endoscopy and bleeding ulcers. JAMA 1989;262:1369–1372.

Ohta S, Yukioka T, Ohta S, et al. Hemostasis with endoscopic hemoclipping for severe gastrointestinal bleeding in critically ill patients. Am J Gastroenterol 1996;91:701–704.

Steffes CP, Sugawa C. Endoscopic management of nonvariceal gastrointestinal bleeding. World J Surg 1992;16:1025–1033.

Sugawa C. Endoscopic diagnosis and treatment of upper gastrointestinal bleeding. Surg Clin North Am 1989;69:1167–1183.

Sugawa C. Injection therapy for the control of bleeding ulcers. Gastrointest Endosc 1990;36:S50–S52.

Sugawa C, Fujita Y, Ikeda T, Walt AJ. Endoscopic hemostasis of bleeding of the upper gastrointestinal tract by local injection of ninety-eight percent dehydrated ethanol. Surg Gynecol Obstet 1986;162:159–163.

Sugawa C, Joseph AL. Endoscopic interventional management of bleeding duodenal and gastric ulcers. Surg Clin North Am 1992;72:317–334.

Sugawa C, Joseph AL. Management of nonvariceal upper gastrointestinal bleeding. In: Endoscopic Surgery. Greene FL, Ponsky JL (eds.). Philadelphia: W B Saunders, 1994, pp. 125-140.

Sugawa C, Steffes CP, Nakamura R, et al. Upper GI bleeding in an urban hospital. Ann Surg 1990;212:521–527.

43.2.2-5. Upper Gastrointestinal Endoscopy—Therapeutic

Timothy M. Farrell, M.D.
John G. Hunter, M.D.

43.2.2. Endoscopic polypectomy

A. Indications

Polypectomy is less commonly applied in the upper GI tract than in the colon, because the majority of upper GI polyps are submucosal or inflammatory in origin, and true adenomas are unusual. Although few of these lesions have malignant potential, biopsy of dominant masses is indicated to exclude early gastroesophageal malignancy.

B. Technique

A **diathermy snare** is effective for esophageal or gastric lesions amenable to excisional biopsy.

1. Use a forward-viewing endoscope.
2. Pass the snare loop over the polyp and tighten the snare around its stalk.
3. Excise the lesion with a blend of cutting and coagulation electrocautery.
4. Gastric polyps may be less pedunculated and therefore require a two-channel endoscope for their manipulation and excision (see Chapter 42, Diagnostic Upper Gastrointestinal Endoscopy).
5. **Endoluminal gastric surgery** may be an alternative for excision of gastric lesions not amenable to snare excision (see Chapter 21, Gastric Resections).
   a. This employs laparoscopic instruments and techniques to work within the stomach.
   b. Trocars are placed through the abdominal wall into the stomach. The number and orientation of trocars depends on the position of the pathology.
   c. While a flexible endoscope may be used to guide endoluminal surgery, a rigid laparoscope introduced through an intragastric trocar optimally facilitates the procedure.

d.   Resection of mucosa-based polyps is facilitated by submucosal injection of saline to elevate the lesion.

e.   Submucosal lesions may be "shelled out" and the mucosa closed over the defect.

43.2.3. Dilatation

A. Indications

Upper gastrointestinal strictures are dilated to improve passage of food and saliva. Dilatation should be preceded by a precise diagnostic evaluation, including biopsies, to detect the underlying etiology and to **exclude unrecognized malignancy**. Dilatation is routinely applied to peptic esophageal strictures, and may also be beneficial in cases of gastric outlet obstruction from ulcer disease or stenosis after gastroenterostomy or pyloroplasty. The objective of esophageal dilatation is to resolve dysphagia. Patients who can accept a 44-French dilator are able to swallow most foods.

B. Technique

1.   **Mercury-filled rubber bougies** are useful in cases of simple, straight strictures.

a.   Maloney dilators have a tapered end, and are well tolerated and easy to use.

b.   The patient may be treated sitting or in the left lateral decubitus position.

c.   Most patients require only topical anesthetic spray; however, small doses of midazolam or meperidine should be available since dilatation may cause discomfort.

d.   Use fluoroscopy liberally, especially for patients with narrow strictures or large hiatal hernias.

e.   Determine the initial caliber of the stricture by passing successively larger dilators until resistance is appreciated.

f.   Dilate the lumen 6 to 10 French beyond this point, using only mild force to advance the dilators.

g.   Schedule repeat sessions at 1- to 3-week intervals until dysphagia is resolved. Overzealous dilatations increase the risk for esophageal perforation.

2.   **Wire-guided dilators** are more rigid than Maloney dilators, and are preferred for tight, tortuous strictures.

a.   Place a guide wire across the stricture and into the stomach using an endoscope.

b.   Pass graded dilators over the wire with fluoroscopic control.

    c.   Do not dilate a stricture more than 6 to 10 French at any one session, with repeat dilations at 1- to 3-week intervals until dysphagia is resolved.

  3.   **Hydrostatic balloons** may be used to dilate upper GI strictures under endoscopic visualization. Since the endoscopist cannot "feel" the stricture, he or she must estimate its diameter. The balloon is inflated with water to a predetermined pressure. Use of progressively larger balloons and multiple procedures are frequently necessary.

43.2.4. Palliation of Upper Gastrointestinal Malignancies

A. Indications

Endoscopic palliation is indicated when resection or other therapy has failed or is impracticable. The most common site is esophageal, and obstruction is the most common indication for endoscopic intervention. Occasionally bleeding or tracheoesophageal fistula require endoscopic control. This section describes several methods currently used for palliation of malignant esophageal obstruction.

B. Techniques

In cases of advanced esophageal cancer with short life expectancy, **dilatation** (see section 43.2.3) alone may afford satisfactory relief of dysphagia. The follow techniques are available when more lasting relief is needed.

  1.   Endoscopic or radiographic placement of rigid plastic or expandable wire **stents** across malignant esophageal strictures will achieve more durable alleviation of symptoms. Both rigid and self-expanding metal stents are available.

    a.   Stents are directed into position over an endoscope or an inner guide tube placed across the stricture.

    b.   Rigid stents are manually pushed into position across the stricture. These stents are more economical, but are accompanied by a 5% to 10% incidence of perforation at placement and a 15% incidence of early migration.

    c.   Rigid prostheses are not easily tolerated for proximal esophageal strictures due to discomfort and airway compression. For these reasons, more expensive self-expanding wire stents have gained popularity.

    d.   Self-expanding wire stents are more easily delivered across tight strictures because of their narrower profile before expansion, and are less prone to migrate since they engage the tumor with outward force.

  e. Problems with tumor ingrowth have been lessened by urethane coating and wire coils.

2. **Laser ablation** of bulky esophageal tumors offers effective palliation of dysphagia in 70% to 80% of patients after 3 to 5 sessions.

  a. Prophylactic antibiotics and under intravenous sedation are useful for most.

  b. Visualize the tumor and direct an endoscopic Nd:YAG or KTP laser at the intralumenal component of a tumor to heat and vaporize the obstructing tissue and restore a 10- to 12-mm lumen.

  c. If the anatomy permits, traverse the tumor with the endoscope and treat during withdrawal. Antegrade treatment is associated with a higher perforation rate.

  d. Complications such as perforation, bleeding, and fistula are reported in 5% to 20%.

43.2.5. **Foreign Body Removal**

A. Indications

Impacted food is the most prevalent esophageal **foreign body** in adults. Sometimes ingestion of carbonated beverages or administration of nitrates or calcium-channel blockers will result in clearance of a retained esophageal food bolus. Otherwise, rigid or flexible endoscopy will allow successful retrieval in 99% of cases.

Swallowed foreign bodies that have cleared the esophagus usually proceed uneventfully through the alimentary tract. Thus most foreign body ingestions that do not result in esophageal impaction can be managed by watchful waiting. Sharp, large, or potentially dangerous foreign objects may need to be removed from the stomach or duodenum.

B. Technique

A rigid endoscope permits better suction and easier fragmentation of the bolus, but a flexible instrument is safer in high-risk patients. Improvements in instrumentation have made fiberoptic endoscopy the procedure of choice for most endoscopists.

1. Most impacted food can be pushed into the stomach with the expectation that it will then pass normally.

2. Retrieve other foreign bodies with snares or foreign body removal forceps.

3. Use a small-caliber fiberscope with an overtube to overcome many of the drawbacks of flexible endoscopy.

4. Grasp smooth or round foreign bodies such as coins with a snare of alligator type forceps.
5. Remove sharp foreign bodies (such as open safety pins) with the point trailing. This may necessitate pushing the object into the stomach where it can be turned around and positioned properly for removal.
6. After removing foreign object, especially impacted food boluses, make a careful search for underlying pathology.
7. Maintain a high index of suspicion for associated perforation. Carefully inspect the mucosal surfaces after removal.

Selected References

Cotton PR, Williams CB. Therapeutic upper gastrointestinal endoscopy. In: Practical Gastrointestinal Endoscopy, 2nd ed. Boston: Blackwell Scientific, 1982:49–61.

Ponec RJ, Kimmey MB. Endoscopic therapy of esophageal cancer. Surg Clin North Am 1997;5:1197–1217.

Schwesinger WH. Laser treatment of esophageal and gastric lesions. Surg Clin North Am 1992;3:581–95.

Wo JM, Waring JP. Medical therapy of gastroesophageal reflux and management of esophageal strictures. Surg Clin North Am 1997;5:1041–53.

43.2.6. Percutaneous Endoscopic Feeding Tube Placement

Carol E.H. Scott-Conner, M.D., F.A.C.S.
Jeffrey Ponsky, M.D., F.A.C.S.

A. Indications

Gastrostomy is indicated as a route for enteral feedings in patients with functioning gastrointestinal tracts who are unable to take oral nutrition. Gastrostomy may be indicated in patients with stroke, dementia, progressive neurologic processes, severe psychomotor retardation, tumors of the upper aerodigestive tract, or severe facial trauma. Patients should demonstrate potential for extended survival with adequate nutrition. Critically ill patients with a low probability of survival are not appropriate candidates for percutaneous endoscopic gastrostomy (PEG) or other invasive methods of feeding tube placement. When the patient's status is uncertain, begin feedings via a nasoenteric feeding tube, and continue this until it is likely that the patient will tolerate an invasive procedure and demonstrates a potential for extended survival.

Three basic routes for gastrostomy creation are now available: traditional surgical gastrostomy, laparoscopic gastrostomy (see Chapter 18, Laparoscopic Gastrostomy), and percutaneous endoscopic gastrostomy (PEG). There are advantages and disadvantages to each method (Table 43.2.6.1).

Two methods of PEG placement (the "push" and "pull" techniques) are in current use and will be described here. A simple modification allows placement of a feeding tube in the jejunum, and will be considered at the end of this section.

Table 43.2.6.1. Advantages and disadvantages of methods of gastrostomy formation

Method	Advantages	Disadvantages
Surgical gastrostomy	• Secure fixation of stomach to anterior abdominal wall • Permanent tract may be created	• Requires laparotomy • May require general anesthesia

Table 43.2.6.1. continued

Method	Advantages	Disadvantages
Laparoscopic gastrostomy	• Less invasive • May achieve secure fixation of stomach to abdominal wall • Visual selection of site of entry onto stomach	• Requires laparoscopic access • May require general anesthesia
PEG	• May be performed under local anesthesia • May be done in the endoscopy suite • Single puncture, no incision	• Requires patent upper gastrointestinal tract • Early dislodgment of tube may require laparotomy • Potential for injury to adjacent viscera unless technique carefully followed

B. The "Push" Technique for PEG Placement

This method utilizes the Seldinger technique to place a Foley catheter in the stomach under endoscopic guidance. The Foley catheter balloon must remain inflated to maintain tube position. Dislodgment of the tube may result if the balloon is inadvertently deflated. The advantage of this method is that the endoscope need be passed just once. Ease of tube dislodgment is a major disadvantage and the authors prefer the "pull" technique for this reason. Kits are available for each method.

1. Two trained individuals are needed: one to perform the upper gastrointestinal endoscopy and the second to perform the PEG insertion. Video-endoscopy allows all members of the team to visualize the procedure.
2. Place the patient on the endoscopy table in the supine position.
3. Prepare the upper abdomen in the usual fashion.
4. Topical anesthesia of the oropharynx may be supplemented with intravenous sedation to allow endoscopy. Local anesthesia will be infiltrated at the PEG site.
5. Introduce the endoscope into the stomach, perform a careful examination, and fully inflate the stomach.
6. Maneuver the endoscope so that its light is seen through the anterior abdominal wall. It may be necessary to turn off the room lights and use the X-illumination function of the video-endoscope to see this. Choose a point on the upper abdomen where the transillumination is

easily seen. This transillumination indicates that the inflated stomach is closely apposed to the anterior abdominal wall without intervening tissue or viscera (for example, the colon). The site will generally be just proximal to the incisura.

7. Gently depress the abdominal wall at the selected site. The endoscopist should easily see the wall indent (Fig. 43.2.6.1).

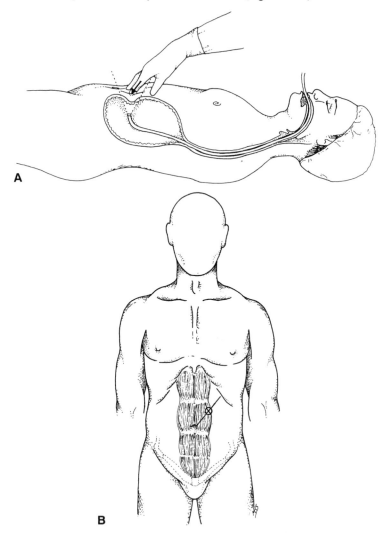

Figure 43.2.6.1. A. Transillumination and finger depression of the abdominal wall confirm juxtaposition of the inflated stomach and the anterior abdominal wall. B. The site selected will generally be approximately halfway between costal margin and umbilicus.

8. Infiltrate the selected site with local anesthesia.
9. Use a #11 blade to make a skin incision 3 to 4 mm in length.
10. Remove the needle, guide wire, dilator, and sheath from the kit. Confirm that the Foley catheter passes easily through the sheath. Test the balloon of the Foley catheter.
11. Thrust the needle through anterior abdominal wall and well into the stomach.
12. Pass the guide wire through the needle and remove the needle.
13. Pass the dilator over the guide wire, followed by the sheath. Firm but gentle pressure and a twisting motion facilitate their passage. The technique is the same as that used for percutaneous insertion of venous catheters. Endoscopic visualization confirms passage of needle, wire, dilator, and finally the sheath into the stomach.
14. Occasionally the dilator or sheath will tent up the mucosa of the stomach rather than entering the stomach. The endoscopist can apply counterpressure with the closed tip of a biopsy forceps, or increase the insufflation of the stomach. The sheath must fully enter the stomach.
15. Lubricate the Foley catheter and slide it into the stomach through the sheath. Peel away the sheath and remove it. Inflate the balloon of the Foley catheter. Pull the catheter back until the stomach is just barely indented by pressure of the balloon and secure the catheter in place. Too much tension on the catheter may lead to pressure necrosis of the gastric wall; too little may allow leakage around the tube.

C. The "Pull" Technique for PEG Placement

1. Prepare the patient and select a site for PEG placement as described in section B, items 1 to 8.
2. Make the skin incision a bit longer, generally around 1 cm in length. This appears to decrease the incidence of infection around the tube site, as the tube will be pulled through mouth, esophagus, and stomach before exiting the skin.
3. The endoscopist should position an open polypectomy snare against the anterior stomach wall at the expected entry site.
4. Take the needle, braided suture, and catheter from the kit and confirm that all are in good working condition. The needle may have a short sheath over it.
5. Thrust the needle through the small skin incision and into the stomach. The needle should enter the stomach through the polypectomy snare. If the snare does not encircle the needle at this point, allow the endoscopist to reposition the snare. If the needle carries a sheath, confirm that the sheath has entered the stomach and withdraw the needle.
6. Look carefully at the braided suture and note that one end is doubled back upon itself, essentially sharply folded on itself. Insert this end through the needle (or sheath) and into the stomach.

7. Withdraw the needle. Allow the endoscopist to lasso the braided suture. The endoscopist should tighten the snare and withdraw endoscope, snare, and braided suture out through the patient's mouth (Fig. 43.2.6.2). Maintain control of the end of the braided suture so that it is not pulled completely into the stomach. The braided suture will generally have a knot or metal clip as a safeguard.

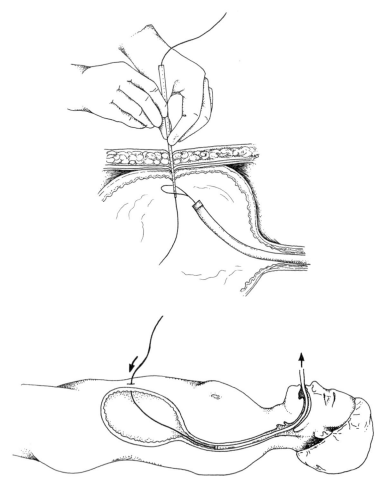

Figure 43.2.6.2. The braided suture is snared by the endoscopist and will be drawn back through the esophagus to exit through the mouth.

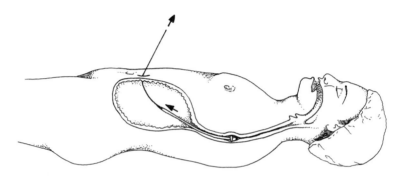

Figure 43.2.6.3. The PEG tube is pulled back into the stomach. Endoscopic verification of placement is essential.

8. The PEG catheter is then handed off to the endoscopist. The PEG catheter has a tapered end that terminates in a suture loop. The endoscopist passes one loop through the other in such a fashion that the PEG catheter is securely fastened to the braided suture. The catheter is generously lubricated with water-soluble lubricant.
9. Gently but firmly pull the braided suture back through the abdominal wall. The PEG catheter will follow (Fig. 43.2.6.3). Resistance will be encountered as the flange of the PEG catheter enters the esophagus, and again as the tapered portion of the PEG catheter exits the abdominal wall.
10. After the tapered portion exits the anterior abdominal wall, the rubber tube of the catheter will be seen. Some catheters have marks or are otherwise identifiable. Continue to pull gently but firmly until resistance indicates that the bumper of the PEG tube is engaged on the stomach wall.
11. The endoscopist should then reinsert the endoscope and again visualize the entry site. Visual confirmation of adequate position of the bumper, which should be snug but not tight against the gastric wall, is the final maneuver prior to securing the catheter (Fig. 43.2.6.4).

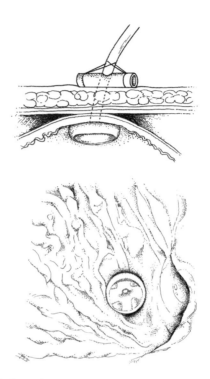

Figure 43.2.6.4. Endoscopic verification of adequate positioning of the bumper, which should be snug but not tight against the gastric wall.

D. Endoscopic Placement of Jejunal Feeding Tubes

Small caliber feeding tubes may be placed through the pylorus under endoscopic guidance. The tube may be a nasoenteric feeding tube, or may be placed adjacent to or through a PEG.

1. Visualize the tube with an endoscope positioned in the stomach. Grasp the tube with an alligator forceps.
2. Advance the endoscope and feeding tube through the pylorus under direct vision.
3. Try to advance the tube as far into the duodenum as possible.
4. Position the patient with the head of the bed elevated and left side down.
5. Allow gravity to carry the tube farther down into the jejunum.

E. Selected References

Gauderer MWL, Ponsky JL, Izant R. Gastrostomy without laparotomy: a percutaneous endoscopic technique. J Pediatr Surg 1980;15:872–875.

Ponsky JL, Aszodi A. Percutaneous endoscopic jejunostomy. Am J Gastroenterol 1984;79:113–116.

Ponsky JL, Gauderer MWL. Percutaneous endoscopic gastrostomy: a nonoperative technique for feeding gastrostomy. Gastrointest Endosc 1981;27:9–11.

44. Complications of Upper Gastrointestinal Endoscopy

Brian J. Dunkin, M.D.

A. General Considerations

Flexible upper gastrointestinal endoscopy is a safe procedure with a complication rate well below 2%. The incidence of complications increases when biopsy, polypectomy, or other invasive diagnostic or therapeutic maneuvers are performed.

Proper preparation for esophagogastroduodenoscopy (EGD) begins with a thorough history and physical examination. Both physician and patient should understand the indications for the procedure and possible complications. Patients who undergo EGD are frequently older and may have multiple medical problems or be taking medications that increase the risk of complications. General risk factors include advancing age, history of cardiac disease, or history of chronic obstructive pulmonary disease. Specific problems that are likely to be encountered and the manner in which they increase risk are given in Table 44.1.

Table 44.1. Medical problems that may increase the risk of EGD

Medical problem	Nature of complication
Valvular heart disease	Bacterial endocarditis
Diabetes	Hypoglycemia (due to NPO status)
Liver disease	Oversedation (inability to metabolize narcotics and benzodiazepines)
Depression	Hypertensive crisis (monoamine oxidase inhibitors react with meperidine)
Renal insufficiency	Oversedation, seizures (inability to excrete normeperidine, a meperidine metabolite)
Cardiac dysrhythmias	Dysrhythmia, hypotension
Chronic obstructive pulmonary disease	Hypoxemia, carbon dioxide retention
Bleeding diatheses	Bleeding

1. **Cardiopulmonary complications:** Although the overall complication rate is low, 40% to 46% of serious complications are cardiopulmonary, related to hypoxemia, vasovagal reflexes, and relative hypotension.

   a. **Hypoxemia** is common. Up to 15% of patients experience a decrease in oxygen saturation below 85% during EGD.

      i. **Cause and prevention**: This is due to sedation and to encroachment upon the airway.

      ii. **Recognition and management**: Routine monitoring of oxygen saturation gives the diagnosis. Supplemental oxygen should be administered, but may result in carbon dioxide retention if chronic obstructive pulmonary disease is present. Constant observation by a second individual who monitors vital signs, oxygen saturation, and level of consciousness (and reminds the patient to take periodic deep breaths) can help minimize this problem. A jaw thrust maneuver, performed by this assistant, will often improve airflow and oxygen saturation.

   b. **Bradycardia**

      i. **Cause and prevention:** The vasovagal reflex can trigger bradycardia and hypotension. Pretreatment with atropine combats the bradycardia, but the resulting tachycardia may increase myocardial oxygen demand. Patients who are taking beta-blockers may be unable to manifest a tachycardia in response to pain and hypovolemia. This relative bradycardia then contributes to hypotension (see below).

      ii. **Recognition and management:** Continuous ECG monitoring allows early recognition. Atropine is generally the drug of choice. Further management should follow advanced cardiac life support (ACLS) protocols.

   c. **Hypotension**

      i. **Cause and prevention:** Hypovolemia, cardiac dysrhythmias, myocardial ischemia, drug interactions, and oversedation are all potential causes. Monitoring, adequate hydration, and attention to medications and level of sedation are all crucial. Take a careful history, including medication usage, prior to EGD.

      ii. **Recognition and management:** Periodic blood pressure checks during the procedure and in the recovery phase will allow early detection. Administer a fluid bolus and search for other treatable causes (e.g., bradycardia).

   d. **Endocarditis, infection of prostheses (including joint prostheses):** Both diagnostic and therapeutic EGD have been demonstrated to cause bacteremia. The significance of this is not entirely clear, but certain groups of patients are considered at risk and should receive antibiotics prior to endoscopic procedures (Table 44.2). Carefully seek any past history of endocarditis, valvular heart disease, or recent valve or joint replacement surgery. An acceptable **prophylactic regimen** for these high-risk patients is 2 gm of parenteral ampicillin and 1.5 mg/kg gentamicin (up to 80 mg) 30 minutes before the procedure. This should be followed by a single dose of oral amoxicillin 1.5 g 6 hours after the procedure. One gram of parenteral Vancomycin may be substituted for the ampicillin in patients allergic to penicillin.

Table 44.2. American Society for Gastrointestinal Endoscopy (ASGE) recommendations for antibiotic prophylaxis for endoscopic procedures

Patient Condition	Procedure	Antibiotic Prophylaxis
Prosthetic valve, Hx endocarditis, systemic-pulmonary shunt, synthetic vascular graft <1yr old	Stricture dilation, varix sclerosis, ERCP for obstructed biliary tree	Recommended
	Other endoscopic procedures including EGD and colonoscopy (with or without biopsy or polypectomy), variceal ligation	Insufficient data to make firm recommendation; endoscopists may choose on case-by-case basis
Cirrhosis and ascites, immunocompromised patient	Stricture dilation, varix sclerosis, ERCP for obstructed biliary tree	Insufficient data to make firm recommendation; endoscopists may choose on case-by-case basis
	Other endoscopic procedures including EGD and colonoscopy (with or without biopsy or polypectomy), variceal ligation	Not recommended

ERCP, endoscopic retrograde cholangio pancreatography

2. **Medications that cause bleeding diatheses:** Many medications have the potential to cause bleeding problems. A list of common medications, problems, and suggestions for management is given below.
    a. **Aspirin:** aspirin irreversibly poisons platelets and the effect lasts until new platelets replace the affected platelets. With an average life span of 10 days in the circulation, a significant replacement effect can be noted after about 7 days. Aspirin should be stopped 1 week prior to the procedure if possible. If therapy is performed, aspirin should not be restarted for another 14 days.
    b. Other nonsteroidal antiinflammatory drugs (NSAIDs) also inhibit platelet function, but the effect is variable and reversible. **Piroxicam** (Feldene) has an effect similar to aspirin in duration.

Most other NSAIDs can be stopped 48 hours prior to the procedure.

c. **Warfarin** is another drug commonly encountered in the EGD patient. As in open surgery, there is no consensus as to its peri-procedure management. Anticoagulated patients undergoing diagnostic EGD alone are not at increased risk for bleeding. Those undergoing therapeutic EGD, however, may be. There are basically four options for management of anticoagulated patients undergoing therapeutic EGD: stop the warfarin with no heparin coverage, stop the warfarin with heparin coverage, continue warfarin at the usual dose, or continue at a reduced dose. In deciding which option to choose, it is important to assess the patient's risk for a thromboembolic complication off anticoagulation and to be clear on the indications for a therapeutic EGD. Patients at highest risk for thromboembolism are those with mechanical heart valves, coronary artery disease with persistent exertional angina, overt arterial disease at more than one site, and those with a history of a thromboembolic event while anticoagulated. The risk-benefit ratio of the four anticoagulation options must be individualized for each patient.

d. **Ticlopidine** (Ticlid) is commonly given to patients with cardiovascular problems. It retards platelet aggregation. A single dose will effect the platelets for 4 to 36 hours. The bleeding time is maximally increased after 5 to 6 days of therapy and will take 4 to 8 days to normalize after stopping the drug. The drug should therefore be managed the same as aspirin. In an emergency situation, the time to normalization of the bleeding time can be decreased to less than 2 hours by administering intravenous methylprednisolone.

e. **Dipyridamole** (Persantine) is a coronary vasodilator. There is no evidence that it increases the risk of bleeding from therapeutic endoscopy.

3. **Transmission of infection:** Strict adherence to proper cleansing procedures is important to avoid iatrogenic transmission of bacterial or viral infection.

a. *Pseudomonas aeruginosa* infections caused by contaminated scopes or water bottles have been frequently reported and have a high mortality rate.

b. *Salmonella*, *Helicobacter*, and *Mycobacterium* contamination have also been documented.

c. Viral infections have not been documented convincingly, and to date there has been no evidence of colonization of an endoscope with HIV and no reports of transmitting HIV to a patient from a contaminated scope.

4. **Aspiration:** Topical anesthesia, gastric distention, and sedation all increase the risk of aspiration during EGD. Yankauer suction must be available in case the patient vomits during endoscopy. Patient position is important: the left lateral ducubitus position with the head

slightly elevated reduces the risk of aspiration. Patients requiring emergent endoscopy or a supine position for the procedure (e.g., PEG placement) are less able to protect their airway. Consider intubation for patients undergoing EGD for bleeding or foreign body removal.

5. **Complications of conscious sedation:** Take a careful history with attention to patient allergies, medications, and comorbidities. Use the smallest amount of sedation that will provide the desired effect. Narcotics and benzodiazepines in combination are more likely to produce cardiopulmonary complications than either drug given alone. Flumazenil (reversibly inhibits benzodiazepines) and Narcan (reversibly inhibits opiate analgesics) should be readily accessible before the start of the procedure. Remember that these drugs have a shorter half-life than the benzodiazepine or narcotic being inhibited. **Therefore, a patient who is awake and responsive after receiving Narcan or flumazenil may again become unresponsive when the drug wears off.**

B. Complications of Diagnostic EGD

Mechanical complications of diagnostic EGD include esophageal perforation and dislodgment of teeth.

1. **Esophageal perforation:**
   a. **Cause and prevention:** The cervical esophagus is the area most likely to be perforated. Risk factors include anterior cervical osteophytes, Zenker's diverticulum, esophageal stricture or web, or a cervical rib. Most cervical esophageal perforations occur during rigid endoscopy, or with blind passage of a flexible endoscope. Gentle passage under direct visual control is the best way to prevent perforation. Perforation can occur at any level where there is a stricture or other pathology. Retching with an overinsufflated stomach and the endoscope occluding the gastroesophageal junction (GEJ) can result in Mallory-Weiss tears or esophageal perforation. Avoid this by adequate sedation, limiting insufflation, and removing the endoscope from the GEJ if the patient starts to retch.
   b. **Recognition and management:** Cervical pain, crepitus, and cellulitis are all signs of a high esophageal perforation. Distal perforations cause chest pain. The diagnosis is confirmed by water-soluble contrast esophagram. **Cervical esophageal perforations** can usually be managed with antibiotics and withholding oral intake, or by cervical exploration and drainage. Rarely is primary repair or diversion necessary. **Distal esophageal perforation** may require immediate surgical drainage or repair.

2. **Dislodgment of teeth or dentures:**
   a. **Cause and prevention:** Avoid this problem by removing any dentures before introducing the scope. Place a bite block to protect the teeth and the instrument.
   b. **Recognition and management:** The problem is usually recognized by the patient. Obtain a PA and lateral chest x-ray to exclude aspiration. Remove aspirated foreign bodies immediately (bronchoscopy). Ingested teeth will pass without incident. Ingested dental appliances may or may not depending on size. Repeat endoscopy and removal may be needed (see Chapter 43.5, Foreign Body Removal).

C. Complications of Therapeutic EGD

1. **Therapeutic endoscopy for nonvariceal bleeding** is associated with few complications. The major risk is **precipitation of bleeding** from a nonbleeding ulcer. Complications of specific modalities used for control of bleeding are listed below:
   a. **Injection therapy:** Bleeding peptic ulcers can be controlled with the injection of epinephrine or a sclerosant. Plasma epinephrine levels increase four- to five-fold within minutes of injection of **epinephrine**, but return to baseline within 20 minutes. These levels may be higher in patients with liver disease. Only one case of **asymptomatic hypertension and ventricular tachycardia** has been reported after epinephrine injection. Sclerosing agents can (rarely) cause **full-thickness necrosis, obstructive jaundice**, and **intramural hematoma**.
   b. **Cauterization (thermal therapy):** Heater probe, multipolar probe, and laser all have low rates of treatment-induced bleeding and perforation. Monopolar cautery is generally avoided because of a high incidence of full-thickness injury.
   c. **Other modalities:** Early experience with the argon plasma coagulator has been associated with no morbidity. Little data are available concerning the safety and efficacy of endoscopic clips.
2. **Therapeutic EGD for variceal bleeding** has become commonplace with approximately a 90% success rate at controlling the initial bleeding episode. The primary complications are stricture, perforation, and bleeding.
   a. **Variceal banding:** The incidence of stricture (0%), perforation (0.7%), and bleeding from ulceration at the banding site (2.6–7.8%) are all lower than with sclerotherapy. Chest pain is common after EVL and may be related to esophageal spasm. Historically, EVL had the additional risk of requiring the use of an overtube to facilitate multiple passes of the endoscope. This is not needed with multiband ligators.

b. **Variceal sclerotherapy:** Complications occur in 20% to 40% of cases with a 1% to 2% mortality. The most common complications are stricture formation (11.8%), perforation (4.3%), bleeding from ulceration at the injection site (12.7%), and pneumonia (6.8%). Chest pain, pleural effusions, pulmonary infiltrates and bacteremia each occur in 44% to 50% of patients.

3. **Dilatation of strictures** is primarily performed for esophageal lesions. Dilatation of nonesophageal lesions is becoming more frequent and is associated with a very low complication rate. This section concentrates on the complication of esophageal dilatation. There are two methods of dilatation: endoscopic placement of a guide wire across the stricture followed by advancement of a dilator, and transendoscopic balloon dilatation. It is unclear if any particular dilatation technique is best to avoid complications. The risk of developing a complication from endoscopic dilatations is more dependent on the underlying pathology than the technique of dilatation, provided proper technique is followed (see Chapter 43.3). **Perforation** is the most common complication, with an overall incidence of 0.2% for all techniques and pathology (Table 44.3). Esophageal dilatation results in **bacteremia** in up to 50% of patients; prophylactic antibiotics should be given to prevent endocarditis (see section A above). **Hematemesis** occurs in 1% to 1.5% of patients but is usually self-limited; hemorrhage requiring transfusion is rare.

Table 44.3. Type of stricture and risk of perforation following dilatation

Type of stricture	Risk of perforation
Benign	Unknown
Malignant	9–24%
Radiation induced	0–3.6%
Caustic	0–15.4% (0.8%/dilatation)
Anastomotic	0%
Achalasia	0–6.6%

4. Endoscopic placement of **esophageal stents** is most commonly performed for palliation of obstructing tumors and is often preceded by dilatation. Complications can occur from dilatation or from the stent itself. The stents can cause erosion with perforation, bleeding, migration, tumor ingrowth with recurrent obstruction, food impaction, and aspiration. Stents placed in the very proximal or distal esophagus are associated with the highest rates of complication. Stents in the **cervical esophagus** can cause difficulty with swallowing and predispose to aspiration. Those across the **GEJ** cause gastroesophageal reflux with esophagitis and aspiration. The risk of **aspiration** is minimized

by maintaining the patient in a "head-up" position. **Esophagitis** is managed with H$_2$-blocker therapy or proton pump inhibitors. **Recurrent obstruction** is treated with laser or argon plasma coagulator ablation of the tumor ingrowth, or placement of a second stent through the first.

D. Complications of Percutaneous Endoscopic Gastrostomy and Jejunostomy

Large cumulative retrospective studies have reported that 10% to % of both adult and pediatric patients have at least one complication following PEG placement.

Pneumoperitoneum is a frequent occurrence after percutaneous gastrostomy. This may be the result of air escaping around the puncturing needle. Routine x-ray films are unwarranted. Air in the abdominal cavity has been shown to last for up to 5 weeks after PEG placement. Patients found to have pneumoperitoneum after gastrostomy must be clinically evaluated. In the absence of abdominal tenderness, leukocytosis, or fever, there is no need for further evaluation.

Good **skin care** is important after gastrostomy. It is common to see a foreign body reaction around the tube with some exudate or granulation tissue. Swab the exudate away with hydrogen peroxide and leave the site open to air. Cauterize granulation tissue with silver nitrate. Avoid occlusive dressings; these may lead to skin maceration.

Other more significant complications are enumerated below.
1. **Wound infections** are common.
    a. **Cause and pevention:** Contamination with oral and gastric flora contribute to the incidence of wound infection (particularly with a "pull" technique). Wound problems can also result from excess tension on the tube (causing pressure necrosis) and a small skin incision (which fails to allow egress of bacteria). The incidence is decreased with a single prophylactic dose of cefazolin.
    b. **Recognition and mnagement:** Signs and symptoms of wound infection include erythema around the gastrostomy tube site several days after the procedure, local tenderness, slight edema of the skin, low-grade fever, and leukocytosis. Incision and drainage of the area under local anesthesia most often resolves the problem. Failure to identify and treat this problem at an early stage can result in **necrotizing infections of the abdominal wall** and death.
2. **Buried bumper syndrome** (extrusion of the head of the tube from the gastric lumen into the subcutaneous tissue):
    a. **Cause and prevention:** Excessive tension is the main cause. Do not tighten up the bumper in an attempt to prevent leakage around the tube, and do not place dressings under the skin anchoring device. At all times, avoid excess pressure and tension.

b.   **Recognition and management:** This may cause wound infection or leakage of gastric juice and feedings into the peritoneal cavity or subcutaneous tissues. Remove the gastrostomy tube, place the patient on nasogastric suction, and treat the patient with parenteral antibiotics until the gastrostomy tract inflammation and skin necrosis resolve.

3.   **Leakage of feedings** into the peritoneal cavity is one of the most serious complications.

a.   **Cause and prevention:** this is usually the result of separation of the gastric and abdominal walls and often is due to necrosis of the gastric wall due to excessive tension on the catheter. Premature dislodgment of the tube (before a tract has formed) or attempt at reinsertion of a dislodged tube may result in malposition and a similar problem.

b.   **Recognition and management:** Patients who develop abdominal tenderness, fever, or leukocytosis should be evaluated for leakage and the resultant peritonitis. This is done by instilling water-soluble contrast material into the gastrostomy tube under fluoroscopic guidance. Intraperitoneal extravasation indicates something has gone awry. If the contrast study indicates that the head of the tube remains in the stomach and that the extravasation is around it, the tube can usually be salvaged by inserting a nasogastric tube, placing the PEG to drainage, and administering intravenous fluids and antibiotics. If the contrast study reveals complete separation of the gastric and abdominal walls with dislodgment of the tube from the stomach, the tube should be pulled from the abdominal wall and the above treatment instituted. A patient whose PEG has been pulled out inadvertently less than 2 weeks from the time of insertion should be treated similarly. If at any time the patient's condition begins to deteriorate or signs of peritonitis worsen, exploratory laparotomy with operative repair should be performed.

4.   **Gastrocolic fistula** has rarely been known to occur after percutaneous gastrostomy.

a.   **Cause and prevention:** This may be due to puncture of the colon at the time of gastrostomy or pinching of the colon between the gastric and abdominal walls with subsequent necrosis of the colonic wall and fistula formation. It is prevented by careful technique. Laparoscopic visualization (described in Chapter 8) may be useful.

b.   **Recognition and management:** This complication usually becomes apparent after several weeks with the development of severe diarrhea following feedings. It may be documented with an upper gastrointestinal series or barium enema. In nearly all cases, the condition may be treated by removing the gastrostomy tube. The fistula closes rapidly once the tube is removed.

5.   **Progressive enlargement of the stoma** around the gastrostomy tube may occur in some patients.

a. **Cause and prevention:** Excessive tension, poor nutritional status, and excess movement of the tube at skin level can cause this problem. As previously mentioned, avoid excess tension. Minimize tube mobility by securing the tube or using a stabilizing device.

b. **Recognition and management:** The problem is easily recognized by leakage of gastric juice and feedings around the tube. Replacing the gastrostomy tube with a larger size only provides a short-term solution, as the tract generally continues to enlarge. A better solution is to remove the tube entirely and allow the tract to close. When the tract contracts, insert a new, smaller tube.

6. **Neoplastic seeding** (to skin around the gastrostomy tube) has been reported when PEG placement for both oropharyngeal and esophageal cancers. This is not an issue when the gastrostomy is placed for palliation in a patient with limited life span. It should be kept in mind when gastrostomy placement is planned prior to neoadjuvant therapy. There may be advantages to using an introducer technique in this setting, but this has not been tested.

E. Selected References

Arrowsmith J, Gerstman B, Fleisher D, et al. Results from the American Society for Gastrointestinal Endoscopy/U.S. Food and Drug Administration collaborative study on complication rates and drug use during gastrointestinal endoscopy. Gastrointest Endosc 1991;37:421–427.

ASGE Position Statement: The recommended use of laboratory studies before endoscopic procedures. Gastrointest Endosc 1993;39:892.

ASGE recommendations for antibiotic prophylaxis for endoscopic procedures. Gastrointest Endosc 1995;42(6):633.

Cook DJ, Guyatt GH, Salena BJ, et al. Endoscopic therapy for acute nonvariceal upper gastrointestinal hemorrhage: a meta analysis. Gastroenterology 1992;102:139.

Jain NK, Larson DE, Schroeder KW, et al. Antibiotic prophylaxis for percutaneous endoscopic gastrostomy. A prospective, randomized, double-blind clinical trial. Ann Intern Med 1987;107:824–828.

Lee JG, Lieberman DA. Complications related to endoscopic hemostasis techniques. Gastrointest Endosc Clin North Am 1996;6(2):305–321.

Marks JM. Esophagogastroduodenoscopy. In: Complications of Endoscopic and Laparoscopic Surgery. Prevention and Management. Ponsky JL (ed.). Philadelphia:Lippincott-Raven, 1997, pp. 13–28.

Ponsky JL, Dunkin BJ. Percutaneous endoscopic gastrostomy. In: Textbook of Gastroenterology, Yamada T, (ed.). Philadelphia: Lippincott-Raven, 1997.

Silvis SE, Nebel O, Rogers G, et al. Endoscopic complications. Results of the 1974 American Society of Gastrointestinal Endoscopy Survey. JAMA 1976;235:928.

45. Small Bowel Enteroscopy

Charles H. Andrus, M.D., F.A.C.S.
Scott H. Miller, M.D.

A. Indications

Small bowel endoscopy (enteroscopy) is generally used when other diagnostic modalities are inadequate.

1. **Occult GI bleeding** is the most common indication.
   a. 5% of GI bleeding is undiagnosed after esophagogastroduodenoscopy (EGD), colonoscopy, and contrast radiographic studies. Enteroscopy has been reported to be successful diagnosis in 26% to 75% of these cases. The most commonly identified source is an angiodysplasia.
   b. Enteroscopy may be used preoperatively as well as intraoperatively to guide treatment. It provides localization of the bleeding source.
2. Evaluation of **small bowel tumors or polyps**
   a. Familial adenomatous polyposis
   b. Gardner's syndrome
   c. Peutz-Jeghers syndrome
   d. Lymphoma or carcinoma
3. Assessment other small bowel pathology
   a. **Crohn's disease**—The endoscopic mucosal involvement is difficult to visualize due to associated stricture formation.
   b. **Celiac disease**—In the endoscopic diagnosis of the loss or reduction in folds for the diagnosis of subtotal villous atrophy: sensitivity 88%; specificity, 83%; positive predictive value, 65%; negative predictive value, 95%.
   c. **Sprue**

B. Technique of Enteroscopy

Several methods of small bowel endoscopy are available. Push and sonde techniques are described here, followed by a discussion of intraoperative endoscopy.

1. **Push enteroscopy:** This is the easiest and quickest of the methods, but can only reach 60 cm beyond the ligament of Treitz.

a. Use a pediatric colonoscope (135–145 cm) or a flexible entero-scope (165–200 cm).

b. Employ a stiff overtube to straighten the scope from the mouth to the pylorus into the short (lesser curve) position in the stomach and prevent curling.

c. This technique requires two individuals: one to control the enteroscope deflection and one to control overtube placement and stability and forward advancement of the scope.

d. Advance the enteroscope through the mouth and esophagus to just beyond the gastroesophageal junction.

e. Advance the overtube over the scope into the proximal stomach.

f. Advance scope and overtube together through the pylorus.

g. Advance the enteroscope through the lumen of the small bowel under direct vision. Attempt to telescope the enteroscope through the small bowel as far as possible.

h. Completely evaluate the small bowel mucosa during enteroscope withdrawal.

2. **Sonde enteroscopy**

a. A 5-mm-diameter, 275-cm scope (e.g., model SSIF VIII, Olympus Corp. Ltd, Tokyo, Japan) is inserted transnasally and introduced through the pylorus by a piggyback technique with a pediatric colonoscope.

b. The scope has two internal channels:
   i. one for air inflation of the small bowel
   ii. one for balloon inflation
   iii. no channel for biopsies or brushes

c. The technique consists of the placement of the scope through the pylorus with subsequent insufflation of the balloon and distal progression by peristalsis.

d. The distal position of the scope is confirmed by fluoroscopy. The average transit time through the entire small bowel is ~6 hours.

e. Once the scope reaches its most distal position, it is withdrawn with small bowel insufflation and the small bowel mucosa is examined during this withdrawal phase.

f. Unfortunately, complete examination of the bowel during withdrawal is impossible due to the inability to steer this scope and the variability to control the rate of withdrawal through the telescoped bowel.

3. **Mayo Clinic sonde technique** (prototype sonde small bowel enteroscope: Olympus, SIF VI KAI: 267.5 cm)

a. The enteroscope is introduced orally through an insertion tube and is positioned by fluoroscopy near the pylorus.

b. The scope is introduced through the pylorus under direct vision.

c. A guide wire is inserted through the inner channel (2 mm diameter) and the scope is advanced over the guide wire under fluoroscopic control.

    d.   The average duration of the procedure is ~4.5 hours. Approximately 85% of the reported procedures by this technique have reached the mid- to distal ileum.

    e.   Although a 2-mm channel is present, it is difficult to pass any instrument through the channel.

4. **Intraoperative enteroscopy**

    a.   This technique is considered the best and most complete method of endoscopic small bowel evaluation.

    b.   Formal laparotomy is performed and adhesions (if present) are lysed so that the small intestine can be freely manipulated from the ligament of Treitz to the ileocecal valve.

    c.   Two trained individuals cooperate. One manipulates the bowel through the surgical incision. The second serves as endoscopist.

    d.   The endoscopist passes a standard colonoscope through the mouth into the stomach.

    e.   The surgeon manually directs the scope through the pylorus and around the sweep of the duodenum while the endoscopist advances the endoscope.

    f.   With continued advancement of the scope by the endoscopist, the surgeon manually telescopes the small bowel over the scope and it is advanced to the ileocecal junction.

    g.   With the operating room lights darkened, the scope is slowly withdrawn, with the rate of small bowel examination controlled by the surgeon. Manual occlusion proximal and distal allows insufflation of a selected segment without distention of the entire small bowel (Fig. 45.1). Ectasias and bleeding sites can be visualized by both the endoscopist directly and by the surgeon by transillumination.

5. **Biopsy and sampling techniques**

    a.   When a pediatric or standard colonoscope are employed by the push technique, standard endoscopic biopsy forceps and brushes can be utilized.

    b.   When the sonde-type scopes are employed, a biopsy channel is absent or extremely small, preventing easy passage of biopsy, brush, or laser fibers.

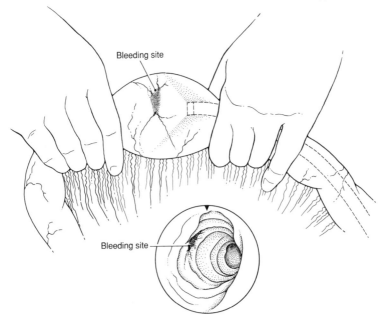

Figure 45.1. Manual compression proximal and distal to a selected segment allow insufflation. The lesion is visualized both by the endoscopist and by transillumination. Reprinted with permission from Scott-Conner CEH and Dawson DL. Operative Anatomy (Lippincott-Raven Publishers, Philadelphia, PA, 1993).

C. Complications

1. **Epistaxis**
   a. **Cause and prevention**: Epistaxis can be caused by prolonged nasal irritation and may be minimized by frequent lubrication during the passage of the enteroscope.
   b. **Recognition and management**: Although easily recognized, complete prevention may not be possible.
2. **Pancreatitis**
   a. **Cause and prevention**: This is theorized to result from prolonged irritation to the ampulla of Vater. No prevention is known.
   b. **Recognition and management**: Pancreatitis is documented by standard chemical serologic markers. It is managed according to severity.
3. **Perforation**
   a. **Cause and prevention**: Forceful or blind advancement of the overtube may cause perforation. Advancement under direct vi-

sion to and through the pylorus is the best way to prevent such an occurrence.

b. **Recognition and management**: Intestinal perforation can be recognized by the radiologic identification of free air and most probably will require operative management.

4. **Inability to advance the scope or to confirm the diagnosis**: By sonde methods, only 50% to 75% of the mucosa is visualized on the average, while by the push technique only 60 cm distal to the ligament of Treitz can be reached. In approximately 50% of patients who come to enteroscopy it is not possible to definitively diagnose the site of GI bleeding.

D. Selected References

Axon ATR. Small bowel and duodenum: enteroscopy. In: Annual of Gastrointestinal Endoscopy 1989. Cotton PB, Tytgat GNJ, Williams CB (eds.). London: Current Science, 1989, pp. 35–37.

Lobo AJ, Axon ATR. Endoscopy of the small bowel and duodenum. In: Annual of Gastrointestinal Endoscopy 1991. Cotton PB, Tytgat GNJ, Williams CB (eds.). London: Current Science, 1991, pp. 33–39.

Schuman BM. Endoscopy of the small bowel and duodenum. In: Annual of Gastrointestinal Endoscopy 1989. Cotton PB, Tytgat GNJ, Williams CB (eds.). London: Gower Academic Journals, 1988, pp. 29–35.

Shinya H, McSherry C. Endoscopy of the small bowel. Surg Clin North Am 1982;62:821–824.

Waye JD. Enteroscopy. In: Annual of Gastrointestinal Endoscopy 1992. Cotton PB, Tytgat GNJ, Williams CB (eds.). London: Current Science, 1992, pp. 61–65.

46.1. Endoscopic Retrograde Cholangiopancreatography

Harry S. Himal, M.D.

A. Indications

For a long time examination of the extrahepatic biliary tree and pancreatic duct was possible only at the time of laparotomy. In 1968 McCune, a surgeon and his colleagues first reported the endoscopic visualization of the common bile and pancreatic duct. Since then, innovations and improvements in technology have resulted in the technique of endoscopic retrograde cholangiopancreatography (ERCP) becoming indispensable in the diagnosis of diseases of the biliary tree and pancreatic duct. The development of compute tomographic scans, endoscopic ultrasonography, percutaneous transhepatic cholangiography, and magnetic resonance imaging has not diminished the importance of ERCP. ERCP is used for three major purposes: visualization of the ampulla of Vater, radiographic study of the common bile duct (cholangiography), and radiographic study of the pancreatic duct (pancreatography). Specific indications are listed in Table 46.1.1, and representative radiographs are shown in Figures 46.1.1–46.1.6.

Table 46.1.1. Indications for ERCP

• Visualization of ampulla of Vater
Adenomas
Carcinoma
Surveillance in patients with polyposis syndromes
• Cholangiography (Figs. 46.1.1–46.1.4)
Cholestatic jaundice of unknown cause
Choledocholithiasis
Cholangitis
Carcinoma of the bile duct
Bile duct stricture
Bile duct injury
• Pancreatography (Figs. 46.1.5–46.1.6)
Chronic pancreatitis
Pancreatic carcinoma
Pancreatic ascites
Pancreatic pseudocyst
Pancreatic trauma
Gallstone pancreatitis

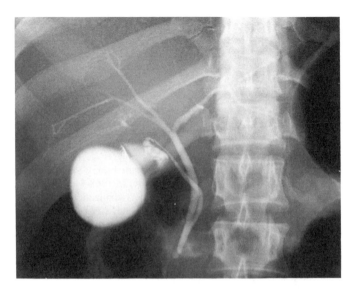

Figure 46.1.1. Normal cholangiogram obtained at ERCP. Note that gallbladder is also visualized.

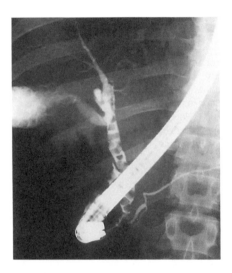

Figure 46.1.2. ERCP performed in patient with cholestatic jaundice in whom the differential diagnosis included both drug-induced and mechanical causes of jaundice. The cholangiogram demonstrates stones within the common bile duct.

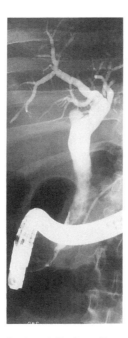

Figure 46.1.3. Common bile duct full of small stones and debris in a patient with cholangitis. Endoscopic sphincterotomy and removal of stones and debris resulted in clinical improvement.

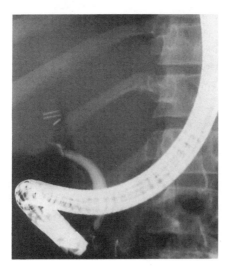

Figure 46.1.4. Common bile duct injury in a patient who had undergone laparoscopic cholecystectomy. Clips are seen across the proximal common bile duct.

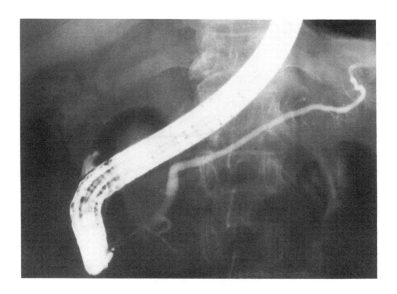

Figure 46.1.5. Normal pancreatogram obtained at ERCP.

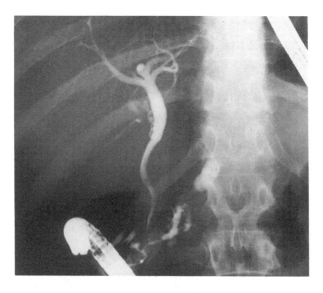

Figure 46.1.6. Pancreatic duct in a patient with chronic pancreatitis demonstrating dilatation and strictures. The common duct is also visualized and demonstrates extrinsic compression by the pancreatic mass.

B. Facilities and Equipment

ERCP requires the following facilities and equipment:
1. An x-ray room capable of both fluoroscopy (to visualize which duct has been cannulated) and film or digital radiography. A room dedicated to ERCP is most convenient (Fig. 46.1.7).
2. The ERCP endoscope is a side-viewing instrument that allows accurate visualization of the ampulla of Vater (Fig. 46.1.8). Videoendoscopy is now considered standard for ERCP.
3. A variety of different catheters are used to cannulate the ampulla (Fig. 46.1.9).

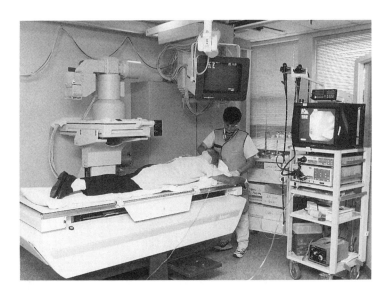

Figure 46.1.7. X-ray facilities to carry out ERCP include fluoroscopy. Note the position of the patient, endoscopic cart, and fluoroscopic monitor.

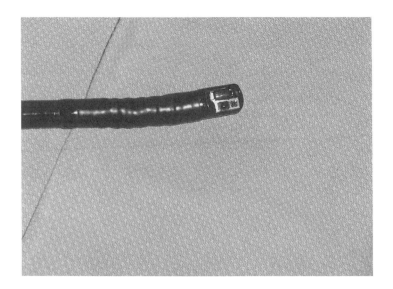

Figure 46.1.8. The side-viewing endoscope used for ERCP allows en face visualization, biopsy, and cannulation of the ampulla of Vater.

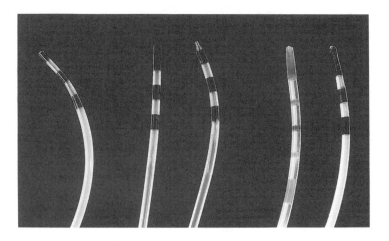

Figure 46.1.9. Catheters used for cannulation of ampulla of Vater.

C. Patient Preparation

1. **Explain the technique and possible complications** to the patient and obtain informed consent. A knowledgeable, informed patient will cooperate with the endoscopist so that the procedure can be done quickly and safely.
2. The patient is **kept NPO for 6 hours prior** to the procedure. Diabetic patients on insulin should have an intravenous drip started.
3. If therapeutic ERCP (papillotomy, biopsy, stone extraction) may be required, evaluate the **coagulation status** of the patient. This is particularly important in jaundiced patients.
4. Patients with possible biliary obstruction, cholangitis, or choledocholithiasis should receive antibiotics directed at common biliary flora.
5. Anesthetize the oropharynx with topical anesthetic. The author prefers Xylocaine 4%.
6. Place a secure intravenous catheter in the right hand or arm.
7. Position the patient prone with the head turned to the right (Fig. 46.1.5).
8. Analgesia and conscious sedation facilitate the procedure (see Chapter 41). The author's preference is for meperidine 25 to 50 mg IV with diazemuls 5 to 10 mg IV.
9. Appropriate monitoring includes pulse oximetry, heart rate, and blood pressure (see Chapter 41).
10. As soon as the endoscope is within the duodenum, give Buscopan (hyoscine butylbromide) 20 to 40 mg IV or glucagon HCl 1 mg IV to decrease duodenal peristalsis.

D. Passing the ERCP Scope — Normal Anatomy

1. Introduce the endoscope gently through the mouth guard into the mouth and oropharynx. This is essentially a blind procedure, which is greatly facilitated by having the patient swallow.
2. Pass the endoscope gently down the esophagus into the stomach.
3. Once in the stomach, advance the endoscope toward the pylorus (Fig. 46.1.10). The side-viewing endoscope sometimes makes it difficult to traverse the stomach and identify the pylorus. Persistent maneuvering, combined with shortening of the endoscope by withdrawing to eliminate redundancy in the stomach, will ultimately prove successful. Frequently the presence of bile in the distal stomach will lead one to the pylorus, which is usually close by.
4. Use gentle rotation and pressure to pass the endoscope through the pylorus into the proximal duodenum (Fig. 46.1.11).
5. Turn the "up and down" and "right and left" dials both to their maximum clockwise extent and lock these controls.

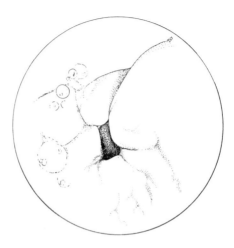

Figure 46.1.10. View of pylorus. Bubbles indicating bile provide a clue to the location of the distal stomach when orientation of the side-viewing endoscope is difficult.

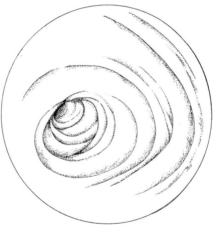

Figure 46.1.11. View of the proximal duodenum.

6. Shorten the endoscope by pulling back. The ampulla of Vater should then be centrally visualized (Fig. 46.1.12). Make small adjustments in the locked dials so that the ampulla of Vater is seen en face.
7. Biopsy of the ampulla or selective cannulation of the pancreatic and common bile ducts may then be performed (Fig. 46.1.13).

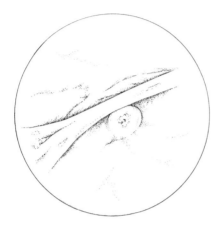

Figure 46.1.12. Endoscopic visualization of the ampulla of Vater. A transverse fold of mucosa overlying the ampulla is frequently seen, as shown here.

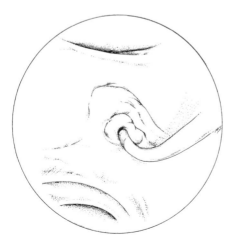

Figure 46.1.13. Cannulation of ampulla of Vater.

8. The orifice of the pancreatic duct is at the 1 o'clock position and the orifice of the common bile duct at the 11 o'clock position. Introduce the cannula into the orifice of the ampulla of Vater and gently inject 1 to 2 ml of 50% Hypaque dye (or alternative contrast medium in patients allergic to Hypaque) while monitoring passage of contrast under fluoroscopy to identify the ductal anatomy. Further technical details of cannulation, cholangiography and pancreatography are given in Chapter 47.

E. Selected References

Bilbao MK, Dotter CT, Lee TG, Katon RM. Complications of endoscopic retrograde cholangiopancreatography (E.R.C.P.). Gastroenterology 1976;70:314–320.

Calleti G, Brocchi E, Agostini D. Sensitivity of endoscopic retrograde pancreatography in chronic pancreatitis. Br J Surg 1982;69:507–509.

Cameron JL. Chronic pancreatic ascites and pancreatic pleural effusions. Gastroenterology 1978;74:134–140.

Frick MP, Feinberg SB, Goodale RL. The value of endoscopic retrograde cholangiopancreatography in suspected carcinoma of the pancreas and indeterminate computer tomography results. Surg Gynecol Obstet 1982;155:177–182.

Gaisford WS. Endoscopic retrograde cholangiopancreatography in the diagnosis of jaundice. Am J Surg 1976;132:699–704.

Ghazi A, Washington M. Endoscopic diagnosis and management of diseases of the pancreas and hepatobiliary tract. Probl Gen Surg 1990;7:1610–1674.

Himal HS. The role of E.R.C.P. in laparoscopic cholecystectomy related cystic duct stump leaks. Surg Endosc 1996;10:653–655.

Himal HS, Lindsay T. Ascending cholangitis: surgery versus endoscopic or percutaneous drainage. Surgery 1990;108:629–634.

Kozarek R, Gannan R, Baerg R, Wagonfeld J, Ball, T. Bile leak after laparoscopic cholecystectomy: diagnostic and therapeutic application of endoscopic retrograde cholangiopancreatography. Arch Intern Med 1992;152:1040–1043.

Kullman E, Borch K, Lindstrom E, Ansehn S, Ilse I, Anderberg B. Bacteremia following diagnostic and therapeutic E.R.C.P. Gastrointest Endosc 1992;38:444–449.

Laraja RD, Lobbato VJ, Cassaro S, Reddy S. Intraoperative endoscopic retrograde cholangiopancreatography (E.R.C.P.) in penetrating trauma of the pancreas. J Trauma 1986;6:1146–1147.

Low DE, Mioflikier AB, Kennedy JK, Stiver HG. Infectious complications of endoscopic retrograde cholangiopancreatography. Arch Intern Med 1980;140:1076–1077.

McCune WS, Shorb PE, Moscowitz H. Endoscopic cannulation of the ampulla of Vater: a preliminary report. Ann Surg 1968;167:752–756.

Neoptolemos JP, Carr-Locke DC, London NJ, Bailey IA, James D, Fossard DP. Controlled trial of urgent endoscopic retrograde cholangiopancreatography and endoscopic sphincterotomy versus conservative treatment for acute pancreatitis due to gallstones. Lancet 1988;2:979–983.

O'Connor M, Kolars J, Ansel H, Silvis S, Vennes J. Preoperative endoscopic retrograde cholangiopancreatography in the surgical management of pancreatic pseudocysts. Am J Surg 1986;151:18–24.

Oi L. Fiberduodenoscopy and endoscopic pancreatocholangiography. Gastrointest Endosc 1970;17:59–62.

Sherman S, Lehman GA. E.R.C.P. and endoscopic sphincterotomy induced pancreatitis. Pancreas 1991;6:350–367.

Skude G, Wehlin L, Maruyama, T, Ariyama J. Hyperamylasemia after duodenoscopy and retrograde cholangiopancreatography. Gut 1976;17:127–132.

Vennew JA, Bond JH. Approach to the jaundiced patient. Gastroenterology 1983;84:1615–1619.

46.2. Surgically Altered Anatomy and Special Considerations

Maurice E. Arregui, M.D., F.A.C.S.

A. Billroth II

Successful passage of the endoscope with cannulation of the ampulla is only achieved in 50% to 85% of patients with Billroth II anastomoses (in contrast to the 90% success rate that can be attained in patients with normal anatomy). This is due to both the difficulty in maneuvering through a variably long or angled afferent limb and the unusual position of the papilla once it is reached. Some endoscopists prefer to use a pediatric colonoscope or gastroscope, others prefer to use the duodenoscope. Specialized papillotomes are often required for therapeutic maneuvers. The indications for performing ERCP in patients with a Billroth II anastomosis are identical to those in patients with normal anatomy.

1. The **room setup**, **patient position**, topical anesthesia, sedation, and monitoring are the same as that used for patients with normal anatomy.
2. It is often useful **pass a gastroscope first** to better familiarize oneself with the anatomy.
3. **Enter the stomach** and identify the gastrojejunal anastomosis.
4. Pass the scope into one of the orifices.
5. It is often difficult to tell which is the afferent limb without fluoroscopy. Therefore, as the scope is passed, **check the position with fluoroscopy**.
6. If the scope goes into the pelvis, it is in the efferent limb. Bring the scope back into the stomach and enter the second orifice.
7. Once the afferent limb is entered, maneuver the scope in a fashion similar to that used to maneuver a colonoscope through a tortuous sigmoid colon. Advance the scope for a distance and then retract it in an attempt to shorten the loop of jejunum. Sharp angles may be difficult to get around and the shortening maneuver often helps to decrease an accentuated angle created by insufflating the bowel or excessive stretching of the bowel limb with the endoscope.
8. **Check the trajectory of the scope** with fluoroscopy to be certain that it is headed for the right upper quadrant (Fig. 46.2.1). An antecolic Billroth II may be more difficult to maneuver than a shorter retrocolic anastomosis.

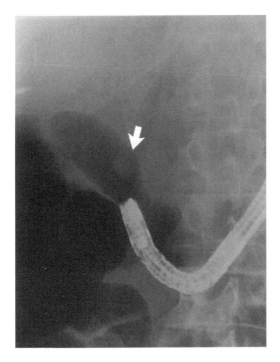

Figure 46.2.1. X-ray showing a gastroscope in the afferent limb of a Billroth II. Insufflation of the duodenum shows a blind ending limb in the right upper quadrant. The ampulla (arrow) is seen in this air duodenogram.

9. Once the **proximal duodenum** is entered, identify the blind proximal end and slowly pull the scope back until the papilla is identified.
10. Many prefer using the side-viewing **duodenoscope**. Passage with either scope is the same but because of the difference in perspective, passage of the duodenoscope is slightly more difficult.
    a. Because the papilla is viewed from below, the orientation and perspective is different.
    b. Rather than a typical en face papilla with the common bile duct oriented at the 11 to 12 o'clock position, the papilla is seen in the right upper portion of the viewing area with the common bile duct orifice at the 6 o'clock position. (Fig. 46.2.2).
11. If a gastroscope or pediatric colonoscope is used, the papilla is oriented in a more tangential position in the lower left of the screen. Cannulation of the common bile duct with a straight-viewing scope is often very straightforward as the scope is often oriented in line with the common bile duct. A standard diagnostic cannula is used.

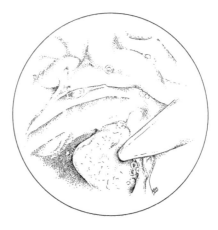

Figure 46.2.2. View of the ampulla through a duodenoscope. Cannulation requires positioning the catheter at a 6 o'clock location.

12. **Cannulation** with a duodenoscope can be more difficult due to the unusual orientation of the common bile duct orifice at 6 o'clock. (Fig. 46.2.3). Because of the curve of the duodenoscope, the cannula tip has a tendency to curve toward a more 12 o'clock to 9 o'clock position. A wire through the tip of the cannula may provide a straighter trajectory to allow cannulation at the 6 o'clock postion.

13. **Technique of sphincterotomy:** (See also Chapter 48) Once successful cannulation is performed and a need for sphincterotomy is established, the orientation of the duodenoscope and the papilla creates a challenge for the endoscopist.

    a.   The advantage of the duodenoscope is the ability to maneuver the papillotome.

    b.   Because of the orientation of the scope and the papilla compounded by the upward deflection of a standard papillotome, specialized sphincterotomes and techniques are often employed. For example, a Billroth II papillotome bows the wire outward, which allows orientation of the cutting wire toward the 6 o'clock position when using the duodenoscope.

    c.   Alternatively, place a 7-French stent in the common bile duct and use a needle papillotome to cut the papilla over the stent.

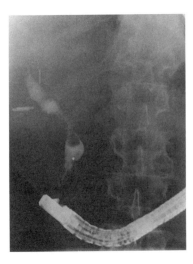

Figure 46.2.3. Cannulation of the bile duct using a duodenoscope. Contrast injection reveals a common bile duct stone.

B. Choledochoduodenostomy

Sump syndrome (characterized by cholangitis, liver abscess, or recurrent pancreatitis) is the most common indication for evaluation of a choledochoduodenostomy. Treatment consists of removal of debris and stones and possible sphincterotomy.

1. Either a thin-caliber gastroscope or a side-viewing duodenoscope may be used.
    a. Advance the gastroscope into the second portion of the duodenum. If the anastomosis is not stenotic, the scope can be advanced in directly. The technique is no different than standard gastroscopy.
    b. Pass the side-viewing duodenoscope as during standard ERCP.
2. Debris can be retrieved through the choledochoduodenostomy or the ampulla
    a. If the choledochoduodenostomy is the route chosen, advance a gastroscope or small-caliber pediatric scope through the anastomosis.
    b. Pass wire baskets or balloon catheters through the channel of the scope to retrieve the stones or debris.
    c. If the anastomosis is stenosed, balloon dilation may be required prior to passage. No attempt should be made to use a sphincterotome to enlarge the anastomosis as bleeding or perforation could result.

d. Alternatively and preferably, the duodenoscope can be used to cannulate the common bile duct through the ampulla and sphincterotomy carried out using standard technique. Debris is removed with a balloon catheter or a wire basket. Performing a sphincterotomy may improve the dependent drainage and thereby reduce the chances for recurrence of the sump syndrome.

C. Choledochojejunostomy

Endoscopy is performed to evaluate bleeding or obstruction at the site of the anastomosis.

1. Use a **colonoscope or enteroscope**. Pass the scope in standard fashion through the pylorus and into the third portion of the duodenum. As in passage in a patient with a Billroth II anastomosis, the jejunum may be difficult to advance due to the length and sharp angles encountered. Maneuver the scope in a to-and-fro manner to try to keep the length of the jejunum short. As in colonoscopy, pressure over the left upper quadrant or to the left of the umbilicus may prevent excess looping of the scope.

2. **Endoscopic treatment:** If the anastomosis is widely patent, the scope can be passed into the biliary tree, which is usually dilated in this group of patients (Fig. 46.2.4). If the anastomosis is narrowed, balloon dilation may be required for entry into the bile ducts.

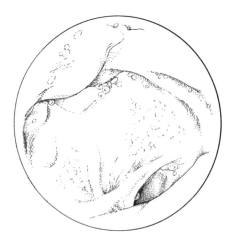

Figure 46.2.4. Endoscopic view of a choledochojejunal anastomosis in a patient who had a gastrointestinal bleed. A laparoscopic side-to-side choledochojejunostomy was performed 2 months previously for an unresectable distal cholangiocarcinoma causing obstructive jaundice.

D. Selected References

Cotton PB, Williams CB. Practical Gastrointestinal Endoscopy, 2nd ed. Oxford, UK: Blackwell Scientific, 1982.

Marbet UA, Staider GA, Faust H. Harder F, Gyr K. Endoscopic sphincterotomy and surgical approaches in the treatment of the "sump syndrome". Gut 1987;28:142–145.

Osnes M, Rosseland AR, Aabakken L. Endoscopic retrograde cholangiography and endoscopic papillotomy in patients with a previous Billroth-II resection. Gut 1986;27:1193–1198.

Siegel JH. Endoscopic Retrograde Cholangio-Pancreatography, 1st ed. New York: Raven Press, 1992.

Siegle JH, Yatto RP. ERCP and endoscopic papillotomy in patients with a Billroth II gastrectomy: report of a method. Gastrointest Endosc 1983;29:117–118.

47. Cannulation and Cholangiopancreatography

David Duppler, M.D., F.A.C.S.

A. Cannulation and Cholangiopancreatography

1. After identifying the papilla, make certain that the patient is adequately sedated to minimize movement and the duodenum adequately paralyzed to stop peristalsis.
2. Keep the tip of the scope deflected to the right—this will usually aid in holding the proper position in the duodenum.
3. Observe the papilla for a few moments. Attempt to identify the orifice, and the likely orientation of the common bile duct and pancreatic duct. Usually, there is one orifice for both the pancreatic and bile ducts, with the ducts sharing a common channel of varying length. Occasionally, there are two orifices, the more superior of which is the orifice of the bile duct.
4. Advance the cannula toward the papilla with a combination of advancement of the cannula with the right hand, change in angle of the catheter using the elevator, and change in the position of the scope using the deflection wheels or by torquing the instrument. It is generally best to cannulate the duct of interest first. If this is the pancreatic duct, the cannula should approach the orifice of the papilla nearly at a right angle to the duodenal wall with the catheter approaching in a left-to-right orientation. For common bile duct cannulation, the cannula should be oriented in a more cephalad direction and approached from a right-to-left position (Figs. 47.1 and 47.2).

    a. In most situations, the pancreatic duct is the easier of the two ducts to cannulate. Once the cannula is within the orifice, inject a small amount of dye under fluoroscopic control. In opacifying the pancreatic duct, it is crucial to avoid distention of the pancreatic ductal system. Overinjection of the pancreatic duct (as evidenced by opacification of the secondary and tertiary branches of the duct) or repeated cannulations of the duct increase the risk of postprocedure pancreatitis.

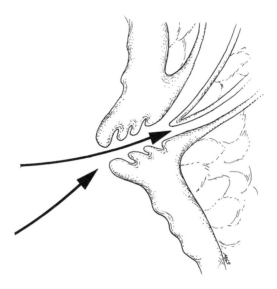

Figure 47.1. The proper cannulation angle for the pancreatic duct is nearly at right angles to the duodenal wall, while bile cannulation requires a more cephalad orientation.

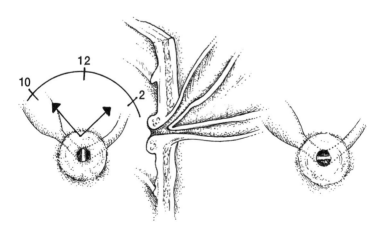

Figure 47.2. The septum separating the orifices to the pancreatic and bile ducts can be oriented in any direction from horizontal to vertical. When the papilla is viewed en face, the course of the bile duct is usually toward the 10 o'clock position and the pancreatic duct toward the 2 o'clock position, although some variation exists.

b. Bile duct cannulation is usually facilitated by advancing the scope past the papilla and deflecting the tip upward. This "tucked under" position often aligns the cannula with the axis of the common bile duct (Fig. 47.3). Direct the cannula toward the 10 to 12 o'clock position on the papilla. As the cannula enters the orifice of the papilla, lift the cannula with the elevator to advance the catheter along the roof of the papilla. This increases the likelihood of elective cannulation of the common bile duct (Fig. 47.4). Manually curving the cannula in a more cephalad orientation prior to its insertion will also enhance common bile duct cannulation, whereas leaving the catheter straight usually facilitates pancreatic duct cannulation.

c. If these maneuvers do not allow for selective cannulation of the appropriate duct, switching to a different type of cannula is sometimes helpful. A tapered tip cannula is often helpful when the orifice of the papilla is quite small. A sphincterotome can be used to obtain a greater cephalad orientation of the catheter for selective bile duct cannulation (Fig. 47.5).

d. Although injection of dye under fluoroscopic control with the cannula impacted at the papilla will often opacify the desired duct, free cannulation of the pancreatic duct usually can be facilitated by advancing the catheter toward the 2 o'clock direction on the papilla. Withdrawing the scope slightly will also make the cannula approach a 90-degree angle with the duodenal wall, which will also improve the chances of free cannulation of the pancreatic duct.

e. Free cannulation of the common bile duct is also often facilitated by withdrawing the scope slightly after the common bile duct has been opacified with contrast. This allows the catheter to change directions within the papilla, as the common bile duct often becomes more horizontal within the duodenal wall. If the sphincterotome is used for cannulation, this can also be accomplished by lessening the tension on the cutting wire, which will straighten the tip of the sphincterotome within the papilla. As the scope is withdrawn, it is sometimes necessary to slightly withdraw the cannula back into the scope to prevent excessive pressure on the papilla. Free cannulation of either duct can also be facilitated by the passage of a floppy-tipped guide wire, although care must be taken to avoid the use of excessive force with guide wires as this can lead to false passages and perforations.

5. In opacifying the common bile duct, make the injection under fluoroscopic control and obtain exposures throughout the injection to provide both early filling and later phases. This facilitates detection of small stones and other more subtle abnormalities.

6. In a patient with an obstructed system, it is often helpful to attempt to aspirate bile initially to try to relieve some of the pressure within the system before adding contrast. This is especially important in a patient who may have cholangitis.

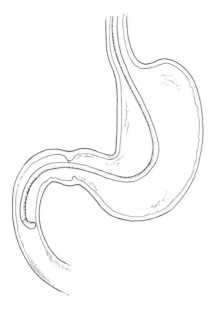

Figure 47.3. The "tucked under" position is usually obtained by advancing the endoscope slightly and deflecting the tip upward.

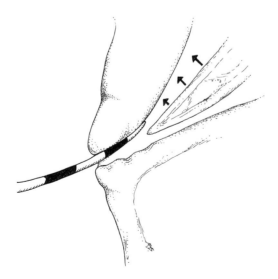

Figure 47.4. Lifting the cannula to insert it along the "roof" of the papilla increases the likelihood of entry into the bile duct.

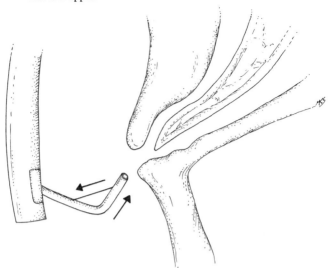

Figure 47.5. Sometimes bile duct cannulation requires orientation of the cannula in a cephalad direction. This can be accomplished by using a sphincterotome. Tightening the cutting wire bows the cannula upward and produces a more cephalad orientation for the tip of the cannula.

B. Special Considerations and Situations

1. **Duodenal diverticula** often make it more difficult to locate the papilla. The papilla is generally located along the inferior edge of the diverticulum, although it is occasionally located within the diverticulum itself.

   a. When two diverticula are present, the papilla is often located on the isthmus of tissue between the diverticula. Once again, time should be spent locating the papilla and observing it to identify the orifice.

   b. If the papilla cannot be identified, it is probably within the diverticulum. It can sometimes be brought into view by suctioning some of the air out of the duodenum, using the cannula to probe the edge of the diverticulum, putting pressure on the right upper quadrant of the patient's abdomen, or changing the patient's position. If the papilla is located within the diverticulum and cannot be easily approached with the cannula, it can sometimes be pulled outside the diverticulum with the cannula or with the use of a sphincterotome. Occasionally, if the diverticulum is large, the tip of the scope can be placed within the diverticulum to facilitate cannulation.

2. **Periampullary tumors** may distort the anatomy of the papilla. Patience is required to search the area slowly to identify the papillary

orifice, which can be significantly elevated or depressed by the tumor. The tumor also can distort the normal path of the pancreatic and bile ducts within the papilla, making free cannulation more difficult. Gentle probing of the tumor with the cannula will often lead to cannulation, but aggressive and forceful probing should be avoided as this will lead to bleeding and edema, which will further obscure the anatomy.

3. An **impacted stone within the papilla** will often turn the orifice of the papilla in a caudad orientation. This will usually require the "tucked under" position for successful cannulation.

4. **Cannulation of the minor papilla** may be indicated when the diagnosis of pancreas divisum is suspected or when a tumor involving the head of the pancreas precludes opacification of the proximal pancreatic duct.

    a. The minor papilla is usually located 1 to 3 cm proximal to the major papilla and slightly to the right.

    b. Approach the minor papilla at right angles to the duodenal wall using a tapered or ultra-tapered catheter.

    c. Once again, care should be taken to not overdistend the pancreatic ductal system.

5. **Precut papillotomy:** If selective cannulation of the common bile duct is not possible with all of the previously mentioned maneuvers, consideration should be given to performing a precut papillotomy. This is a blind maneuver in which the sphincter is cut prior to radiographic visualization. This procedure is associated with an increased risk of bleeding and pancreatitis. It should only be used in cases where access to the common bile duct is considered mandatory, such as in patients with jaundice or cholangitis.

    a. Insert a precut papillotome or a needle-knife papillotome into the papillary orifice and make small, 1- to 2-mm cuts in the direction of the 10 to 12 o'clock position.

    b. In general, the precut sphincterotomy should not extend more than 5 mm and then repeated attempts should be made at obtaining a selective cannulation of the common bile duct.

    c. Avoid injection of dye in the impacted position after precut sphincterotomy, as this increases the risk of developing an intramural injection.

    d. Precut sphincterotomies should only be performed by endoscopists with significant experience in standard sphincterotomy.

6. Multiple attempts at cannulation often result in enough papillary trauma to induce edema and occasionally bleeding. This further decreases the likelihood of successful cannulation. If this has occurred or if there has been an intramural injection of contrast, it is best to terminate the procedure with plans to repeat it 2 to 3 days later. One can expect an approximate 50% success rate with this second procedure. If unsuccessful, referral of the patient to a more experienced endoscopist or the use of other modalities for evaluating the pancreaticobiliary system should be considered.

48. Therapeutic ERCP

Gary C. Vitale, M.D., F.A.C.S.

A. Biliary Sphincterotomy

1. **Selective cannulation of bile duct**: Before endoscopic sphincterotomy, the common bile duct must be selectively cannulated with passage of the opacifying cannula or a guide wire up into the duct (deep cannulation). A wire-guided sphincterotomy is performed with the sphincterotome over a guide wire. This helps keep the sphincterotome from twisting and also allows the operator to advance the instrument in and out of the papilla during the course of the sphincterotomy.

2. **Positioning the sphincterotome**: Place the sphincterotome in the orifice of the papilla with the wire coming in contact with the papilla at the 11 o'clock to 12 o'clock position. Cutting in this position reduces pancreatitis and bleeding (Fig. 48.1).

3. **Cutting the papilla**: Bow the sphincterotome by tightening the wire. Using a blended current, with more cutting current than coagulation, apply short bursts of current, allowing the sphincterotome wire to cut slowly through the ampullary sphincter.

    a. The complete sphincterotomy should extend just to the inferior margin of the suprapapillary duodenal fold.

    b. To avoid the "zipper effect" in which the sphincter is cut too fast risking bleeding and perforation, the sphincterotome should not be bowed too tightly by the nurse during the sphincterotomy. It should be bowed just enough to press lightly into the tissue, letting the current do the cutting.

4. **Transhepatic-guided sphincterotomy**: In cases in which the sphincterotome or the guide wire cannot be advanced into the bile duct, a transhepatic wire can be placed percutaneously into the duodenum. This wire can then be grasped endoscopically and brought out through the operating channel of the scope. A sphincterotome can then be passed over the guide wire and positioned for a standard sphincterotomy.

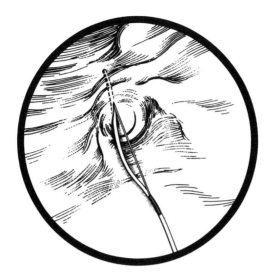

Figure 48.1. Positioning the sphincterotome.

5. **Precut sphincterotomy**: In selected cases, a precut sphincterotomy may be performed. The precut knife is used to directly cut the papilla to gain access to the biliary tree. There are two techniques used. In the first, the cut is made beginning at the orifice of the ampulla and is extended superiorly along the apex of the ampulla. In the second, the cut is begun on the superior aspect of the infundibulum (bulge) of the papilla and extended inferiorly with short, deepening cuts into the papilla. The principal risk in either of these techniques is perforation, and thus it should be performed by experienced endoscopists and even then only sparingly, in cases with definite therapeutic indications.

B. Pancreatic Sphincterotomy

1. Perform a **biliary sphincterotomy** before pancreatic sphincterotomy to facilitate access to the pancreatic duct.

2. **Selective cannulation of the pancreatic duct**: Insert a guide wire into the pancreatic duct and confirm position under fluoroscopy. Pass the sphincterotome over the wire into the orifice of the pancreatic duct.

3. **Cutting the pancreatic ductal septum and sphincter**: Depending on the variable anatomy, there may be a short or long septum between the pancreatic duct and the bile duct within the ampulla. There is an additional muscular sphincter specifically encircling the orifice of the pancreatic duct. In some cases, pancreatic septoplasty may be sufficient to allow free flow of pancreatic juice. In other cases, the cut must be extended further into the pancreatic ductal orifice to ablate the muscular sphincter. This is particularly true when the indication for pancreatic ductal sphincterotomy is papillary hypertension with recurrent pancreatitis as its clinical manifestation. Direct the sphincterotome in an orientation toward the 1 o'clock position. Cutting proceeds as described above (section A).

C. Biliary Tract Stone Removal

1. **Basket stone removal**: Stones may be removed from the bile ducts and intrahepatic biliary radicals using a standard stone basket.

   a. Insert the basket into the bile duct, open it, and engage the stone. The assistant can open and partially close the basket, while the operator jiggles the catheter in order to trap stones. The catheter can be withdrawn in the open position, and stones often will pop out.

   b. Larger stones can be individually engaged and removed after securing the basket around them.

   c. Apply traction in the axial direction of the bile duct in removing a stone so as not to further cut the apex of the sphincterotomy with the wire of the stone basket during stone extraction. Perforation may result if the wire of the stone basket cuts the apex of the sphincterotomy.

2. **Balloon stone extraction**: For smaller stones, a balloon stone extractor can be used to pull stones through the sphincterotomy.

   a. Insert the balloon catheter through the sphincterotomy and inflate the balloon above the stone.

   b. As the catheter is retrieved, the stone is pulled into the duodenum.

3. As an alternative to sphincterotomy, **the sphincter can be dilated** first using a longitudinal hydrostatic dilating balloon, with balloon stone extraction of small stones following. While this method avoids sphincterotomy, it may be associated with a higher incidence of pancreatitis and cannot be unequivocally recommended at this time.

4. **Mechanical lithotripsy**: For larger stones, lithotripsy is often necessary to fracture the stone before extracting it. Extracting a very large stone through the sphincterotomy risks either perforation or stone entrapment. If the stone becomes entrapped in the distal bile duct with the basket still around it, a surgical procedure may be necessary to disengage it. The mechanical lithotripter functions by tightening the wire basket around the stone against a metal sheath using a hand crank.

5. **Electrohydraulic and candela laser lithotripsy**: When mechanical fracture of the stones is not successful, one may employ electrohydraulic or pulsed-dye laser techniques. In each of these approaches, a catheter is passed under direct vision into the bile duct and placed in direct contact or close proximity to the stone before applying the energy. The mother-daughter scope is often used for this, as it allows for direct vision of intrabiliary stones. Direct visualization with a daughter scope is necessary to reduce the risk of common bile duct injury from poor positioning of the catheter, particularly if the electrohydraulic lithotriptor is used. After the stone is fractured, the pieces can be extracted using conventional techniques.

6. **Extracorporeal lithotripsy** has also been used for fracture of large common bile duct stones with some success. This is most often necessary for occlusive stones that do not allow passage of a basket or balloon. In these cases, if a guide wire can be passed above the stone, a stent may be placed to relieve obstruction. Treatment can then be performed with extracorporeal lithotripsy or gallstone dissolving agents prior to another ERCP attempt at stone extraction.

7. **Intrahepatic stones**: Intrahepatic stones may be extracted using stone basket or balloon stone extraction methods described above in many cases. When the stones are larger, a mother-daughter scope can be used with intrahepatic lithotripsy. For multiple, large intrahepatic stones, it is often better to use a percutaneous transhepatic approach. With this method, a percutaneous transhepatic tract is developed and dilated to the diameter of a choledochoscope with a working channel. Percutaneous choledochoscopy is then performed with fracture and extraction of intrahepatic stones. Electrohydraulic or candela laser lithotripsy is often necessary as an adjunct procedure for successful stone clearance in these cases.

D. Pancreatic Duct Stone Removal

Stones in the pancreatic duct should be removed when possible. In some cases, stones are a result rather than a cause of the disease process and removing them may not always improve a patient's course of recurring pancreatitis. There are good data, however, that complete stone clearance improves patient outcome with regard to chronic pain.

1. Stones may be removed with a combination of stone basket and balloon. The stone basket is often necessary to fracture the stones, which are frequently soft, and the balloon can clear the fragments.

2. Some stones are embedded in the wall of the duct or are located at junctions or angulated curves in the duct, which makes them inaccessible to the basket or balloon.

3. Large stones often will obstruct the duct making extraction impossible. In these cases, a guide wire should be passed above the stone and a 5-French (Fr) stent passed if at all possible. Extracorporeal lithotripsy can then be performed to fracture the stone followed by endoscopic stone fragment extraction.

E. Biliary Stenting

1. **Stent selection**: Polyethylene stents are available in 7-Fr, 10-Fr and 11.5-Fr diameter.

   a. For short-term stenting of 30 days or less or in cases of difficult access in which changing to a larger diameter working channel scope could compromise access, the 7-Fr-stent is appropriate.

   b. For longer term stenting, indications such as cancer, the 10 Fr or 11.5 Fr is a better choice. These larger stents remain open significantly longer than the 7-Fr stents in randomized trials. There is no significant difference between the longevity of the 10-Fr and the 11.5 Fr stents.

   c. Metallic self-expanding stents are indicated for longer term cancer stenting indications and last for a mean of approximately 1 year. These stents are nonremovable and may limit some treatment options later in the course of disease, and thus should be used selectively.

   d. Nasobiliary stents can be used for temporary stenting situations when repeat opacification of the biliary tract is desirable.

2. **Stent insertion**: For the 10-Fr and 11.5-Fr stents, a wire-guided stent introducer is passed above the level of the stenosis over which the stent is pushed into position. The 7-Fr stents are placed directly over the guide wires and pushed into place. Metallic stents are initially 7-Fr prior to deployment and are positioned over a guide wire across the stenosis. They are released by retracting a plastic sleeve, which holds the stent in its stretched, compressed configuration. Upon release, the stent shortens and assumes its full diameter of 8 to 10 mm. Nasobiliary stents are introduced over a guide wire into the biliary tree above the level of obstruction and then are brought out through the nasopharynx.

3. **Stent change**: Polyethylene stents can be changed electively every 3 to 4 months, or one can wait until serum bilirubin and liver enzyme levels indicate impending obstruction prior to changing the stent. Stent exchange is usually a simple process, except in cases of long or very high level strictures. In those cases, it is wise to pass a guide wire through the stent prior to removing it through the scope using a special stent retriever designed for this purpose. Polyethylene stents can be exchanged repeatedly over time allowing the biliary system to remain patent indefinitely. Metallic stents when obstructed cannot be replaced, but a second plastic or metallic stent can be passed through the center of the original stent restoring biliary patency. Newer stent designs incorporating a Silastic sleeve over the mesh may reduce tumor and granulation tissue ingrowth, thus, improving patency and facilitating recannulation.

F. Pancreatic Duct Stenting

1. **Stent options**: Smaller stents of 5 Fr or 7 Fr are used in the pancreatic ducts. These stents have multiple side holes and phlanges and are more specifically designed to facilitate pancreatic duct drainage. Metallic stents have been used for benign pancreatic strictures, but their use in that clinical setting remains experimental.

2. **Stent insertion**: Stent insertion is accomplished over a guide wire that has been placed in the pancreatic duct. Balloon dilatation of strictures prior to stent placement may be necessary to allow stent placement. Stents are left in place for shorter intervals than in the biliary system. As noted above, simultaneous clearance of pancreatic duct stones improves long-term results.

G. Endoscopic Drainage of Pancreatic Pseudocysts

1. **Pseudocyst identification**: Location of the pseudocyst adjacent to the gastric or duodenal wall by computed tomography (CT) is essential. During endoscopy, indentation by the cyst of the gastric or duodenal wall confirms location. Endoscopic ultrasound can be used to further identify the pseudocyst from the endoscopic view. Wall thickness is determined from the scan and should be less than 1 cm to consider endoscopic drainage. Patients with associated masses in the pancreas or with pancreatitis of unclear etiology may have tumors such as pancreatic cancer with associated pancreatitis and pseudocyst, serous cystadenoma or lymphoma. Adequate biopsy or a direct operative approach is mandatory in these patients.

2. **Technique of endoscopic pseudocyst drainage**:

    a. At the apex of the bulge of the cyst into the gastric or duodenal lumen, a small area of mucosa is coagulated with the precut knife.

    b. In the center of this area, a direct puncture of the cyst is made using cutting or blended current.

    c. A guide wire is passed into the cyst, and an opacifying cannula is passed over the guide wire and contrast injected to confirm cyst size and position compared to the CT scan.

    d. A biopsy of the pseudocyst wall is taken at some point in the process of draining the cyst. A sphincterotome is then passed into the cyst, and the opening enlarged. Care is taken to use a combination of cutting and cautery to avoid bleeding at the site of the cyst-enterostomy.

    e. A polyethylene stent is placed into the cyst in selected cases. If the pseudocyst is in communication with the pancreatic duct, or if the duct is obstructed, a stent should be placed to allow longer term drainage. Also, if the cyst wall is thick or if a small opening has been made due to risk of bleeding, a stent should be placed to ensure that the cyst-enterostomy remains open until the cyst resolves. The stent should remain in place until the cyst has resolved by CT and there is demonstration of a patent pancreatic duct. The stent may be left indefinitely if there is obstruction of the mid-portion of the pancreatic duct with the tail of the pancreas draining into the stomach or duodenum via the stent. In younger, healthy patients operative intervention should be considered in cases of complete duct occlusion and recurrent/persistent cyst or pancreatitis following stent removal.

H. Selected References

Barkun AN, Barkun JS, Fried GM, et al. Useful predictors of bile duct stones in patients undergoing laparoscopic cholecystectomy. Ann Surg 1994;220:32–49.

Binmoeller KF, Soehendra N, Liguory C. The common bile duct stone: Time to leave it to the laparoscopic surgeon? Endoscopy 1994;26:315–319.

DeIorio AV Jr, Vitale GC, Reynolds M, Larson GM. Acute biliary pancreatitis: the roles of laparoscopic cholecystectomy and endoscopic retrograde cholangiopancreatography. Surg Endosc 1995;9:392–396.

Fan TS, Lai ECS, Mok FPT, et al. Early treatment of acute biliary pancreatitis by endoscopic papillotomy. N Engl J Med 1993;328:228–232.

Freeman ML, Nelson DB, Sherman S, et al. Complications of endoscopic biliary sphincterotomy. N Engl J Med 1996;335:909–918.

Grace PA, Williamson RCN. Modern management of pancreatic pseudocysts. Br J Surg 1993;80:573–581.

Huibregtse K. Complications of endoscopic sphincterotomy and their prevention [Editorial]. N Engl J Med 1996;335:961–962.

Pitt HA, Venbrux AC, Coleman J, et al. Intrahepatic stones. The transhepatic team approach. Ann Surg 1994;219:527–535.

Scholmerich J, Lausen M, Lay L, et al. Value of endoscopic retrograde cholangiopancreatography in determining the cause but not course of acute pancreatitis. Endoscopy 1992;24:244–247.

Vitale GC. Advanced interventional endoscopy. Am J Surg 1997;173:21–25.

Vitale GC, George M, McIntyre K, et al. Endoscopic management of benign and malignant biliary strictures. Am J Surg 1996;171:553–557.

Vitale GC, Larson GM, Wieman TJ, Cheadle WG, Miller FB. The use of ERCP in the management of common bile duct stones in patients undergoing laparoscopic cholecystectomy. Surg Endosc 1993;7:9–11.

Vitale GC, Stephens G, Wieman TJ, Larson GM. The use of ERCP in the management of biliary complications following laparoscopic cholecystectomy. Surgery 1993;114:806–814.

49. Complications of ERCP

Morris Washington, M.D.
Ali Ghazi, M.D.

A. Pancreatitis

1. **Cause and prevention:** Pancreatitis is the most common complication following ERCP. While hyperamylasemia may be seen in up to 60% of patients after ERCP, clinical pancreatitis occurs in approximately 5%. The incidence is the same for both diagnostic and therapeutic procedures. The severity of post-ERCP pancreatitis in the majority of cases is mild to moderate and self-limited. Unfortunately, however, fatal necrotizing post-ERCP pancreatitis is reported. Post-ERCP pancreatitis is more common in younger patients and has its highest incidence in patients having ERCP for suspected sphincter of Oddi dysfunction (19%).

    a. The exact **mechanism** that initiates post-ERCP pancreatitis is still unproven, but it is believed by most to be mechanical in nature caused by an increase in pancreatic intraductal pressure with release of pancreatic enzyme from acini into the pancreatic parenchyma. This increased intraductal pressure may result from the following:

       i. Difficulty with cannulation leading to overmanipulation of the papilla of Vater causing trauma and spasm of the sphincter of Oddi.

       ii. Repeated injection into the pancreatic ductal system in an attempt to access the bile duct.

       iii. Overzealous injection of contrast media into the pancreatic ductal system resulting in a complete outline of the pancreas on x-ray known as acinarization.

       iv. Injury to the papilla of Vater from the electrocautery used during endoscopic sphincterotomy (ES).

       v. Placement of large endobiliary stents without an ES causing obstruction of the pancreatic duct orifice.

    b. **Prevention:** Intuitively, better technique during cannulation and ES should lower the incidence of post-ERCP pancreatitis; however, this has been difficult to study and document. Neverthe-less, the following technical considerations may be helpful in the prevention of post-ERCP pancreatitis:

i.   Selective cannulation to avoid injection into the pancreatic ductal system if a pancreatogram is not required.

ii.   Use only a few milliliters of contrast to fill the main pan-creatic ducts of Wirsung and Santorini.

iii. A 50-cc syringe to inject contrast media delivers less hy-drostatic pressure than a syringe of lesser volume and thus may avoid inadvertent overfilling of the pancreatic ductal system.

iv.   If the initial cannulation of the bile duct has been difficult and therapeutics are required, then maintain access with the use of a guide wire.

v.   During ES use more cutting than coagulation current to de-crease the amount of edema and tissue injury.

vi.   Early precut sphincterotomy using a needle knife sphinc-terotome on difficult bile duct cannulations, but this is controversial and requires particular endoscopic skill.

vii. There have been many attempts at pharmacologic preven-tion of post-ERCP pancreatitis using atropine, glucagon, calcitonin, steroids, and somatostatin; all of which have shown limited efficacy in experimental and clinical trials. Recently, however, Gabexate, a protease inhibitor, has been shown to decrease the severity of post-ERCP pan-creatitis if given intravenously for 30 to 90 minutes prior to the procedure and continued for 12 hours thereafter. Addi-tional clinical trials are needed to further document its effi-cacy prior to general use.

2. **Treatment:** Most cases of post-ERCP pancreatitis are mild to mod-erate in severity and will resolve with modest treatment. Restriction of oral intake and intravenous fluids until the symptoms abate and the serum amylase and lipase normalize is usually all that is required. In a minority of patients the pancreatitis may be more severe with the establishment of several Ranson's criteria and phlegmon develop-ment on imaging studies. Oral intake should be restricted in these patients, parenteral nutrition instituted, and serial sonograms ob-tained to assess the degree of pancreatic inflammation. Pseudocyst may develop in the acute phase and take several weeks to resolve. Avoid the temptation of starting oral intake prematurely, leading to an exacerbation. Sonographic evidence of resolution of the phlegmon or pseudocyst should be established prior to oral intake. Large pseu-

docysts that persist with therapy longer than 6 to 8 weeks will require internal drainage. This can be accomplished surgically via cystogastrostomy or cystojejunostomy. Persistent symptomatic cysts in the tail of the pancreas can be treated with resection. Some pseudocysts can be drained internally via an endoscopic approach (see Chapter 50). Endoscopic ultrasound may help to determine the feasibility of endoscopic drainage. Percutaneous drainage should be avoided because of the high incidence of prolonged catheter drainage.

Death from post-ERCP pancreatitis is fortunately a rare occurrence. These patient develop necrotic pancreatitis frequently with infection. Dynamic CT scanning will demonstrate a large amount of devitalized pancreas. The patients appear severely toxic and frequently have positive blood cultures. Exploration with pancreatic debridement and necrosectomy will be required as a lifesaving measure. These patients often require repeated debridement as the inflammatory process progresses.

B. Cholangitis

1. **Cause and prevention:** The overall incidence of cholangitis following ERCP is low (0.1%). Cholangitis following ERCP in patients with nonobstructed biliary systems is exceedingly rare and therefore antibiotic prophylaxis is not indicated in these patients. When cholangitis does occur following ERCP it almost always occurs in jaundiced patients with obstructed biliary systems. Patients at particular risk for cholangitis are those patients undergoing stenting for malignant biliary strictures, patients having combined percutaneous endoscopic procedures and in patients who have had failed biliary drainage. Antibiotic prophylaxis has been shown to lower the incidence of cholangitis in these patients following ERCP. Piperacillin, which is secreted in the bile, has been particularly effective.

    Cholangitis following ERCP can be completely prevented by timely relief of the biliary obstruction. This can be accomplished using ERCP therapeutics or surgical intervention. If surgical intervention is chosen, prior coordination between the endoscopist and surgeon is important to effect a timely relief of the biliary obstruction.

2. **Treatment:** Once cholangitis is established, immediate drainage is indicated. At this point the patient must be considered to have an undrained abscess and therefore every hour counts. If the patient is allowed to progress to septic shock, then a high mortality will result.

C. Hemorrhage

1. **Cause and prevention:** Clinically significant bleeding following endoscopic sphincterotomy (ES) is reported to occur in 2% of cases. Minor bleeding (oozing) is not uncommon and will stop spontaneously provided that the patient has normal coagulation parameters. In patients with obstructive jaundice it is important that the prothrombin time (PT) be checked prior to ES since these patients will frequently have elevation secondary to impaired vitamin K absorption. If ES can be delayed for a few days, the PT can be easily corrected with vitamin K given subcutaneously. If ES must be done urgently, fresh frozen plasma must be given until the PT is corrected. Patients that are taking antiplatelet medication (e.g., aspirin, persantine) should have them discontinued 7 to 10 days prior to ES. If ES cannot be delayed, a bleeding time should be done and if abnormal corrected with platelet transfusion.

   While it is again difficult to document what role technique has in preventing clinically significant bleeding following ES, it has been reported that endoscopists who perform ES more frequently have a lower rate of complications. The following technical considerations may be helpful:

   a. ES should be made as close to the 12 o'clock position as possible to avoid duodenal vasculature.
   b. A blended cutting current should be used that has some cautery effect.
   c. ES should be made slowly in sequential steps instead of one uncontrolled cut.
   d. Tailor the size of the ES to the need; e.g., only a small ES is needed to extract small stones or insert large endobiliary stents.
   e. Do not forcefully extract large stones; use a mechanical lithotriptor.

2. **Treatment:** As mentioned earlier, minor oozing after ES is not uncommon and will usually stop spontaneously with observation. Pulsatile (arterial) bleeding after ES is of more concern. If the bleeding is not so brisk as to impair endoscopic visualization, it may also stop spontaneously or can be treated by injection of the bleeding point with epinephrine solution. A few milliliters of 1:10,000 epinephrine solution delivered using a variceal injection device may be helpful.

   Brisk arterial bleeding that obscures endoscopic visualization must be treated more aggressively. The patient should be admitted to the ICU for close monitoring. A baseline Hgb/Hct and type and crossmatch should be obtained. Two large-bore IV catheters should be placed for infusion of crystalloid and blood products. An arterial line and Foley catheter should be inserted. If there is evidence of brisk active bleeding manifested by tachycardia, hematemesis, hematochezia, and a falling Hgb/Hct, intervention is required. If an experienced interventional radiologist is available, celiac arteriography with selective embolization of the bleeding branch of gastroduodenal artery may avoid operative intervention. However, if embolization fails or is unavailable and the bleeding continues, operative intervention must be undertaken prior to the onset of hypovolemic shock. The patient should be explored through a midline incision and the duodenum fully kocherized. A duodenotomy in the second portion of the duodenum will allow access to the papilla of Vater. The bleeding can be controlled with a suture ligature, being careful not to stenose the sphincterotomy. If the patient is stable, possibly then attention can be turned to surgical correction of the problem for which the ES was being done. Otherwise, a T-tube should be placed, the duodenotomy closed in two layers, and a drain placed.

D. Perforation

1. **Cause and prevention:** Perforation following ES is uncommon and occurs in approximately 0.3% of cases. The patient frequently will complain of abdominal and back pain. There may be associated fever and leukocytosis. The perforation is usually retroperitoneal and hence abdominal x-rays will demonstrate retroperitoneal air. Intraperitoneal (free air) is unusual and perforation in another area of the GI tract should be entertained. The mistaken diagnosis of pancreatitis is sometimes made, leading to delay in recognition and management. The following technical considerations may help to avoid this complication:
   a. Use sphincterotomes with short cutting wire lengths (20–25 mm).
   b. Do not extend the ES beyond the transverse duodenal fold that lies proximal to the papilla of Vater.
   c. As mentioned earlier tailor the length of ES to the need.
2. **Treatment:** If recognized early, perforations as a result of ES can be managed conservatively with good success. A nasogastric tube should be inserted and broad-spectrum antibiotics with adequate gram-negative coverage administered. The patient should be fol-

lowed closely and improvement should be expected in 12 to 24 hours. If the patient's condition fails to improve with signs of ongoing sepsis, operative intervention should be undertaken. The patient should be explored through a midline incision and the duodenum fully kocherized, revealing the site of the perforation posteriorly. Depending on the degree of inflammation and induration of the tissues, either primary closure or an omental patch should be done. Depending on the adequacy of the repair, a pyloric exclusion procedure should be considered. This can be accomplished by performing a gastrotomy, closing the pylorus with absorbable suture, gastrojejunostomy, and T-tube drainage. A drain should be placed and consideration should be given to placement of a gastrostomy and feeding jejunostomy.

E. Rare Complications

There are rare complications of ERCP that can occur. Some of which are unique to ERCP and others which can occur with any upper GI endoscopic procedure. They are listed here so that one may have a general knowledge of them.

1. Esophageal perforations
2. Mallory-Weiss tears
3. Hepatic and splenic hematomas
4. Bile duct perforations by guide wires
5. Stone extraction basket entrapment
6. Stent loss within the bile duct

G. Selected References

Arcidiacono R, Gambitta P, Rossi A, Grosso C, Bini M, Zanasi G. The use of long acting somatostatin analogue (octreotide) for prophylaxis of acute pancreatitis after endoscopic sphincterotomy. Endoscopy 1994;26:715–718.

Byl B, Deviere J, Struelens MJ, et al. Antibiotic prophylaxis for infectious complications after therapeutic endoscopic retrograde cholangiopancreatography: a randomized, double-blind, placebo-controlled study. Clin Infect Dis 1995;20:1236–1240.

Cavallini G, Tittobello A, Frulloni L, Masci E, Mariana A, DiFrancesco V. Gabexate for the prevention of pancreatic damage related to endoscopic retrograde cholangiopancreato-graphy. N Engl J Med 1996;26:961–963.

Flemmer M, Oldfield EC 3rd. Prophylax or perish? Am J Gastroenterol 1996;91:1867–1868.

Freeman ML, Nelson DB, Sherman S, Haber GB. Complications of endoscopic biliary sphincterotomy. N Engl J Med 1996;335:909–918.

Ghazi A, Washington M. Endoscopic diagnosis and management of diseases of the pancreas and hepatobiliary tract. Curr Probl Surg 1990;7:161–174.

Lo AY, Washington M, Fischer MG. Splenic trauma following endoscopic retrograde cholangiopancreatography. Surg Endosc 1994;8:692–693.

Pasricha P. Prevention of ERCP-induced pancreatitis: success at last. Gastroenterology 1997;112:1415–1417.

Schneider J, Barkin J. Gabexate for prevention of pancreatic damage related to endoscopic retrograde cholangiopancreatography. Gastrointest Endo 1997;45:447–448.

Tarnasky PR, Cunningham JT, Hawes RH, et al. Transpapillary stenting of proximal biliary strictures: Does biliary sphincterotomy reduce the risk of postprocedure pancreatitis? Gastrointest Endosc 1997;45:46–51.

50. Diagnostic Choledochoscopy

Bruce V. MacFadyen, Jr., M.D., F.A.C.S.

A. Intraoperative

1. **Indications:** Intraoperative choledochoscopy is performed at the time of laparoscopic or open cholecystectomy with common duct exploration, or when common duct exploration is performed as an isolated procedure. The major indications are listed in Table 50.1.
2. **Preparation, equipment, and room setup (laparoscopic):**
   a. When choledochoscopy is performed during laparoscopic biliary surgery, the standard laparoscopic cholecystectomy room setup, patient position, and trocar sites are used. Place an additional 5-mm trocar in the mid-right subcostal abdominal wall and use this for access into the common bile duct (CBD). A sixth 5-mm trocar is frequently inserted in the upper midline between the umbilical and subxiphoid ports in order to perform CBD exploration (CBDE) and choledochoscopy using a two-handed surgical technique.
   b. The surgeon stands at the patient's left side and the video monitors are placed over the right and left shoulders as in laparoscopic cholecystectomy.

Table 50.1. Indications for intraoperative choledochoscopy

Indication	Purpose
• Filling defect(s) on operative cholangiogram	• Visualize and remove stone(s)
• Bile duct stricture on operative or preoperative cholangiogram	• Visualize and obtain biopsy/brush cytology
• Polypoid filling defect on cholangiogram	• Visualize and obtain biopsy/brush cytology
• Evaluate common duct after mechanical removal of CBD stones	• Assure completion of stone removal

c. A second camera is attached to the choledochoscope and using a video mixer, the monitor displays a simultaneous split image from the laparoscope and the choledochoscope.

d. **Passing the scope (laparoscopic)**

a. **Transcystic:** When the operative cholangiogram (performed through the cystic duct) indicates that choledochoscopy is required, first advance a 0.035" guide wire through the cholangiocatheter into the cystic duct, common bile duct, and into the duodenum.

  i. Remove the cholangiocatheter and advance a 5-mm trocar with a plastic seal (instead of a valve) over the guide wire into the right subcostal area.

  ii. Pass rigid or balloon dilators over the wire to dilate the cystic duct to 5 mm. Sometimes the valves of Heister prevent advancement of the wire or dilator into the bile duct. In this case, it may be necessary to make another 2-mm opening in the cystic duct 7 to 10 mm from its entry into the bile duct. However, in most cases, if the cystic duct can be dilated to 5 mm, passage of the choledochoscope easily occurs. The smaller flexible choledochoscope with an outside diameter of 3 mm and a 1.2-mm accessory channel is preferred for the transcystic approach.

  iii. Backload the 0.035" guide wire through the accessory channel of the choledochoscope where a special dual valve is used on the exit port, thus allowing a pressurized saline solution to be infused through the choledochoscope channel to maximize bile duct visualization. At the same time, instruments can be advanced through the accessory channel for biopsy, stone removal, lithotripsy, and cytology.

b. **Alternative technique via choledochotomy:** Another alternative is to open the CBD longitudinally for 5 mm at its midportion, thus eliminating the resistance from the valves of Heister. Direct access to the common bile duct is performed when CBD stones are greater than 5 mm in diameter, when visualization of the upper bile ducts is necessary, and when the choledochoscope cannot be advanced through the cystic duct. The length of the choledochotomy should be no longer than the diameter of the choledochoscope or the largest stone because significant leakage of the pressurized saline solution in the common bile duct can occur, thus decreasing visualization.

  i. Place a 5-0 prolene stay suture on each side of the choledochotomy and use these to keep the incision open.

    ii.   Pass a rubber tip grasper through the upper midline trocar and use this for manipulation of the endoscope into the bile duct. This type of grasper minimizes injury to the outer sheath of the choledochoscope.

    iii.   Complete the common duct exploration as previously described (Chapter 14.2).

  e.   **Passing the scope (open):** Perform a Kocher maneuver to allow the distal bile duct to be straightened. Insert the choledochoscope into the choledochotomy. Cross the stay sutures over the choledochoscope to allow the bile duct to distend with saline. Pass the scope proximal and distal under visual control. Generally the scope must be removed and reinserted to reverse the direction from proximal to distal or vice versa.

  f.   **Technical points for performing choledochoscopy by either route:** The bile duct must be continuously flushed with saline during choledochoscopy. Saline provides distention and is the viewing medium. It also serves to flush away blood or debris.

  a.   Keep the lumen of the bile duct in the center of the field. If the picture becomes red, the scope may be impacted against the bile duct wall. Pull the scope back 1 to 2 cm and deflect the tip until the lumen is in the center of the screen.

  b.   In the transcystic technique, visualization of the distal bile duct can be readily performed but proximal duct visualization is only successful in 10 to 20% of the cases because of the angulation of entry of the cystic duct into the CBD. If proximal bile duct visualization is crucial, a choledochotomy should be performed.

B. Postoperative Choledochoscopy

Postoperative choledochoscopy is most commonly performed when retained common duct stones are seen on a postoperative cholangiogram. Possible routes of access to the common duct include percutaneous (through the T-tube tract), peroral (mother-daughter scope technique during ERCP), and transhepatic. Each will be described briefly here. Fluoroscopy is needed for all three methods.

  1.   **Percutaneous via T-tube tract**

    a.   Insertion of the choledochoscope into the CBD can be performed percutaneously when the T-tube tract has matured for 5 to 6 weeks.

    b.   Position the patient supine.

    c.   The surgeon stands on the patient's right side, with the video monitor directly opposite.

    d.   Prep and drape the right upper quadrant of the abdomen around the T-tube exit site in the standard manner. Intravenous sedation is given.

    e.   Pass two 0.035" guidewires through the T-tube into the CBD and then into the duodenum under fluoroscopic guidance. One wire is the guiding wire and the second wire is a safety wire that can maintain access to the duct should the first wire become dislodged.

    f.   Remove the T-tube over the wires. Using one of the wires as a guide, insert a 5 mm dilating balloon and expand it to dilate the tract.

    g.   After complete tract dilation, backload one 0.035" guide wire through the accessory channel of the choledochoscope and advance the endoscope into the CBD.

    h.   Proximal CBD visualization can be accomplished by withdrawing the 0.035" wire and deflecting the endoscope tip toward the bifurcation of the common hepatic duct. Since the endoscope tip deflection ranges from 90° to 120°, visualization of the upper bile ducts can be accomplished.

    i.   When choledochoscopy has been completed and the endoscope removed, reinsert a 12- to 14-French T-tube or straight catheter into the CBD over the wire and remove both wires.

2. **Peroral cholangioscopy**

    a.   This technique is performed using a therapeutic duodenoscope and a small "baby" scope inserted through the accessory channel of the duodenoscope using a fluoroscopic guide wire. There are two therapeutic duodenoscopes that can be used for this technique. The largest one has an outside diameter of 15 mm and an accessory channel of 5.5 mm, which allows the passage through its accessory channel of a 5-mm cholangioscope with an accessory channel in the "baby" scope of 2.2 mm. A smaller therapeutic duodenoscope has an outside diameter of 11.5 mm and an accessory channel of 4.2 mm and allows the passage of a 3-mm cholangioscope with a 1.2-mm accessory channel. The diagnostic and therapeutic accessories for the smallest cholangioscope are limited to a cytology brush, a four-wire helical basket, and an electrohydraulic lithotripsy (EHL) fiber.

    b.   The patient is sedated and the duodenoscope passed as described in Chapter 48 (ERCP).

c.   The endoscope and fluoroscopic monitors are placed opposite the surgeon on the patient's left side in the prone position.

d.   Visualize the papilla and position it so that the longitudinal axis is in the center of the video monitor.

e.   Insert a tapered papillotome through the duodenoscope channel into the papillary orifice at the 11 o'clock to 12 o'clock position in order to visualize the CBD. (If the papillotome is advanced into the papilla at the 3 o'clock position, the pancreatic duct will be injected.)

f.   Perform a 7- to 10-mm papillotomy at the 11 o'clock to 1 o'clock position of the papilla, being careful not to cut through the transverse duodenal fold (which may produce perforation of the duodenum).

g.   After this is done, advance a 0.035" guide wire through the papillotome high into the biliary radicals. Withdraw the papillotome from the duodenoscope, leaving the wire in place.

h.   Backload the guide wire through the 3-mm cholangioscope and advance the daughter scope through the duodenoscope accessory channel. This part of the procedure requires an assistant to hold the duodenoscope in position and the surgeon advances the daughter endoscope over the wire. Take care not to cause sharp angulation of the daughter scope at the duodenoscope accessory port, which can cause breakage of the fiberoptic bundles. Additionally, the duodenoscope should lie in the shortest route to the papilla so as to more easily advance the daughter scope.

i.   As the choledochoscope exits the accessory channel, the elevator of the mother scope is left completely open so that the daughter scope can be advanced out of the mother scope into the duodenum and then into the CBD over the wire, thus avoiding breakage of the cholangioscope. In addition, any movement of the duodenoscope can cause potential breakage of the daughter scope.

j.   Once the daughter scope is in the CBD, remove the guide wire and use pressurized saline to irrigate the bile duct in order to maintain visualization. Since the daughter scope channel is small (1.2 mm), only a cytology brush, lithotriptor fiber, and a three- or four-wire spiral basket can be used. Biopsy forceps are not yet available for the smallest daughter endoscope at this time.

k.   Once the choledochoscope has been removed, use the papillotome catheter to obtain a completion cholangiogram for documentation.

3. **Transhepatic choledochoscopy**
   a. Position the patient supine, give intravenous sedation and inject local anesthesia into the skin for needle access into the right or left lobe of the liver.
   b. Pass a needle into the ductal system under fluoroscopic guidance. For access to the right or left hepatic duct, the surgeon stands on the patient's corresponding left or right side and the TV and fluoroscopy monitors are facing the surgeon.
   c. Dilate the tract to 5 mm using a dilating balloon. Tract dilatation can be done in one procedure or serially every 2 to 3 days over a 2-week period using Amplatz dilators.
   d. Finally, a 22- to 24-French Amplatz dilator sheath is inserted to keep the liver tract open during the insertion of the choledochoscope. The same two-wire technique for T-tube tract access is used as for the T-tube tract technique, and the choledochoscope is advanced into the left or right hepatic and common hepatic ducts through the sheath. The left and right hepatic ducts, common hepatic and common bile ducts can be visualized.

C. Biopsy and Brush Cytology Techniques

The technique for biopsy and brush cytology is similar for the choledochoscope and cholangioscope except that there is not a biopsy forceps for the 3-mm cholangioscope.

1. It is important to visualize all the bile ducts that can be safely cannulated, to ensure completeness of examination. Bile duct tumors are frequently multicentric.
2. Note tumor size and length. In addition to biopsy and cytology, bacterial and fungal cultures may be appropriate.
3. Perform at least six biopsies of the tumor or stricture in all quadrants.
4. Perform brush cytology on the tumor and in all quadrants of a stricture after the biopsy has been done. Three to four passes of the brush over the tumor in different areas are necessary to ensure adequate sampling.
5. Obtaining a successful diagnosis in the bile duct using these techniques is only 60 to 80% whereas in the stomach or colon, similar techniques are 95% accurate.

51. Therapeutic Choledochoscopy and Its Complications

Raymond P. Onders, M.D.
Thomas S. Stellato, M.D.

A. Therapeutic Choledochoscopy

1. **Stone retrieval** (see also Chapter 14.1, Laparoscopic Common Bile Duct Exploration: Transcystic Duct Approach).

   a. The simplest method is to **flush** the stones through the ampulla under direct visualization. This is usually aided by the administration of 1 mg of glucagon given intravenously. By advancing the choledochoscope against the stones and directing the stone to the ampulla, bile duct stones can at times be forced through the ampulla and into the duodenum.

   b. The second method to remove stones that are visualized with the flexible choledochoscope is with the use of a straight **four-wire basket.**

      i. Advance the basket beyond the stone and then slowly withdraw it until the stone is in the basket.

      ii. Close the basket to entrap the stone. Visually verify stone capture.

      iii. Pull the basket up to the scope and withdraw scope, basket, and stone as a unit.

      iv. Repeat this process until all visualized stones are removed and a completion cholangiogram shows a clear duct.

   c. When stones are larger than the junction between the cystic and common bile duct, vigorous attempts to remove them can injure the duct. In these cases **lithotriptors**, introduced through the working port of the choledochoscope, can deliver an energy source to fragment the calculus. Mechanical lithotriptors are used to crush the stones but are difficult to use if the stone is adherent to the wall of the duct or if the stone is lodged in the ampulla. Electrohydraulic and pulse dye laser lithotriptors deliver an energy beam to break up the stones when placed in direct contact with the stones. If inadvertent bursts of energy strike the bile duct wall instead of the stone, then there may be damage to the tissue causing perforation. It is important to make sure the electrohydraulic lithotriptor is firmly in contact with the stone when power is applied. After the stones are broken up they can then be removed by the previously mentioned techniques.

B. Complications of Choledochoscopy

1. **Bile leak**
   a. **Cause and prevention**: Bile may leak from the cystic duct stump, the choledochotomy site, or from an unrecognized injury to the common bile duct. If choledochoscopy was performed via the cystic duct, the cystic duct may have been dilated or damaged during instrumentation. In this situation, the closure of the cystic duct stump should not be performed with clips but rather with a suture loop or some other type of suture ligation. The most common reason for a leak is a partial or complete obstruction of bile flow across the ampulla because of a retained stone or edema.
   b. **Recognition and management**: If a closed suction drain was placed, the presence of bile in the drain would signify a biliary leak. The drain may be adequate to control the biliary fistula. In patients with a T-tube in which a biliary complication is suspected, a T-tube cholangiogram should be performed expeditiously. This may demonstrate a normal system (no leak), an obstruction without leakage, leakage without obstruction or a dislodged T-tube. In those patients without a T-tube, a hepatic 2, 6-dimethyliminodiacetic acid (HIDA) scan is an easy and noninvasive way to confirm if there is a leak. Once a leak is recognized, the source of it needs to be identified. This can be done through an endoscopic retrograde cholangiography (ERC). If the reason for the leak is a retained stone, this can then be removed endoscopically. If the leak is via the cystic duct stump, then an endoscopically placed transampullary biliary stent would allow for decompression and healing. Small bile leaks and collections recognized promptly will not require drainage if the leak is controlled with an endoprosthesis. If the collection is

significant, it can be drained percutaneously by CT or ultrasound guidance.

2. **Bleeding**
   a. **Cause and prevention**: Inflamed bile ducts can be quite friable and bleed when manipulated. To prevent bleeding it is necessary to be as gentle as possible with guide wires, baskets, and the choledochoscope. Bleeding from the edges of the choledochotomy can be annoying and rarely serious. Guy sutures at the site of the bleeding can control the bleeding and assist with access to the common bile duct. If there appears to be a fair amount of oozing during surgery, it would be better to place a T-tube for decompression and flushing in the postoperative period. A rare complication is a fistula formation between the hepatic artery or portal structures and the bile duct secondary to perforation during the instrumentation by wires, baskets, etc. To prevent this complication, the baskets, balloons, and guide wires all need to be visualized with the choledochoscope or with fluoroscopy while being manipulated.
   b. **Recognition and management**: Bleeding can be recognized postoperatively as either a blood through the T-tube or as an upper or lower GI hemorrhage. If the bleeding is significant it can be localized to the biliary tract by blood from the T-tube or if endoscopy shows blood coming from the ampulla. Bleeding can be further localized and treated by angiography if a branch of the hepatic artery has fistulized to the biliary system.

3. **Perforation**
   a. **Cause and prevention**: Manipulation of wires and baskets through the choledochoscope can result in perforations of the common bile duct or duodenum. Observing the baskets and wires through the choledochoscope or with fluoroscopy as they are being placed can prevent this problem. A second camera and a video mixer (picture in picture) allows the entire operating team to view the proceedings, which may decrease the risk of perforation or not recognizing that a perforation has occurred.
   b. **Recognition and management**: The injury can be seen on completion cholangiogram or present as a bile leak postoperatively. If the injury can be visualized, then it can be sutured. Small leaks from the common bile duct can be managed as described above. An injury to the duodenum that cannot be visualized laparoscopically will necessitate converting to an open operation for definitive repair.

4. **Pancreatitis**

   a. **Cause and prevention**: Excessive and forceful flushing of contrast when the ampulla is obstructed can cause reflux into the pancreatic duct with resultant pancreatitis. This can also occur when high-pressure water is infused through the choledochoscope in an obstructed system. This complication cannot always be avoided, but the use of gentle manipulation of the distal common bile duct and avoiding unnecessary instrumentation of the ampulla can help decrease its incidence.

   b. **Recognition and management**: The patient will present with excessive nausea and pain postoperatively and with an elevated amylase and lipase. The usual treatment regimen of bowel rest usually suffices and this process will be self-limited. A more serious problem exists if the pancreatitis is secondary to a retained stone. This scenario should be considered if the pancreatitis fails to improve and/or if the hepatic enzymes progressively increase. In severe cases of pancreatitis secondary to a retained stone, an ERCP and stone removal may be indicated.

5. **Retained common bile duct stones**

   a. **Cause and prevention**: It is difficult to pass the choledochoscope into the proximal common hepatic and intrahepatic ducts and therefore it is crucial to obtain a completion cholangiogram under fluoroscopy to prevent this problem.

   b. **Recognition and management**: If it is recognized intraoperatively, then the choledochoscope can be replaced to attempt further removal of the stones. If the stone is in the proximal ducts and the exploration was done via the cystic duct, it may be necessary to divide the cystic duct to better position the passage of the scope into the proximal ducts. This is usually the last maneuver because once the cystic duct is divided it is very difficult to replace the scope. The other option for retained stones is to convert to a laparoscopic choledochotomy, which can allow a larger choledochoscope (4.5 mm) to be placed and a better angle for passing the scope into the proximal ducts. Postoperatively retained stones can present with pain, pancreatitits, cholangitis, or asymptomatic jaundice. If a T-tube was used, the stones can be removed percutaneously through the T-tube tract. A postoperative ERC can also be used to identify and treat most retained stones.

6. **Stricture of the common bile duct**

   a. **Cause and prevention**: Excessive manipulation of a small common bile duct with a large choledochoscope through a choledochotomy can result in a difficult to close choledochotomy with a T-tube. Common duct explorations are the leading causes of Bismuth level I strictures. This can be prevented by preferentially using a transcystic method of exploration, not performing a choledochotomy on a small duct, not using electrocautery on the duct, and using meticulous suturing when closing the choledochotomy. If unable to do this, a postoperative ERC may be preferential to a bile duct exploration.

b. **Recognition and management**: This difficult problem can be a late complication from laparoscopic CBDE and is recognized by elevated liver enzymes and diagnosed with ERC. The treatment includes endoscopic balloons, stent placement, and more definitive biliary enteric anastomosis.

7. **Damaging the choledochoscope**

a. **Cause and prevention**: The manipulation of a fine and fragile choledochoscope across the peritoneal cavity can easily damage the scope, which can be quite expensive to repair. Care must be utilized in handling the scope with laparoscopic instruments and in placing the scope through a trocar. Many times it is often better to place the scope through a separate port and use a long flexible "peel-away" sheath from a Cordis-type introducer set.

b. **Recognition and management**: The damage is usually recognized when the scope is examined after the procedure and the protective sheath is noted to be cracked, which can limit its ability to be sterilized.

C. Selected References

Hunter JG, Soper NJ. Laparoscopic management of bile duct stones. Surg Clin North Am 1992;72:1077–1097.

Petlin JB. Laparoscopic approach to common duct pathology. Am J Surg 1993;165:487–491.

Phillips EH, Rosenthal RJ, Carrol BJ, et al. Laparoscopic transcystic common bile duct exploration. Surg Endosc 1994;8:1389–1394.

Sandosal BA, Goettler CE, Robinson BA, O'Donnel JK, Adler LP, Stellato TA. Cholesintigraphy in the diagnosis of bile leak after laparoscopic cholecystectomy. Am Surg 1997;63:611–616.

Strasberg SM, Hertl M, Soper NJ. An analysis of the problem of biliary injury during laparoscopic cholecystectomy. J Am Coll of Surgeons 1995;180:101–125.

Trus TL, Hunter JG. Laparoscopic bile duct techniques. Semin in Laparosc Surg 1995;2:118–127.

52. Flexible Sigmoidoscopy

John A. Coller, M.D.

A. Indications

The flexible sigmoidoscope is now the standard device for evaluation of the distal large bowel. Flexible sigmoidoscopy is used for screening of asymptomatic patients. When neoplastic polyps are found in the distal colon during **asymptomatic screening**, the entire colon must subsequently be examined. Flexible sigmoidoscopy may also be used to investigate symptoms referable to the distal large bowel, but is not a substitute for complete colon evaluation (for example, for workup of an iron deficiency anemia).

B. Instrumentation

Two principal 65-cm flexible sigmoidoscopic imaging systems are currently available.

1. The older style instrument is the **flexible fiberoptic sigmoidoscope**. A fiber bundle carries the illumination light down the shaft and a second fiber bundle carries the image back to the eyepiece.

2. The second instrument is an electronic **videoscope**. The light is carried down by a fiber bundle but the image is registered on a CCD chip at the tip of the scope. Although a great number of traditional fiberscopes remain, they are gradually being replaced by video technology. As with other endoscopes, the video system provides better image quality, reliability, image capture, annotation, and printing.

3. Both the fiberoptic and videoscopes require thorough mechanical cleansing and high-level disinfection of external surfaces and internal channels. A **sheathed videoendoscope system** has been developed that addresses some of the elements of scope cleansing. The use of a sheath may prolong examination time slightly, but significantly decreases downtime.

C. Patient Preparation

Adequate bowel preparation is essential for more than simple accuracy reasons. Any residual that is more substantive than a thin aspiratable liquid prolongs the examination, contributes to discomfort by requiring greater air insuflation, and adds to the risk a injury. Formed stool, once adherent to the viewing lens can be very tenacious, requiring blind removal of the instrument. Stool coating the mucosa obscures surface morphology and vasculature. A pool of opaque liquid between folds may be much deeper than apparent and consequently harbor a significant lesion beneath the surface. Fecal residue has a tendency to adhere to an abraded or demucosalized surface more readily than to the surrounding normal epithelium. Consequently, all stool-coated surfaces must be exposed if one is to clear the examined area with confidence.

Either cathartic, lavage, or enema preparation can be used for flexible sigmoidoscopy preparation. Preparation with a hypertonic sodium phosphate (Fleets, CB Fleet Co., Inc., Lynchburg, VA) enema is simple and safe in most patients. Symptomatic hyperphosphatemia and hypocalcemia can occur in children or patients with renal insufficiency.

Flexible sigmoidoscopy is an office procedure. Sedation is rarely needed.

D. Technique of Flexible Sigmoidoscopic Intubation

1. Flexible sigmoidoscopy does not require special positioning, but most right-handed physicians find the **left lateral decubitus** position most convenient.
2. Perform a **digital examination** with a well-lubricated gloved finger. This lubricates the anal canal and confirms that there are no lesions of the distal rectum. Carefully palpate the prostate (in male patients) and the posterior ampulla of the rectum, an area that may be difficult to visualize with the endoscope.
3. **Grasp the control housing** of the scope with the left hand, so that the thumb can manipulate the deflection controls and the second and third fingers can activate the air and suctions channels. Grasp the distal end of the scope with the right hand, apply lubricant to the shaft (not the lens).
4. Use the index finger of the right hand to **stabilize the deflection mechanism** (bendable tip). Gently insert the scope. The complete de-

flection mechanism, about 10-cm, must be inserted before the dial controls become effective.

5. After obtaining a view of the rectum, **position the right hand** on the shaft about 10- to 15-cm from the anal verge. Use the right hand to maintain shaft position, manipulating the deflection controls with the left hand. Greater speed and efficiency will be attained if the endoscopist avoids jumping the right hand back and forth between the shaft and the dials.

6. **Intubation** is performed using a combination of tip deflection, shaft torque, and shaft advancement/withdrawal, along with air insufflation and removal (see Chapter 40, Endoscope Handling).

    a. Two concentric dials control **tip deflection**. The larger outer dial deflects the distal 10 cm of scope nearly 180 degrees in either the up or down direction. The smaller dial does the same in the left-right direction. When both dials are maximally applied, the tip of the scope will overdeflect, well beyond 180 degrees. Judicious use of tip deflection greatly facilitates finding the lumen. However, once 90 degrees of deflection have been applied, the deflection mechanism begins to impede forward advancement of the scope. The leading edge of the scope is no longer the tip of the scope but rather the sharply angled shaft of the deflection tip itself (Fig. 42.2), and the colon deforms rather than permitting scope passage. Severe tip deflection, when necessary, should be restricted to finding the lumen, flattening the angle as much as possible before further advancement.

    b. **Shaft torquing** permits the partially deflected tip to press against a fold and ease into the lumen ahead. This is particularly useful when there is considerable circular muscular hypertrophy associated with diverticular disease in the sigmoid. When the full length of the scope has been inserted into a redundant sigmoid, **clockwise** torquing tends to straighten the loop whereas **counterclockwise** torque usually accentuates the redundancy.

    c. **Shaft advancement** is obviously necessary in order to obtain maximum intubation with the flexible sigmoidoscope. Incorporate torque and tip deflection as the scope is advanced. Rather than simply pushing the scope ahead, it is more effective to advance and withdrawn the shaft in a repetitive rhythmic fashion covering 10 to 15 cm (**dithering**). This shortens the colon by reefing it back onto the shaft of the scope.

7. **Insufflate air** to visualize the lumen, but avoid excess insufflation. Unnecessary distention increases patient discomfort and accentuates the angulation between fixed loops of colon. Since there is continu-

ous air flow to the control button, a lazy finger blocking the air vent can result in a great deal of unnecessary insufflation.

8. There are **three general approaches** to complete intubation using the flexible sigmoidoscope: intubation by elongation, intubation by looping, and intubation by dither-torquing.

    a. **Intubation by elongation**, the most basic approach, simply means advancing the shaft of the scope until there is no longer any scope left to advance. In some circumstances, such as after anterior resection, when all left colon redundancy has been removed the scope may be able to be maximally inserted with minimal manipulation of the control dials. More often, however, this approach will result in substantial stretching of the sigmoid colon into a large bow with the tip of the scope reaching only the sigmoid-descending junction (Fig. 52.1).

        i. To advance further, direct the deflection tip of the scope proximally into the distal descending colon lumen.

        ii. Reduce the elongated sigmoid by clockwise torquing while withdrawing scope shaft. The net result is to reef the sigmoid onto the shaft of the scope.

        iii. After reducing the sigmoid, advance the shaft while maintaining clockwise torque.

    b. **Intubation by looping** takes advantage of a redundant sigmoid and manipulates it into position (Fig. 52.2).

        i. After reaching the rectosigmoid, apply counterclockwise torque during shaft advancement. The proximal sigmoid will be directed toward the right side of the lower abdomen and pelvis.

        ii. This creates an **alpha loop** (name derived from resemblance to Greek letter alpha). The sigmoid-descending junction can then be approached in a horizontal direction, thus flattening the angle that has to be negotiated with the deflection tip of the scope.

        iii. Once the deflection tip has been positioned at the mid- or distal descending colon, reduce the loop by **simultaneous clockwise torque and shaft withdrawal**. As the loop is removed, the tip of the scope will extend more proximally as the colon accordionizes onto the scope even though some shaft is being withdrawn.

        iv. Once the sigmoid is straight, advance the shaft while maintaining clockwise torque.

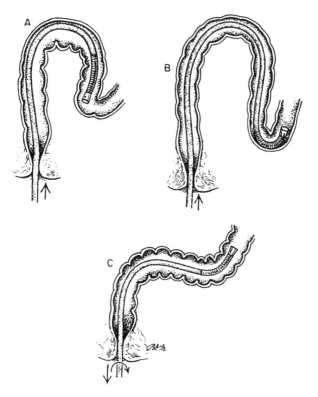

Figure 52.1. Intubation by elongation. A. The sigmoidoscope is advanced to the proximal sigmoid. B. Severe tip deflection prevents further advancement resulting in sigmoid elongation. C. Clockwise torquing and shaft withdrawal accordionizes the sigmoid.

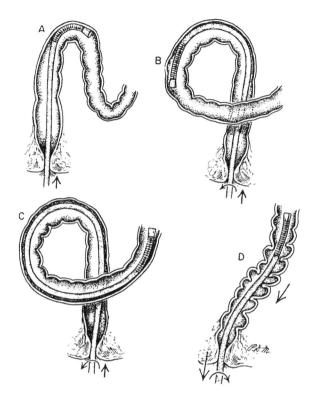

Figure 52.2. Intubation by looping. A. The sigmoidoscope is advanced to the distal sigmoid. B. Counterclockwise torquing during further advancement loops the proximal sigmoid in front of the distal sigmoid. C. The looped sigmoid flattens the angle at the distal descending colon. D. Clockwise torquing and shaft withdrawal accordionizes the sigmoid.

    c.   Intubation by **dither-torquing** attempts to minimize stretching or deforming of the colon. The colon is shortened and reefed during intubation, rather than after a large loop has been produced. Synchronous use of a back-and-forth movement with the shaft while torquing left and right is very effective in showing the way to the lumen while encouraging the colon to accordianize onto the scope (Fig. 52.3). This avoids the development of a large and often uncomfortable loop. When the sigmoid is tightly nested in the pelvis, dither-torquing method is usually the only way the intubation can be accomplished.

i.   Move the right hand (on the shaft) in a figure-of-eight–like motion and apply clockwise torque during a few centimeters of withdrawal.

ii. Continue this repetitive motion, attempting to bring the colon down onto the scope rather than pushing the scope into the colon.

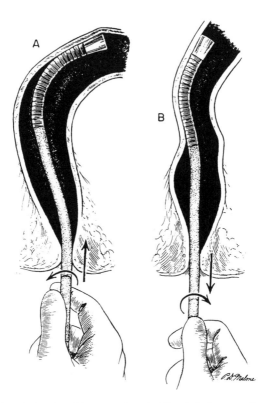

Fig. 52.3. Intubation by dither-torquing. A. The shaft is torqued counterclockwise while advancing the shaft 10- to 15-cm. B. The shaft is torqued clockwise while withdrawing the shaft 10- to 15-cm. Repetition of this cycle encourages the sigmoid to accordianize onto the sigmoidoscope.

    iii.   Advance additional scope only when there is no further progress. Use gentle tip deflection towards the lumen. Severe deflection will prevent accordianization of the colon.

E. Biopsy

Biopsy forceps are used to obtain tissue specimens. The forceps can either have a simple cup for single specimen retrieval or a cup with a central spire upon which two or three specimens are gathered. **Avoid the use of electrocautery** (hot biopsy forceps, snare) in the absence of complete mechanical bowel preparation to reduce hydrogen and methane gas concentrations. Always ensure a clear view of the lumen when passing the biopsy forceps through the channel, in order to avoid perforation of the bowel wall (particularly in diverticular bowel).

F. Complications

Intubation may be difficult in the presence of extensive diverticulosis or pelvic adhesions. A dense population of large-diameter diverticular orifices in association with circular muscular hypertrophy can confuse identification of the lumen. Do not proceed with shaft advancement in the absence of a clear view of the lumen. If the next proximal fold cannot be clearly identified through the prospective opening, one is more likely peering into a diverticulum rather than the lumen.

Pelvic adhesions may severely limit the degree of manipulation that one can apply to the sigmoid and descending colon. Prior gynecologic surgery, a history of peritoneal sepsis, and radiation injury are often responsible for severe adhesive formation. If the colon between the rectosigmoid and the distal descending colon is fixed into tightly nested loops, intubation may not be possible.

Persistence or the application of undue force may result in perforation. This complication is quite rare when proper technique is used.

G. Selected References

Coller JA. Technique of flexible fiberoptic sigmoidoscopy. Surg Clin North Am 1980;60:465–479.

Harrington L, Schuh S. Complications of Fleet enema administration and suggested guidelines for use in the pediatric emergency department. Pediatr Emerg Care 1997;13(3):225–226.

Helikson MA, Parham WA, Tobias JD. Hypocalcemia and hyperphosphatemia after phosphate enema use in a child. J Pediatr Surg 1997;32(8):1244–1246.

Preston KL, Peluso FE, Goldner F. Optimal bowel preparation for flexible sigmoidoscopy—are two enemas better that one? Gastrointest Endosc 1994;40(4):474–6.

Rothstein RI, Littenberg B. Disposable, sheathed, flexible sigmoidoscopy: a prospective, multicenter, randomized trial. The Disposable Endoscope Study Group. Gastrointest Endosc 1995;41(6):566–72.

53. Therapeutic Flexible Sigmoidoscopy

Irwin B. Simon, M.D., F.A.C.S.

A. Polypectomy

Polypectomy is the major therapeutic maneuver performed at flexible sigmoidoscopy. Snare polypectomy is used for medium and large polyps. Small polyps (less than 4–5 mm) may be removed with the hot biopsy forceps. Identification of polyps during screening flexible sigmoidoscopy should prompt full colonoscopy to exclude the presence of other lesions above the reach of the flexible sigmoidoscope.

1. **Snare polypectomy**: pedunculated polyps are ensnared at their stalk, and sessile polyps are ensnared within normal mucosa lateral to the polyp. The snare is tightened and monopolar electrocautery is used to coagulate and transect the polyp at the level of the snare.

    a. Push the snare out the distal tip of the sigmoidoscope.

    b. Open the snare well proximal to the lesion. Open the snare fully regardless of lesion size, to obtain better control for placement of the snare.

    c. Withdraw the snare to position the plastic sheath at the base of the polyp or lesion.

    d. Close the snare slowly until the tissue is visualized and felt to give resistance.

    e. Set the electrocautery to apply primarily coagulating current. Minimal if any cutting current should be required.

    f. Apply cautery slowly and in short bursts.

    g. When the polyp is large, minimize the risk of electrocautery complications by two means:

        i. Move the snare tip slowly back and forth to avoid prolonged contact with the wall of the colon with concentration of current at one place.

        ii. Deliberately place the broad surface of the polyp against the colon wall to maximize the surface area over which the electric current is distributed.

2. **The hot biopsy forceps** utilizes monopolar cautery to destroy the base of a minute polyp while preserving the architecture of the specimen within the biopsy jaws. The specimen may then be examined histologically.

B. Dilatation of Anastomotic Strictures and Control of Bleeding

1. **Anastomotic strictures** within reach of the flexible sigmoidoscope may be therapeutically dilated by use of pneumatic balloon dilators in a fashion identical to that of colonoscopy.
2. **Control of bleeding** has previously been less emphasized and felt to be impractical in flexible sigmoidoscopy and colonoscopy. More recent studies have shown that endoscopic evaluation of the lower GI tract in the setting of acute bleeding is feasible and of value from both a diagnostic as well as therapeutic standpoint.

    a. **Injection sclerotherapy** is most commonly used. Generally sodium tetradecol or ethanolamine oleate are used. Absolute alcohol injection is not recommended. This agent has caused full-thickness necrosis and perforation of the colon wall.

    b. **Monopolar cautery** may be cautiously applied in a short burst. The very tip of a closed snare may be extended beyond the plastic sheath to allow for a controlled application of current in a desired location.

    c. **Heater probe** may be used to apply heat directly over a source of bleeding. The technique is similar to application of a branding iron. It is best utilized in cases of small angiodysplasias.

    d. The **BICAP** is a bipolar application of electrical current. It is generally considered safer than monopolar current. The current path flows between two electrodes, thus limiting stray current and the risk of full thickness burn that may occur with monopolar electrocautery.

    e. **Lasers** may be utilized in a therapeutic fashion but are often not available in the office setting where flexible sigmoidoscopy is most often performed. Lasers must be of a frequency that yields low depth of penetrance. They are best utilized in cases of bleeding angiodysplasia.

C. Removal of Foreign Bodies

Foreign body removal from the rectum and colon has become more common today. The embarrassed patient may give minimal history, but usually knows it is there. 70% to 80% of swallowed foreign objects will pass spontaneously and do not require removal. In contrast, foreign objects that have been inserted through the anus frequently will not pass due to size and associated sphincter spasm, thus requiring endoscopic extraction.

First obtain an abdominal x-ray series to assess that the foreign body is within reach of the flexible sigmoidoscope and to rule out a perforation. Perforation changes the procedure to an operative procedure. If removal by flexible sigmoidoscopy is felt to be feasible:

1. First apply **topical anesthetic** to the anal sphincter to help break the reflexive sphincter spasm.
2. **Consider the size** of the object. Spinal anesthesia allows wide sphincter dilatation for removal of large or rounded objects.
3. Try to **obtain a duplicate** of the foreign object. Careful analysis may yield the solution as to what instrument will allow the best purchase and the most secure/safest orientation to remove the object.
4. A large snare is usually the best tool for sigmoidoscopic retrieval.
5. Use an overtube for multiple objects or objects with leading edges.
6. Turn sharp objects such that the leading edge becomes a trailing edge.
7. Repass the scope after foreign body removal to assess for injury such as bowel wall perforation or laceration that may have occurred during removal.

D. Complications of Flexible Sigmoidoscopy

1. **Missed diagnosis**
   a. **Cause and prevention:** The diagnosis may be missed as a result of failure to recognize the pathologic finding. Formal training and experience are the key to avoiding this complication.
   b. **Recognition and management:** This is difficult because the complication is truly one of omission. The diagnosis may be missed due to failure to recognize the indication and thus failure to perform the procedure. A classic example would be to attribute bright red blood per rectum to hemorrhoids, rather than do-

ing the endoscopic evaluation needed to diagnose cancer of the rectum or sigmoid colon.

2. **Complications of the bowel preparation** may arise and include electrolyte imbalance and cardiac effects, hypovolemia, and solitary rectal ulceration resulting from enema insertion.

   a. **Cause and prevention:** pay careful attention to the overall status of the patient. Avoid the 4-L polyethylene glycol solutions in those patients with poor functional status. Such patients may require a 2- or 3-day prep to avoid fluid imbalance. For flexible sigmoidoscopy, most patients can be prepped with simple enemas. Even then, the patient and/or nurse must be attentive to technique to avoid local trauma.

   b. **Recognition and management:** Poor skin turgor, obvious dyspnea, or cardiac dysrhythmias signal fluid and electrolyte abnormalities. New onset of anorectal pain should prompt careful examination of the anorectal region during the procedure. Solitary rectal ulcers are managed by bulking agents, topical anesthetics, and careful hygiene.

3. **Anorectal trauma due to scope insertion**

   a. **Cause and prevention:** Anal injury may result in painful fissures. Causes include inadequate lubrication and reflexive sphincter spasm at scope insertion. Avoid this by careful and gentle digital pressure on the perineal body just prior to and at the insertion of the scope. This causes reflex relaxation of the anal sphincter, minimizing the risk of trauma.

   b. **Recognition and management:** Acute bleeding and pain with blood on the insertion tube should make this issue suspect. This should be followed by careful anorectal examination during the procedure. The management includes bulking agents, topical anesthetics, and keeping tissues dry to promote healing.

4. **Perforation** is the most common and most morbid complication of therapeutic flexible sigmoidoscopy.

   a. **Cause and prevention:** Immediate perforation may result from electrocautery injury, taking too large a bite with the snare or hot biopsy forceps, traction injury (excessive wall tension during scope manipulation), or blowout of a diverticulum. Delayed perforation occasionally results when wall necrosis from electrocautery is not obvious for several days.

   b. **Recognition and management:** Acute perforation is frequently easy to recognize. The view through the scope shows intraabdominal organs rather than mucosa. Other signs include pain beyond that normally encountered, along with mild to moderate distention. The diagnosis is confirmed by free air on upright or left lateral decubitus film. Suspect delayed perforation in the appropriate setting when pain, leukocytosis, abdominal distention and signs of peritonitis develop several days to even several weeks after flexible sigmoidoscopy. Acute perforations taken to surgery immediately may be managed without creation of a stoma. The amount of time since perforation, degree of spillage of colonic contents, and health status of the patient all factor into the decision to repair the perforation, resect the segment, and whether to create a colostomy. The preparation for flexible sigmoidoscopy may be sufficient for primary repair if the perforation is recognized immediately and the patient taken to the operating room promptly, before much spillage occurs. Either an open or a laparoscopic approach may be used at the discretion of the surgeon.

5. **Hemorrhage** is generally recognized after the procedure is terminated.

   a. **Cause and prevention:** Immediate, visible bleeding is most often due to inadequate cauterization during polypectomy or biopsy. Immediate occult (internal) bleeding occasionally results from mesenteric or splenic capsule tears from overly aggressive endoscope manipulation. Delayed visible bleeding usually occurs around the eighth day when the eschar separates from coagulated site.

   b. **Recognition and management:** At times brisk bleeding is noted immediately, setting the endoscopist into theraputic maneuvers. Otherwise, immediate bleeding may first be recognized by the passage of bright red blood per rectum in the recovery area or unfortunately in the case of flexible sigmoidoscopy, by the patient at home. Tachycardia and hemodynamic are not always obvious. Splenic injury may be noticed by a frightening and rapid instability with possible expanding abdomen. However, it may also go unnoticed until the patient becomes unstable at home. Endoscopic interventions are most commonly applied to hemorrhagic complications. The most common setting would be in postpolypectomy bleeding. Even this is generally self-limited.

      i. If recognized at endoscopy, the bleeding polypectomy site may be immediately recauterized with monopolar cautery or bipolar cautery (BICAP) instrumentations.

    ii. Intervention with injection sclerotherapy is also fast, safe, and strongly recommended. The agents most commonly utilized are sodium tetradecol and ethanolamine oleate. This technique does carry with it the risk of a full-thickness colonic wall necrosis. The volume of any agent utilized should be minimized. Use of absolute alcohol is not recommended due to the significant risk involved for full-thickness necrosis after alcohol-induced desiccation.

    iii. Delayed postpolypectomy bleeding may be suspected in the patient who develops acute lower gastrointestinal bleeding at around 8 days postpolypectomy. The eschar separation classically occurs in this time frame. It is usually self limited and may be managed with intravenous hydration and supportive care. In specific cases, endoscopic interventions as outlined above will usually be successful.

    iv. Surgery is rarely required for postpolypectomy bleeding. When surgery is required, localize the bleeding site accurately before laparotomy. It is rarely feasible to mark the bleeding site preoperatively with vital dye at endoscopy (although this is helpful when it can be accomplished). Colotomy with oversewing of the bleeding point is the simplest maneuver, but is not always possible. The patient may need an anatomic resection to ensure that the site has been removed.

6. **Bacteremia and possible sepsis:** Bacteremia has been demonstrated after colonic manipulation. Antibiotic prophylaxis is recommended for high-risk patients (for example, patients with artificial heart valves or or other implanted prosthetic devices).

7. **Incomplete polypectomy** may be a technical error or deliberate in cases of large sessile polyps. Attention to detail of polypectomy technique is the best prevention. If snare placement does not seem appropriate, it is generally possible to regrasp the polyp as long as electrocautery has not yet been applied. Reapplication of the snare to complete an adequate polypectomy prevents a clinical situation requiring repeat endoscopy. Mark polyps that are too large to completely remove with indigo carmine or other vital dyes to facilitate removal of the proper colonic segment at open or laparoscopic surgery.

8. **Explosion** is far less common with better methods of bowel preparation that prevent accumulation of hydrogen or methane gas. If the prep is not good, it may be prudent to defer use of electrocautery

(scheduling a second procedure if necessary) until an adequate mechanical preparation has been attained.

9. **Glutaraldehyde-induced colitis** results from inadequate washing of endoscopes with ineffective flushing of biopsy/instrument channels. This iatrogenic colitis can be prevented by careful training of endoscopy personnel and attention to detail. Newer methods of endoscope cleansing avoid use of the inciting agent. The colitis generally presents less than 6 hours after flexible sigmoidoscopy. Management is supportive.

10. **Rare and unusual complications:** Though rare, the theoretical possibilities must be known and vigilant attention paid to avoid such occurrences as:

    a. Incarceration of bowel in a hernia.
    b. Incarceration of the flexible sigmoidoscope in a hernia.
    c. Aortic aneurysm rupture.
    d. Creation of a sigmoid volvulus.
    e. Pneumocystoides intestinalis.
    f. Accidental removal of a ureterosigmoidoscopy stoma by mistaking it for a polyp.

E. Selected References

Hayashi K, Urata K, Munakata Y, Kawasaki S, Makuuchi M. Laparoscopic closure for perforation of the sigmoid colon by endoscopic linear stapler. Surg Laparosc Endosc 1996;6:411–413.

Jentschura D, Raute M, Winter J, Henkel T, Kraus M, Manegold BC. Complications in endoscopy of the lower gastrointestinal tract. Therapy and prognosis. Surg Endosc 1994;8:672–676.

Manier JW. Flexible Sigmoidoscopy. In: Gastroenterologic Endoscopy. Sivak MV (ed.). Philadelphia: WB Saunders, 1987, pp. 975–991.

Norfleet RG. Infectious endocarditis after fiberoptic sigmoidoscopy. With a literature review. J Clin Gastroenterol 1991;13:448–451.

Ponsky JL, Mellinger JD, Simon IB. Endoscopic retrograde hemmorhoidal sclerotherapy using 23.4% saline: a preliminary report. Gastrointest Endosc 1991;37:155–158.

Sanowski RA. Foreign body extraction in the gastrointestinal tract. In: Gastroenterologic Endoscopy. Sivak MV (ed.). Philadelphia: WB Saunders, 1987, pp. 321–331.

Simon IB, Lewis RJ, Satava RM. A safe method for sedating and monitoring patients for upper and lower gastrointestinal endoscopy. Am Surg 1991;57:219–221.

Waye JD, Kahn O, Auerbach ME. Complications of colonoscopy and flexible sigmoidoscopy. Gastrointest Endosc Clin North Am 1996;6:343–377.

West AB, Kuan SF, Bennick M, Lagarde S. Glutaraldehyde colitis following endoscopy: clinical and pathological features and investigation of an outbreak. Gastroenterology 1995;108:1250–1255.

Williard W, Satava R. Inguinal hernia complicating flexible sigmoidoscopy. Am Surg
1990;56:800–801.

54. Diagnostic Colonoscopy

Bassem Y. Safadi, M.D.
Jeffrey M. Marks, M.D.

A. Indications

Generally accepted indications for diagnostic colonoscopy are summarized in Table 54.1. Colonoscopy is usually **not indicated** in patients with bright red rectal bleeding when a convincing anorectal source has been found on anoscopy or sigmoidoscopy and when there are no other symptoms suggesting a more proximal source of bleeding. It is also not necessary in upper gastrointestinal bleeding when a source proximal to the colon has been clearly identified. Colonoscopy is generally **not indicated** in the workup of metastatic carcinoma in the absence of symptoms related to the colon. Colonoscopy is indicated for evaluation of unexplained abdominal pain or change in bowel habits **only in select cases**. It is generally **not indicated** in patients with chronic stable abdominal pain or symptoms of irritable bowel in the absence of other indications for colonoscopy.

Table 54.1. Indications for diagnostic colonoscopy

Evaluation of gastrointestinal bleeding
• Hemoccult positive stools
• Hematochezia when an anal or rectal source is not certain
• Melena after excluding an upper GI source
• Unexplained iron deficiency anemia
Surveillance for colon neoplasia
• Following resection of carcinoma or malignant polyp
• When a cancer or neoplastic polyp has been found on screening sigmoidoscopy (provided the results will change treatment plan)
• In high cancer risk patients
- First-degree relatives or multiple family members with colon cancer
- Cancer family syndrome
- Chronic ulcerative colitis with pancolitis greater than seven years or left-sided colitis of greater than ten years

Table 54.1. continued

Inflammatory bowel disease
- Determination of extent of disease
- Confirmation of diagnosis
- Cancer surveillance in chronic ulcerative colitis

Evaluation of
- Clinically significant abnormalities on barium enema
- Clinically significant diarrhea of unexplained etiology
- Suspected ischemic colitis

Intraoperative localization of lesions not apparent at surgery

---

Contraindications to colonoscopy include peritonitis or suspected colorectal perforation, severe acute diverticulitis, fulminant colitis, and hemodynamic instability. **Relative contraindications** include large bowel obstruction and recent myocardial infarction or pulmonary embolus.

B. Preparation and Positioning of the Patient and Room Setup

1. **Bowel preparation** is essential; the entire colon should be cleansed of all fecal matter for an adequate exam and to decrease the risk for potential complications.
   a. Discontinue iron=containing medications or constipating agents.
   b. **Clear liquids** or other residue-free diets for 24 hours.
   c. Four liters of specially balanced electrolyte lavage solution, e.g., **polyethylene glycol-electrolyte (PEG)** given orally, beginning approximately 18 hours prior to the exam. Administer at a rate of 1 to 2 L per hour (8 ounces every 10 minutes). Modifications include sulfate-free PEG lavage solution, which tends to be less salty, and various flavored PEG solutions. Sugars should not be added to the gut lavage as it may cause sodium retention or lead to production of potentially explosive gases. Reglan is occasionally given prior to the prep to prevent the associated nausea and vomiting.
   d. An alternative small-volume regimen of **oral sodium phosphate** (Fleet R Phospho R-Soda). A ~1.5 oz bottle is given orally b.i.d. the day before the colonoscopy. One **small-volume enema** (Fleet enema R) is given the morning of the examination. This regimen has been shown to be as effective, better tol-

erated, and less expensive than the PEG prep. This is a highly osmotic buffered saline laxative that stimulates the small bowel and therefore may cause dehydration and electrolyte imbalance, and transient hyperphosphatemia. Use cautiously in patients with symptomatic congestive heart failure, ascites, or renal insufficiency.

e. Alternatively, the "traditional" bowel prep of **clear liquids** for 2 days and a purge with **oral magnesium** and **enemas** the day before the exam.

f. Do not use mannitol or other fermentable carbohydrates, which could be converted to explosive gases.

2. **The instruments:** The newer generation of colonoscopes that are predominantly used nowadays are **videoscopes.** Light signals pass through a wide-angle lens onto a CCD chip, which in turn transmits them into electronic signals to a video processing unit where the image is reconstructed digitally. This is in contrast to **fiberoptic scopes** where the image is a real image transmitted through the eye piece via fiberoptics (see Chapter 39, Characteristics of Flexible Endoscopes, Troubleshooting, and Equipment Care). Become familiar with the basic components of the endoscope and the video system. Always check the instrument before the examination.

3. **Patient preparation and positioning**

a. Before beginning any endoscopic procedure, review the procedure with the patient, answer questions, ease the patient's concerns, and obtain an informed consent.

b. For patients with high risk of developing infections from bacteremia such as patients with valvular heart disease and prosthetic valves, **endocarditis prophylaxis with antibiotics** is recommended.

4. **The basic room setup** is diagrammed in Fig. 54.1. The patient is in the center of the room in the left lateral position with thigh and legs flexed. The endoscopist stands on the right side of the patient and the assistant on the left. The presence of two video monitors allows both endoscopist and assistant a comfortable view.

5. **Appropriate monitoring** includes continuous EKG, pulse rate, and pulse oximetry monitoring, and intermittent blood pressure recording. Most patients will need supplemental oxygen given via a nasal canula (see Chapter 41, Monitoring, Sedation, and Recovery).

6. **Conscious sedation** is used for most patients. The most popular agents are a combination of a narcotic (e.g., Demerol or morphine sulfate) and a benzodiazepine (e.g., diazepam, midazolam). Titrate

dose to effect and always have reversal agents (naloxone and flumenazil) available.

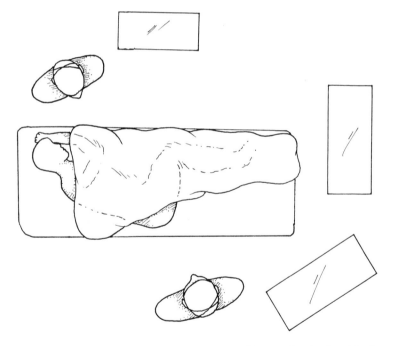

Figure 54.1. Patient position and room setup. A video monitor is placed in the direct line of sight of the endoscopist (at the back of the patient) and the assistant (who stands in front of the patient). Monitoring equipment for EKG, blood pressure, and oxygen saturation are positioned at the foot of the bed.

C. General Principles of Colonoscopy

After ensuring adequate sedation, the exam should always start with a visual inspection of the anus and a digital rectal exam.

1. Place your index finger about an inch from the tip of the scope and **insert the scope** by sliding the tip across the perineal body and into the anus. This reduces trauma to the anal canal. Use plenty of lubricant on the endoscope, but not on the lens. Insert the scope straight without twists.

2. Use **air insufflation** to open the rectum and to visualize the lumen, and from there on advance the scope while keeping the lumen of the colon in view.

3. **General principles** to follow (see Chapter 40, Endoscope Handling):
   a. To maintain maximal control during the colonoscopy keep your right hand on the shaft of the scope and use the left hand to control the suction, irrigation, insufflation, and tip deflection.
   b. Use a combination of simultaneous moves to maneuver your way through the colon.
   c. Torque with the right hand moving clockwise and counterclockwise; push, pull, and jiggle and use the left hand to deflect the tip of the scope up and down, left and right.
   d. Alternatively, a two-operator technique can be used: one operator controls scope deflection while the other advances and withdraws the scope.

4. Pay attention to the following:
   a. Avoid overinsufflation.
   b. Minimize "loop" formation by periodically straightening the colon by jiggling and withdrawing the colonoscope. This facilitates the procedure (Fig. 54.2).
   c. Always try to **keep the lumen in view** and avoid pushing the scope blindly or "sliding by" as this may increase the risk of perforation.

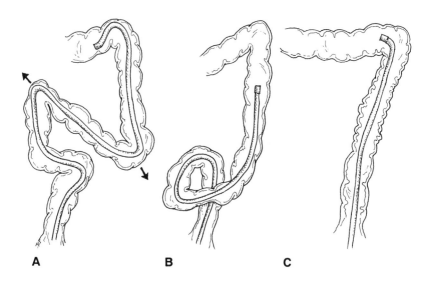

A   **B**   **C**

Figure 54.2 A. Formation of loops in the colon can cause patient discomfort, difficulty in advancing the scope, and may increase the risk of perforation. B. Here an alpha loop has been formed in the sigmoid colon, facilitating passage into the descending colon. Clockwise torque is sometimes necessary to derotate the loop. C. In the early phase of colonoscopy, try to keep the tip of the scope straight or only slightly bent. Use a combination of push, pull, jiggle, and torque to remove the loops and "straighten" the colon. This facilitates passage through the splenic flexure.

D. Passing the Colonoscope —Normal Anatomy

1. **The rectum:** The rectum is characterized by its valves of Houston, which will appear as semilunar folds as soon as you enter the rectal vault. In addition the rectal wall has a prominent submucosal venous plexus and the rectal veins are larger than elsewhere in the colon.
2. **The sigmoid colon:** The sigmoid colon has a high muscular tone and can easily go into spasm. It is tortuous with a semilunar appearance of folds. Diverticulae are common in this portion of the colon and they may mimic the lumen, so be careful advancing. Passage of the scope may be particularly difficult in patients who have had prior

pelvic surgery (e.g., hysterectomy) and in the elderly. In general, avoid overinsufflation and periodically straighten the scope and reduce loops as they form.

3. **The descending colon:** The descending colon has a straight, tubular shape with no haustral markings and has less musculature than the sigmoid colon. Although passage of the scope may be easier here, continue to periodically jiggle back and forth attempting to straighten the scope. "A straight sigmoid is the key to an easy splenic flexure" (Church, 1995).

4. **The splenic flexure:** The splenic flexure will appear as a turn at the end of the descending colon. It has a characteristic blue shadow reflecting the spleen and frequently a strong transmitted cardiac pulsation can be seen. Often, asking the patient to take a deep breath will help making the turn.

5. **The transverse colon:** The transverse colon has a characteristic triangular appearance.

    a. Difficulty in advancing the scope or complaints of pain from the patient are probably caused by a sigmoid loop.

    b. Try to "reduce" the loop in the scope by withdrawing to straighten the sigmoid colon.

    c. Sometimes it is possible to gently "push through the loop" to advance, but be careful as force may cause tears and perforations in the sigmoid colon.

    d. Applying pressure to the left or lower abdominal wall or changing the patient's position may help (supine or prone).

6. **The hepatic flexure**: The hepatic flexure has a characteristic blue liver shadow and there is usually a pool of liquid at the end of the transverse colon.

7. **The ascending colon and cecum:** The ascending colon is also triangular. The three colonic taenia converge at the cecum giving it its characteristic "Mercedes sign" where the appendiceal orifice can be found. The ileocecal valve will appear as a yellowish fold or may look polypoid, and occasionally may look flat. Flowing liquid stool or gas bubbles sometimes can be seen emerging from it. Advancing the scope beyond the hepatic flexure will often lead to a paradoxical movement, i.e., scope moves backward. Pull the scope back and use intermittent suctioning and that will most often push the tip of the scope forward toward the cecum (another paradox). Remember the suction channel is at the six o'clock position on the screen, so tip the scope up as you apply suction to avoid catching the mucosa. Rotating the patient here can also be helpful in advancing the scope. It is very important to ascertain reaching the cecum by clearly identifying the

appendiceal orifice and the ileocecal valve. Other maneuvers include transilluminating the right lower quadrant (RLQ) and seeing indentations on the cecal wall as the RLQ is palpated. The only way to verify reaching the ileocecal valve with 100% confidence is intubating the terminal ileum and visualizing ileal mucosa.

8. **Scope withdrawal:** After complete insertion, withdraw the colonoscope gradually, carefully inspecting the colonic mucosa circumferentially. If an area slips, readvance the scope to get a satisfactory exam. When the rectum is reached, "retroflexing" the scope will provide a view of the lower rectal ampula. After careful inspection straighten the scope and suction excess air in the lumen and withdraw the scope.

E. Passing the Colonoscope —Postsurgical Anatomy

After colon resections, the colon is generally shorter and the colonoscopy is correspondingly easier and less time-consuming.

1. If the sigmoid colon has been resected, the colon will appear straighter.

2. Anastomoses are recognized by either visualizing a suture or staple line with its characteristic whitish linear scar. Occasionally suture or staple material can be seen through the mucosa. Anastomoses may be an end to end (one lumen), side to side (two lumina seen simultaneously) or end to side (one lumen and one blind end). It is very important to recognize the blind end and avoid forceful insertion as this may lead to perforation. This is especially true in stapled low anterior resection anastomoses and stapled colostomy takedowns. A sharp turn is frequently noted in stapled side-to-side, functional end-to-end anastomoses.

3. **Passing scope via colostomy:** This is done with the patient in the supine position. Again, a careful visual inspection and digital exam to the level of the fascia is mandatory before introducing the scope. This will also help in gently dilating the stoma prior to introducing the scope. The remainder of the colonoscopy follows the above-mentioned principles. A problem particular to this situation is air leakage around the stoma, which could compromise insufflation. Applying mild pressure with a gauze around the scope at the stoma level may be helpful.

F. Biopsy

Colonoscopic biopsies are generally mucosal. Submucosal lesions cannot be biopsied using these conventional methods. The cecum and right colon are thin walled, and caution should be exercised when using the hot biopsy technique in that portion of the colon due to increased risk of perforation.

1. **The indications for biopsy** are very broad and guided by their clinical relevance to diagnosis and treatment. In general, biopsies are obtained to check for neoplasia (e.g., carcinoma, adenoma, dysplasia, lymphoma) or colitis (e.g., eosinophilic, ischemic, radiation-induced, infectious, inflammatory bowel disease).

2. **Introduce biopsy forceps** into the scope via the biopsy channel. This may be difficult when the scope is looped and is often facilitated by straightening the scope.

3. Because the forceps exit the scope at the six o'clock position, make an effort to **position the lesion at six o'clock** on the screen to facilitate the biopsy.

4. When random biopsies are needed (such as in ulcerative colitis) it is easiest to **obtain the biopsies from a fold**.

5. Direct the forceps to the target, open the forceps, push in, and close the forceps. Pull abruptly to obtain the specimen.

   a. There are numerous types of biopsy forceps.

   b. Biopsy forceps can be equipped with a spike that holds the first biopsy allowing the forceps to be used for an immediate second biopsy.

   c. In general a **cold biopsy** refers to one done without the use of cautery.

   d. **Hot biopsy** uses cautery and is primarily used for removing small polyps (< 5 mm).

      i. Advantages include the ability to obtain a sample suitable for histologic examination, destroy the residual polyp with the effect of the cautery, and achieve hemostasis.

      ii. Grasp the polyp with the biopsy forceps and pull it away from the bowel wall.

      iii. Push the forceps out until the tip of the insulating sheath is seen to avoid damage to the scope.

      iv. Use medium-strength coagulating current in short bursts until the polyp and 2mm of surrounding mucosa turn white (coagulum).

      v. Pull the forceps and withdraw from the scope.

G. Endoscopic Ultrasound (EUS)

1. **Indications for rectal EUS:** Endoscopic ultrasound (EUS) examination of the rectum has been primarily used for:
    a. **Staging of rectal cancer.** It is useful for selecting tumors for local treatment, selecting patients for neoadjuvant therapy, and predicting patients who may need en bloc resection of other pelvic organs.
    b. **Follow-up of rectal cancer** to monitor local recurrence.
    c. Delineating **perianal fistulaes** and **abscesses** and their relationship to the sphincters.
    d. Imaging internal and external sphincter in the evaluation of incontinence.
    e. Identification of **submucosal** masses.
2. **Indications for colonic EUS:** EUS in colon cancer staging and follow-up has not been as clinically relevant as in rectal cancer for several reasons. Generally, there is no role for neoadjuvant therapy in colon cancer (controversial in T-4 lesions) and local recurrence is uncommon. In addition, EUS of the colon is technically more difficult. EUS **may** have a role in:
    a. Guiding therapeutic plans on large sessile adenomatous polyps whether endoscopic, laparoscopic, or open removal is appropriate.
    b. Differentiating between transmural colitis (Crohn's) and mucosal colitis (ulcerative colitis).
3. **Equipment**
    a. **Radial scanning** EUS scopes are the most popular. They give a circumferential ultrasonic image, producing cross-sectional anatomic sections. The longitudinal extent of the lesion can be determined by carefully moving the instrument in the proximal-distal direction.
    b. **Linear scan** EUS scopes provide a longitudinal section and this instrument must be rotated to delineate the entire circumference of the rectal wall. For acoustic interface, a water-filled balloon surrounds the transducer head. The frequency most commonly used is ~7.5 MHz. (The shorter the frequency, the greater the depth of penetration and the worse the resolution and vice versa.)
    c. **Rectal EUS probes** are either rigid, inserted blindly or via a proctoscope (up to 20 cm), or flexible.

d. The ultrasonic colonoscope is a flexible instrument, forward viewing with a biopsy channel, and a radial scanning method. Alternatively, miniature ultrasound scanners can be mounted on a probe that is inserted into the biopsy channel of an endoscope.

e. Newer scanners have the capability of imaging with color Doppler as well as ultrasound-guided needling. Future-generation probes will allow for three-dimensional intrarectal ultrasonography with computer-generated three-dimensional reconstruction using a continuous pull-through technique with the radial scanner.

4. **General principles of EUS technique**

a. **Bowel prep:** for rectal EUS, bowel preparation with enemas is usually sufficient, whereas a routine bowel prep is necessary for colonic EUS.

b. Start with direct examination by proctosigmoidoscopy or total colonoscopy.

c. Identify the target lesion and determine its distance from the anal verge. Place the EUS probe at that level (for colonic EUS, fluoroscopy may help in localization). Some EUS scopes allow you to identify the lesion through an optical piece. Scanning begins proximal to the lesion.

d. Withdraw the probe slowly to assess the entire length of the GI lumen. Repeat the exam two or three times. Optimal imaging is obtained by the combination of balloon insufflation and water instillation.

5. **Normal findings**

a. Tissues with high levels of collagen (e.g., submucosa) or fat appear hyperechoic, whereas tissues with high water content (e.g., muscle) appear hypoechoic. Using a frequency ~7.5 MHz probe allows visualization of five layers in the rectal wall (Fig. 54.3):

  i.   Hyperechoic/hypoechoic (two layers)—mucosa
  ii. Hyperechoic—submucosa
  iii. Hypoechoic—muscularis propria
  iv. Hyperechoic—perirectal fat

b. Occasionally seven layers can be delineated (separation of inner circular muscle layer and the outer longitudinal muscle layer of the muscularis propria).

c. Normal rectal wall thickness is between 2 and 4 mm.

d. Normal colonic wall is between 2 and 3 mm.

6. At a frequency of 7.5 MHz, the penetration depth of an ultrasound scan is about 3 to 4 cm; therefore, other structures could be visual-

ized with rectal EUS: prostate and seminal vesicles in males, vagina and uterus in females. Urinary bladder can be shown in both sexes, especially if full. Valves of Houston may mimic lesions. Adjacent organs occasionally visualized in colonic EUS include parts of the left and right kidneys, liver, pancreas, and spleen.

7. **The staging of rectal cancers** follows the TNM classification Depth of penetration determines the T stage. In determining the N state, any enlarged lymph node is suspicious. Generally inflammatory nodes are hyperechoic, elongated, and heterogeneous, and have indistinct borders, whereas metastatic nodes are hypoechoic, rounded, sharply demarcated, and homogeneous (Table 54.2).

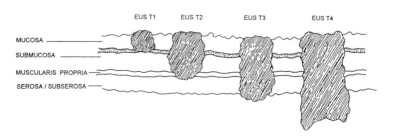

Figure 54.3. System of T (tumor)-staging of rectal cancers based upon endoscopic ultrasound appearance.

Table 54.2. EUS staging of rectal cancers

T staging (Fig. 54.3):

 T1. Tumor confined to mucosa and/or submucosa.
   Does not interrupt the middle hyperechoic layer.
 T2. Invasion of muscularis propria.
   Does not interrupt the outer hyperechoic area.
 T3. Penetration through the muscularis propria into perirectal fat.
   Through the outer hyperechoic area.
 T4. Invasion of adjacent organs.

Stages EUS3 and EUS4 are combined.

N staging:

 N0. LNs not visualized, or hyperechoic.
 N1. LNs hypoechoic or with mixed echo patterns.

8. **Results**
    a. Accuracy is ~88–92% in assessing the depth of invasion, ~69–80% in assessing regional adenopathy with a sensitivity of ~70–80% and a specificity of ~80–90%.
    b. Limitations:
        i. It is difficult to evaluate obstructing lesions.
        ii. Small LNs with micrometastases are difficult to differentiate from normal LNs. Newer scopes with capability of EUS-guided needle biopsy of nodes may increase diagnostic yield.
    c. The **most common misinterpretation** of endosonographic tumor staging is caused by **overstaging**, specifically for T2 tumors. Due to a peritumoral inflammation that appears hypoechoic on ultrasound, a penetration through the wall may be falsely predicted (this may be seen following biopsy).

H. Selected References

ASGE: Preparation of patients for gastrointestinal endoscopy: guidelines for clinical application. Gastrointest Endosc 1988;34(3):32S.
ASGE: Policy and Procedure Manual for Gastrointestinal Endoscopy: Guideline for Training and Practice. May 1997.

Catalano MF. Normal structures on endoscopic ultrasonography: visualization measurement data and interobserver variation. Gastrointest Endosc Clin North Am 1995;5(3):475–486.

Church JM. Endoscopy of the colon, Rectum, and Anus. New York: Igaku-Shoin, 1995.

Golub RW, Kerner BA, Wise WE Jr, et al. Colonoscopic bowel preparations—Which one? Dis Colon Rectum 1995;38(6):594–599.

Hildebrandt U, Feifel G. Importance of endoscopic ultrasonography staging for treatment of rectal cancer. Gastrointest Endosc Clin North Am 1995;5(4):843–849.

Ponsky JL (ed.). Atlas of Surgical Endoscopy. St. Louis: Mosby-Year Book, 1992.

Romano G, Belli G, Rotondano G. Colorectal cancer: diagnosis of recurrence. Gastrointest Endosc Clin North Am 1995;5(4):831–841.

Rosch T, Lorenz R, Classen M. Endoscpic ultrasonography in the evaluation of colon and rectal disease. Gastrointest Endosc 1990;36(2): S33–39.

Senagore AJ. Intrarectal and intra-anal ultrasonography in the evaluation of colorectal patholoby. Surg Clin North Am 1994;74(6):1465–1473.

Silverstein FE, Tytgat GNJ, Hunter J (eds.). Atlas of Gastrointestinal Endoscopy, 2nd. New York: Gower Medical, 1991.

Van Outryve M. Endoscopic ultrasonography in inflammatory bowel disease, paracolorectal inflammatory pathology, and extramural abnormalities. Gastrointest Endosc Clin North Am 1995;5(4):861–867.

55. Therapeutic Colonoscopy, Complications of Colonoscopy

C. Daniel Smith, M.D.
Aaron S. Fink, M.D.
Gregory Van Stiegmann, M.D.
David W. Easter, M.D.

A. Introduction

Polypectomy is the commonest therapeutic maneuver performed at the time of colonoscopy. This technique is described in Chapter 53 (Therapeutic Flexible Sigmoidoscopy). Control of bleeding and removal of foreign objects are also discussed in that section. This section of the manual describes decompressive colonoscopy for Ogilvie's syndrome, reduction of volvulus, band ligation of hemorrhoids, and complications of colonoscopy.

B. Decompressive Colonoscopy for Ogilvie's Syndrome

Acute colonic pseudo-obstruction (Ogilvie's syndrome) is a condition in which the colon becomes massively dilated without apparent mechanical obstruction. Commonly associated conditions are listed in Table 55.1. The cause is unknown but likely to be multifactorial.

The diagnosis is usually straightforward. The predominant clinical feature is abdominal distention developing over 3 to 4 days. Bowel sounds are variably present and the abdomen is generally tense with mild tenderness. Fever and leukocytosis are common. Plain abdominal x-rays frequently reveal massive dilatation of the proximal colon with relatively normal colonic diameter from mid-transverse colon to rectum. Contrast enema is necessary to exclude mechanical obstruction. Radiographic demonstration of perforation mandates urgent laparotomy.

Table 55.1. Conditions associated with Ogilvie's syndrome

Nonabdominal surgery	• Orthopedic surgery
Blunt trauma	
Electrolyte abnormalities	• Hypokalemia • Hypomagnesemia • Hypophosphatemia
Chronic illness	• Renal failure • Diabetes mellitus • Malignancy • Autoimmune disorders • Hypothyroidism
Medications	• Anticholinergic agents • Narcotics • Phenothiazines • Tricyclic antidepressants

Initial therapy includes cessation of oral intake, nasogastric decompression, and correction of fluid and electrolyte abnormalities. All potentially exacerbating medications (such as narcotics) should be discontinued. Prokinetic agents, epidural anesthesia, frequent positional change, or ambulation may promote motility. Serial abdominal examinations and daily abdominal x-rays should be used to monitor response or progression. The cecum is at greatest risk of perforation due to the thin wall and greater circumference. When cecal diameter exceeds 12 cm, or if there is persistence or progression of colonic dilatation despite conservative measures, colonoscopic decompression is indicated.

1. Set up the room and position the patient as for routine colonoscopy.
2. Minimize air insufflation during endoscope passage. The pathologic distention usually facilitates endoscope passage, which is often surprisingly easy.
3. Irrigate frequently with small volumes (50 cc) of saline through the endoscope's suction channel to help maintain channel patency and a good view of the lumen.
4. It is not necessary to reach the cecum with the colonoscope in order to effect colonic decompression, especially if the colon is distended beyond the hepatic flexure.
5. Carefully inspect the mucosa during insertion and withdrawal. Cyanotic or ischemic mucosa may indicate the need for operative intervention. Sometimes bloody drainage is the only sign of proximal ischemia.

6. Use of an overtube for this purpose must be done with care, as the large size and stiff nature of this tube complicate endoscope insertion while increasing the risk of perforation or erosion.
7. After maximal insertion, apply intermittent suction as the endoscope is withdrawn until the colonic lumen collapses. Withdraw the scope in 4- to 5-cm increments, keeping the tip of the scope in the middle of the bowel lumen. This allows decompression of gas and liquid through the suction channel without trapping bowel mucosa.
8. Evaluate the success of decompression by serial abdominal physical and radiographic examination.
9. A nasogastric tube or long intestinal tube may be passed with the colonoscope and left in place after scope removal.

C. Decompressive Colonoscopy for Sigmoid Volvulus

Sigmoid volvulus occurs when a large bowel segment abnormally twists or folds on its mesentery. Volvulus produces a closed loop obstruction with a high mortality unless treated. The diagnosis may be suspected on the basis of clinical presentation and plain abdominal films (which may be diagnostic). Contrast studies confirm the problem by showing the typical bird's beak deformity of the twisted segment.

In the absence of signs of gangrene, the safest initial treatment of sigmoid volvulus is sigmoidoscopic reduction and decompression. This provides assessment of mucosal viability, and more importantly, may decompress the dilated loop and reduce the volvulus. Urgent laparotomy is mandated for suspicion of colonic gangrene (elevated temperature, leukocytosis, abdominal tenderness with peritoneal signs, necrotic mucosa at endoscopy) or inability to reduce the volvulus.

In contrast to sigmoid volvulus, endoscopic reduction and decompression is not effective for cecal volvulus. Although both colonoscopic and barium-assisted reduction of cecal volvulus have been described, successes have been limited and associated with high morbidity due to delays in definitive management. The mainstay of management for cecal volvulus remains prompt laparotomy, at which time the volvulus is reduced.

1. Begin preparing the patient for surgery, so that operative intervention will not be delayed if endoscopic treatment fails.
2. Position the patient in the prone jackknife position. This facilitates decompression by allowing the colon to fall away. The lateral decu-

bitus position is acceptable if the patient cannot tolerate the jackknife position.

3. Because the twist is low in the sigmoid, it can generally be reached with a **rigid sigmoidoscope**. This instrument facilitates decompression, often resulting in a dramatic passage of gas and stool as the volvulus is entered and the segment is decompressed.

   a. Minimize air insufflation during insertion.
   b. Carefully insert the rigid sigmoidoscope until the site of torsion is seen. Thoroughly inspect the mucosa at this point for signs of ischemia or necrosis.
   c. If the mucosa appears intact, gently advance the sigmoidoscope beyond the point of torsion until there is an immediate return of gas and stool from the obstructed loop.
   d. Perform a further limited examination of the bowel mucosa to assure viability, then place a rectal tube well above the site of torsion, secure it to the perianal skin, and leave it for at least 48 hours. This will maintain decompression and facilitate subsequent bowel preparation or further evaluation.
   e. Alternatively, a soft, well-lubricated 40- to 60-cm rectal tube can be gently passed beyond the site of torsion under endoscopic vision to accomplish decompression. Obviously, endoscopic evaluation of mucosal viability may be limited with this tecnique.

4. Points of axial rotation and obstruction beyond the reach of a rigid scope require use of a **flexible sigmoidoscope or a colonoscope.**

   a. Suction and an assistant are critical to safe completion of endoscopic decompression and evaluation.
   b. The colonoscope is passed through the site of torsion, often with gentle air insufflation, as the scope is passed beyond the site of obstruction.
   c. Suction decompression may be facilitated by attaching an external suction device to the colonoscope's biopsy channel, or by attaching a long, soft, 14- to 16-French straight catheter to the colonoscope while advancing past the torsion and into the proximal colon. This tube is then left in place for subsequent decompression.

5. Endoscopic decompression and detorsion is successful in 85% of cases of sigmoid volvulus. A high rate of recurrence argues in favor of elective resection of the redundant segment. Patients in whom endoscopic decompression fails, or in whom nonviable mucosa is seen on colonoscopy, require urgent surgery.

D. Endoscopic Band Ligation Treatment of Internal Hemorrhoids

Indications for treatment of internal hemorrhoids include bleeding and prolapse. Hemorrhoids of grade 1, 2, or 3 are suitable for endoscopic treatment. Band ligation treatment is usually preceded with a Fleet enema. Thorough examination of the anorectum, including anoscopy and flexible sigmoidoscopy/colonoscopy is indicated for most patients with such symptoms.

Patients with external hemorrhoids, some patients with large grade 3 hemorrhoids, and those with grade 4 hemorrhoids are **not suitable** for endoscopic therapy. Caution is indicated in patients who are neutropenic or have compromised immune function. These patients may have a higher risk of impaired healing or septic complications.

1. Place the patient in the **Sims' position** (left lateral decubitus with right knee flexed).
2. Sedation is usually not necessary.
3. Mount the ligating device on the endoscope and pass the endoscope just beyond the dentate line. When using a "see through" ligator, the dentate line is easily visualized as it passes by.
4. Perform ligations 1 cm or more above the dentate line to avoid patient discomfort.
5. The direct approach (Fig. 55.1) is simplest and best tolerated by most patients.
    a. Identify the largest hemorrhoid.
    b. Aspirate it into the ligating cylinder using endoscopic suction, and release the rubber band to produce ligation.
    c. Single-fire instruments require that the endoscope be removed and a second band loaded. Multifire devices do not require this maneuver.
    d. Repeat the ligation for additional hemorrhoids. Up to three ligations are done at one sitting.
    e. Patients with a short anal canal, such as female patients, may be more easily approached with the endoscope retroflexed.
        i.   Insert the endoscope with the attached ligating device into the rectum.
        ii. Retroflex the endoscope within the rectum to visualize the region above the dentate line.
        iii. The cephalad view facilitates visualization and ligation when the anal canal is too short to permit a direct approach.
        iv. The retroflexed approach is best suited to endoscopic ligation done with a multifire device, which does not require

removal and reloading. From one to three ligations are
done at one sitting as described above.

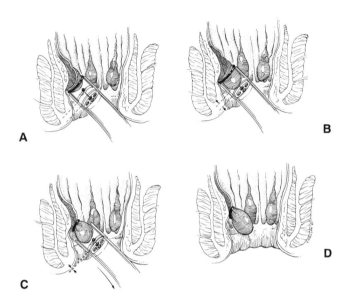

Figure 55.1. Endoscopic ligation of internal hemorrhoids. A. The endoscopist
positions the ligator in contact with the hemorrhoid about 1 cm above the dentate line. B. Endoscopic suction draws the hemorrhoid into the banding cylinder. C. The elastic "O" ring is ejected to ensnare the hemorrhoid. D. the ligated
hemorrhoid.

E. Complications of Colonoscopy

A sure way to compound any complication is to delay its recognition and
treatment. Inexperienced endoscopists are more likely to produce complications—including both technical and judgmental errors. At both the beginning
and end of each procedure, review any risks and unusual events specific to the
individual patient and procedure. For example, is the patient on antiplatelet
medications? Was there any undue difficulty experienced during the procedure?

Instruct the patient and/or guardian of the common presenting symptoms
and signs of complications that can follow an "uneventful" colonoscopy. These
generally include pain, bleeding, sensorium changes, nausea, and abdominal

distention. Any worrisome event should prompt urgent physician contact and an appropriate evaluation.

1. **Bleeding**

    a. **Cause and prevention:** Bleeding, the most common complication following colonoscopy, is usually a result of faulty hemostasis following biopsy. Resections of polyps >15 mm are at particular risk of continued or delayed bleeding. Rarely, bleeding can occur from trauma to hemorrhoidal veins, or from mucosal erosions caused by mechanical trauma. Very rarely, direct mechanical trauma results in splenic rupture. The best ways to prevent these injuries are to (1) anticipate potential problems, (2) correct coagulation disorders prior to <u>and</u> following any biopsy, (3) carefully inspect all biopsy sites minutes after manipulation, (4) not overmedicate the patient (to the state of being unable to report undue pain).

    b. **Recognition and management:** Do not aggressively pursue self-limited bleeding from biopsy sites, lest one risk perforation from the nonindicated use of excessive cautery. Less than 50% of biopsy sites will require additional cautery and/or the injection of 1:100,000 epinephrine. Delayed bleeding, which occurs between hours and 30 days following colonoscopy, requires immediate resuscitation, correction of any coagulation disorders, and, usually, repeat colonoscopy. As arterial embolization is largely contraindicated (the risk of perforation is already high), abdominal exploration must occur if bleeding sites cannot be promptly controlled. If, after replacing fluids and coagulation deficits, the patient has clearly and decidedly stopped bleeding, one may elect to omit repeat colonoscopy so as to minimize the risk of perforation at the biopsy site(s). Unaltered, fresh blood per rectum should raise the suspicion of hemorrhoidal bleeding. Bleeding hemorrhoids require immediate banding, or unusually, open hemorrhoidectomy. Clinical fluid losses and/or shock without an obvious source should raise the concern of an occult splenic rupture. Emergency ultrasound of the abdomen (as for trauma patients) is indicated, and any free fluid should prompt an immediate laparotomy.

2. **Perforation**

    a. **Causes and prevention:** The incidence of perforation following routine diagnostic colonoscopy is approximately 0.8%. This rate doubles following therapeutic procedures. Prior surgery, diverticulitis, or any cause of preexisting intra-abdominal adhesions increase the difficulty of the procedure and the enhance the possibility of a colon perforation. Causes include barotrauma from excessive insufflation, direct mechanical trauma from the scope or its instruments, and perforation from compromised biopsy sites. Oversedation can promote the creation of this deadly complication, i.e., a reasonably alert patient can complain of over-distention and mechanical scope trauma. The rate of perforation increases with the size of any resected lesion and the amount of cautery used. Large lesions should prompt the consideration of staged, partial resections. Miscellaneous causes of perforation include overzealous dilation of strictures, excessive laser ablation, and inappropriate use of biopsy instruments. Manipulations should occur under visual control at all times, and patience and caution are the foundations of any therapeutic procedure.

b. **Recognition and management:** If there has been any departure from a smooth and uneventful colonoscopy, it must be considered that a perforation might have occurred. This is particularly true when the patient complains of, or awakens with, unexpected discomfort. Escalating pain is a very worrisome sign, and should prompt urgent evaluation and abdominal radiographs. An elevated temperature, tachycardia, and/or a leukocytosis add to the specificity of diagnosis. Broad-spectrum antibiotics and fluid resuscitation should be considered at the first suspicion of perforation. Upright chest x-ray and left lateral decubitis films are the standards for detecting free intra-abdominal air. Computed tomography is more sensitive, but also more costly. Intraperitoneal air is absent in ~12% of perforations. Delayed recognition and gross soilage requires a diverting colostomy and washout of the abdomen (note: consider laparoscopy). Early suspicion and no free air on plain radiographs may be managed expectantly with broad-spectrum antibiotics in selected patients. Of note, patients who are "poor surgical candidates" are those who are least likely to survive continued fecal soilage. Whether employing laparoscopy, computed tomography (CT), or other means of diagnosis (e.g., contrast enemas if CT is not available), the decision tree should clearly anticipate what will be required with each finding. For example, if a "confined leak" will be treated expectantly, then computed tomography plays a role. Likewise, if the results of laparoscopic diagnosis or treatment are untrusted, one should not utilize laparoscopy for this situation!

3. **Infection**
   a. **Causes and prevention:** The transmission of infectious material from one patient to another via colonoscopic equipment is certainly possible, but also, fortunately, a rare event. Proper attention to scope preparation, especially the mechanical scrubbing of all ports and instruments, is essential. Even the most hearty spore or virus is reliably rendered harmless with standard soaking protocols. That colonoscopy can and does produce a transient bacteremia is well known. Antibiotic prophylaxis should be given to those with vascular prostheses or valvular abnormalities.
   b. **Recognition and management:** Delayed presentation of vague or confusing symptoms following colonoscopy should prompt a careful history, physical, and review of symptoms. Awareness of this possible iatrogenic complication will facilitate appropriate recognition and management.

4. **Missed diagnosis**
   a. **Causes and prevention:** A most serious "complication" is the failure to diagnose an existing condition that warrants prompt treatment. An inadequate bowel prep can certainly obscure significant colon and rectal neoplasia. The three anatomic "silent areas" of the colon are the cecum, the most distal rectum, and the splenic flexure. Even in experienced hands, the cecum is not adequately visualized in 5% to 10% of cases. Confirmation of reaching the cecum is verified using multiple criteria. Accuracy is nearly 100% when three of the following criteria are met: (1) transillumination of the cecum in the right lower abdomen, (2) convergence of the cecal haustra, (3) identification of the appendiceal lumen, (4) identification and/or cannulation of the terminal ileum, (5) exact recognition of the palpating hand in the right lower abdomen, or (6) the normal progression of intraluminal landmarks (e.g., hepatic flexure and capacious cecum). If doubt persists, fluoroscopy will confirm the exact location of the colonoscope. Careful attention to technique, with meticulous inspection of all potential blind spots including a retroflexed view of the anoderm junction, will minimize the chance of a missed lesion. If the preparation of the bowel is inadequate, thorough washing/irrigation of the retained feces is attempted via the colonoscope. If the visual inspection remains incomplete, then a second exam is indicated at a later date with a more vigorous preparation.

b. **Recognition and management:** Faulty judgment and pride can obscure the realization of an incomplete colonoscopy. Unless complications ensue, if a full diagnostic colonoscopy was initially indicated, then full screening must be accomplished. If necessary, repeat colonoscopy and/or double-contrast barium enema should be scheduled. Good relations and personal communication with radiology colleagues will often secure an "add-on" barium enema exam on the same day as the incomplete colonoscopy, thus sparing the patient a second bowel prep.

5. **Lost specimens**

   a. **Causes and prevention:** It can be difficult at times to retrieve biopsy specimens. This is particularly true for small polyps resected with the snare loop. Careful cleansing of surrounding feces <u>prior</u> to polypectomy, and optimal patient positioning (e.g., rolling the patient on his/her side, abdomen, or back) will prevent many frustrating situations.

   b. **Recognition and management:** If a specimen is not retrieved on initial attempts, a series of maneuvers can be employed. A suction trap is placed in-line. Careful removal of all debris and fecal material with suction is essential to recovering small lost specimens. Often, the small polyp, when found, can be immobilized at the suction port, and the scope removed while constant suction is applied. If the desired specimen is not found upon removal of the scope (following all due diligence), the suction trap is first completely inspected, and second, the suction port of the scope is probed. Next, it is recommended that the diagnostic colonoscopy be completely repeated. Finally, the patient is instructed in the use of a collection "seat" for the home toilet, and (s)he is encouraged to participate in the search by screening all fecal matter over the next 2 days. But clearly, the best hope of retrieving a lost specimen rests with the careful attempts of an experience endoscopist.

6. **Complications of endoscopic hemorrhoid ligation**

   a. **Pain**

      i. **Cause and prevention:** The most common complication of endoscopic ligation for hemorrhoid disease is pain. Severe pain immediately after ligation usually indicates that the site of ligation was too close to the dentate line.

      ii. **Recognition and management:** Recognition is usually easy. If severe pain occurs immediately following endoscopic ligation, an anoscope may be inserted and, using a pointed scissors, the elastic band divided and removed. Repeat endoscopic ligation may then be performed at a more cephalad site if the patient is willing.

b. **Bleeding:** Limited bleeding that occurs from 3 to 6 days after endoscopic ligation treatment is common and the patient should be advised to expect it. Occasionally, breakage or dislodgment of an elastic band in the first 24 to 48 hours following endoscopic ligation is associated with significant (more than 100 ml) bleeding, which may require repeat application of an elastic band or suture ligation via an anoscope to control. The latter complication is uncommon.

c. **Thrombosis of external hemorrhoids** occasionally occurs following band ligation of internal hemorrhoids. Most cases can be managed conservatively with sitz baths and analgesics.

d. **Pelvic sepsis**

   i. **Cause and prevention:** This <u>very</u> rare complication of band ligation has been reported most frequently in younger males and may be devastating. No specific preventative measures have been identified.

   ii. **Recognition and management:** The typical patient develops perineal pain, swelling, inability to urinate, and may have cellulitis, perineal ulceration, or gangrene on examination. These symptoms mandate admission to hospital, computed tomography of the pelvis to rule out other pathology, intravenous antibiotics, examination under anesthesia, and possibly perineal debridement and colostomy. This complication has been reported in a small number of cases over the past two decades. It is wise to inform patients of both the symptoms associated with this complication as well as its rarity as part of the informed consent.

F. Selected References

Ballantyne GH. Review of sigmoid volvulus: history and results of treatment. Dis Colon Rec 1982;25:494–501.

Ballantyne GH, Brandner MD, Beart RW Jr, Ilstrup DM. Volvulus of the colon: incidence and mortality. Ann Surg 1985;202:830–892.

Bat L, Melzer E, Koler M, Dreznick Z, Shemesh E. Complications of rubber band ligation of symptomatic internal hemorrhoids. Dis Colon Rectum 1993;36:287–90.

Branum GB, Fink AS. Ogilvie's syndrome. In Current Surgical Therapy, 6th ed. Cameron JL (ed.). St Louis: Mosby Year Book, 1997.

Brothers TE, Strodel WE, Eckhauser FE. Endoscopy in colonic volvulus. Ann Surg 1987; 206:1–4.

Corman ML. Hemorrhoids. In: Colon and Rectal Surgery. Philadelphia: Lippincott, 1993, pp. 54–116.

Geller A, Petersen BT, Gostout CJ. Endoscopic decompression for acute colonic pseudoobstruction. Gastrointest Endosc 1996;44:144–150.

Jetmore AB, Timmcke AE, Gathright JB, et al. Ogilvie's syndrome: colonoscopic decompression and analysis of predisposing factors. Dis Colon Rectum 1995;35:1135–1142.

Lau WY, Chow HP, Poon GP, Wong SH. Rubber band ligation of three primary hemorrhoids in a single session. A safe and effective procedure. Dis Colon Rectum 1982; 25:336–9.

MacRae HM, McLeod RS. Comparison of hemorrhoidal treatment modalities. A meta-analysis. Dis Colon Rectum 1995;38:687–94.

Rex DK. Colonoscopy and acute colonic pseudo-obstruction. Gastrointest Endosc Clin of North Am 1997;7(3):499–508.

Smith CD, Fink AS. The management of colonic volvulus. In: Current Surgical Therapy, 6th ed. Cameron JL (ed.). St Louis: Mosby Year Book, 1997.

56. Pediatric Gastrointestinal Endoscopy

Thom E. Lobe, M.D.

A. Pediatric Esophagoscopy

1. **Indications**
   a. **Diagnostic esophagoscopy** is performed for the evaluation of caustic ingestion, gastroesophageal reflux, and the diagnostic of specific inflammatory or infectious problems.
   b. **Foreign body removal** by esophagoscopy is indicated whenever the foreign body has been present for more than 48-hours and when it cannot be removed by simple means such as Foley catheter extraction or advancing the foreign body into the stomach with insertion of a bougie.
   c. Strictures due to caustic ingestion or gastroesophageal reflux may need **dilatation.**
   d. **Sclerotherapy of esophageal varices** is performed for control of hemorrhage in patients with portal hypertension.
2. The examination may be performed with either a rigid or a flexible esophagoscope. General anesthesia is commonly used.
   a. **Rigid esophagoscopy** must be done under endotracheal general anesthesia. The patient lies supine on the operating table with the anesthesiologist to the left of the patient's head.
   b. **Flexible esophagoscopy** can be done under general endotracheal anesthesia with the patient supine and either straight or turned with the anesthesiologist sitting to the side of the patient's head (whichever seems most comfortable or convenient).
3. **Rigid esophagoscopy**
   a. Place a roll under the patient's neck to extend the neck and make it easier to pass the rigid scope.
   b. Use a laryngoscope to lift the endotracheal tube anteriorly and to expose the pharyngeal opening so that the esophagoscope can be introduced under direct vision.

    c.   Take care to protect the patient during the introduction of the esophagoscope. Wrap the head with a towel to protect the face and eyes.

    d.   Introduce the esophagoscope with the right hand while using the left hand to guide the esophagoscope and to protect the lips, gums, and teeth.

    e.   Never advance the esophagoscope blindly. Advance the scope only under direct vision and with caution, only as far as necessary to visualize the lesion.

    f.   Use suction liberally to ensure adequate vision.

4. **Flexible esophagoscopy under general anesthesia**

    a.   Use a mouth guard of an appropriate size for the patient (although this may be less necessary in the anesthetized child).

    b.   Confirm that the end of the scope is free to move in all directions during its introduction.

    c.   Use the index finger of the dominant hand to elevate the patient's tongue and mandible.

    d.   Introduce the endoscope into the pharynx and just into the esophagus with the nondominant hand.

    e.   Advance the endoscope gently under direct inspection with gentle insufflation of air. Never advance the esophagoscope blindly.

5. **Flexible esophagoscopy under conscious sedation**

    a.   Sedation may consist of Demerol, 1 to 2 mg/kg and Versed 0.1 mg/kg administered intravenously or its equivalent.

    b.   Monitoring may consist of assessing heart rate, blood pressure, respiratory rate, and oxygen saturation (by pulse oximetry), every 5 minutes during the procedure and every 30 to 45 minutes during the recovery time.

    c.   Position the patient supine. Use the appropriate size of mouth guard to protect the endoscope.

    d.   Passage of the scope proceeds in the same manner described above.

6. **Special considerations**

    a.   **Diagnostic esophagoscopy:** inspect for mucosal abnormalities including hemangiomas and other vascular malformations, esophageal varices, esophagitis, or evidence of gastroesophageal reflux. If the child has ingested caustic material, do not advance the rigid esophagoscope beyond the first indication of injury. If a flexible scope is used, advance the scope through the injured esophagus with caution.

  i.   If biopsies are needed, use a cup biopsy forceps to take su-
       perficial bites.
  ii. Multiple biopsies should be taken for histology, cultures,
       and any special studies.
b. **Stricture**
  i.   Pass a balloon dilator (size depends upon age and size of
       child) through the stricture under direct vision until it is in
       the proper location. Introduce radiopaque contrast into the
       balloon and dilate the stricture under fluoroscopic and di-
       rect visual guidance. Steroid injections in conjunction with
       dilatation are favored by some and can be performed using
       a retractable sclerotherapy needle.
  ii. If the stricture is tight, it may be necessary to pass a string
       or a wire and create a gastrostomy. One end of the string is
       withdrawn through the nose and the other end through the
       gastrostomy. The two ends are tied and left in place. Dila-
       tors can then be passed serially to accomplish gradual
       dilatation.
c. **Foreign body removal**
  i.   **Coins:** Use an alligator or rat tooth grasper with teeth on
       the end of the instrument to catch the rim of the coin. Se-
       curely grasp the coin, edge on, and then remove the entire
       unit (scope, grasper, and coin) together.
  ii. **Sharp objects:** grasp the object by the blunt end and with-
       draw it, or maneuver the sharp end of the object into the
       lumen of a rigid esophagoscope and the scope, grasper, and
       object withdrawn as a unit.
d. **Variceal sclerotherapy** is performed in a manner similar to that
   used for adults.
  i.   Inject 1 to 3 cc of sclerosant into each varix at or just
       proximal to the esophagogastric junction.
  ii. Use a total of about 5 to 10 ml of sclerosant at each ses-
       sion.
  iii. Space sessions at 3- to 6-week intervals.
7. **Complications**
   a. **Perforation**
     i.   **Cause and prevention:** Rigid esophagoscopy beyond the
          cephalad margin of injury from caustic ingestion may re-
          sult in perforation. Minimize the risk by not advancing the
          rigid scope beyond the first recognition of injury. Forceful
          dilatation of an esophageal stricture or forceful removal of
          a foreign body that has been present for more that 48 hours

may result in perforation. The former can be prevented by not being too zealous in attempts at dilatation of tight strictures. The latter may not be preventable.

ii. **Recognition and management:** Blood at the site of injury or stricture should make one suspect of a perforation. A two-view chest x-ray should be taken to search for mediastinal air or pneumothorax. If these images are suspicious, then a contrast esophagram should be performed. Additional management of a perforation depends on the location. In most instances drainage will be required with or without repair of the perforation. A thoracoscopy or a thoracotomy may be required to accomplish this. Rarely, a gastrostomy and a cervical esophagostomy may be required to protect the area of injury. For perforation of the cervical esophagus, a cervical exploration with drainage may be necessary.

b. **Mucosal injury**

  i. **Cause and prevention:** Mucosal injury can occur from forceful dilatation, the removal of a foreign body, or the injection of esophageal varices. All of these maneuvers should be carried out by experienced endoscopists and with care to prevent their occurrence.

  ii. **Recognition and management:** When mucosal injury is apparent, radiographs should be taken to exclude the possibility of a perforation. If there is no perforation, then most of these injuries will heal without any specific therapy.

c. **Extra-esophageal injection of sclerotherapy solution**

  i. **Cause and prevention:** When sclerotherapy is performed, the possibility exists of injecting the solution outside the esophagus, rather than intra- or paravariceal.

  ii. **Recognition and management:** Failure to do a proper injection is immediately apparent. Either the varices blanch or the paravariceal esophageal mucosa swells and blanches to indicate a proper injection. If neither of these occurs, one should be suspicious of a transmural injection and a two-view chest x-ray should be obtained to exclude perforation. In most instances, nothing need be done except observation.

B. Gastroduodenoscopy

1. **Indications**
   a. **Diagnostic gastroduodenoscopy** is indicated for the assessment of inflammatory conditions and suspected gastritis or peptic ulcer disease. Biopsy may be required for diagnosis of *H. pylori* or other infections.
   b. **Foreign bodies** such as coins or sharp objects such as pins or needles often need to be removed using endoscopic snares or graspers.
   c. **Hemorrhage** from the stomach and duodenum can best be assessed by endoscopy.
   d. Assessment of an upper gastrointestinal **mass** can be made by inspection and biopsy depending on the nature of the mass.
   e. **Percutaneous endoscopic gastrostomy (PEG)** tube placement is a useful alternative to open gastrostomy.
2. The examination may be performed under general anesthesia using the same patient position and room setup described above, or may be performed under conscious sedation with appropriate monitoring. In this case, the patient is often placed in a lateral position starting with the left side down.
3. The initial part of the examination proceeds as described for flexible esophagoscopy, above.
4. Upon entering the stomach, retroflex the endoscope to inspect the cardia of the stomach and the gastric side of the gastroesophageal junction.
5. Next, thoroughly inspect the body of the stomach, including the greater and lesser curvature.
6. In the small infant and child, the pylorus is quite high, at about at the level of the gastroesophageal junction. The best way to find this structure is by retroflexing the endoscope and maneuvering the scope back and forth on either side of the incisura.
7. With the pylorus in view, advance the endoscope toward the pyloric opening and into the duodenum.
8. **Special considerations:**
   a. Common causes of upper gastrointestinal bleeding are listed in Table 56.1. When gastritis is found, biopsy to evaluate for *H. pylori*.
   b. Most patients who are scoped for evaluation of pain will prove to have gastritis. Biopsy should be taken to evaluate for *H. pylori*.

Table 56.1. Causes of upper gastrointestinal bleeding in children

- Gastric varices
- Peptic ulcer disease
- Vascular malformations (rare)
- Mallory-Weiss tears (rare)
- Tumors (uncommon)
- Gastritis (common)

9. Removal of foreign bodies from the stomach
    a. Coins may sit in the stomach for prolonged periods and often are adherent if they are multiple.
    b. Use forceps with teeth on the end. This allows the grasper to gain a firm grip on the raised edge of the coin.
    c. Remove sharp foreign bodies blunt end first, to avoid injuring the esophagus on the way out.
10. Percutaneous gastrostomy placement
    a. The techniques are essentially the same as those used in adults.
    b. Take care to avoid injury to colon or small intestine, and consider using laparoscopic visualization to minimize the danger of injury to adjacent viscera.
11. Complications
    a. The complications of **diagnostic gastroduodenoscopy** in children are the same as in adults
    b. **Extragastric placement of PEGs**
        i. **Cause and prevention:** PEG tubes can be placed erroneously in the adjacent colon or small bowel. Minimize the risk by considering alternate techniques in patients with previous abdominal surgery, peritonitis, or tumors. Carefully distend the stomach and choose the site of the PEG tube carefully. When the stomach is distended and illuminated, look for a transverse shadow across the upper abdomen (which may represent a loop of small bowel or colon between the stomach and the abdominal wall). Avoid this problem completely by using a laparoscopic assisted technique.
        ii. **Recognition and management:** This complication may not be recognized immediately. Local peritonitis may develop leading one to suspect the possibility. When gastrostomy feedings result in severe abdominal cramping (with small bowel placement) or diarrhea (colon placement), perform a contrast study to document the position of

the tube. If the complication is discovered late, then all that may be necessary is to remove the tube and allow the tract to seal itself. If the complication is discovered early or if the contrast study suggests intraperitoneal extravasation, then a laparotomy may be required for repair of the injured bowel

C. Sigmoidoscopy

1. **Pediatric sigmoidoscopy** can be used to assess bleeding or a suspected mass in the sigmoid colon. Just as with adults, biopsy or excision of polypoid masses can be performed.

2. In young children, sigmoidoscopy is often performed under general endotracheal anesthesia. Position the patient either in the lateral flexed position with the buttocks over the side of the table, or in the lithotomy position. Conscious sedation may be used in older children. In some children, it may be feasible to perform flexible sigmoidoscopy in the office without sedation.

3. A pediatric Fleets enema or its equivalent should be given to the child before sigmoidoscopy.

4. First introduce a finger into the anus to dilate it and to assess whether there exist any obstructing lesions.

5. **Rigid sigmoidoscopy:** having established that the anus and distal rectum are clear of obstruction, introduce the sigmoidoscope with obturator into the anus. Remove the obturator, close the observation window, and gently introduce sufficient air into the rectum to visualize the lumen. Advance the scope in the direction of the lumen under direct vision. Never force the scope blindly. Inspect the mucosal surface through its entire circumference as the scope is withdrawn.

6. **Flexible sigmoidoscopy** (see colonoscopy, below).

7. During sigmoidoscopy, search for fissures, arteriovenous malformations, foreign bodies, signs of trauma, or mass lesions. **Always remember the possibility of child abuse.**

D. Colonoscopy

1. **Indications:** as with adult patients, colonoscopy is performed for evaluation of suspected infectious or inflammatory colitis, bleeding, or mass lesion above the range of the flexible sigmoidoscope.

2. **Bowel preparation:** A bowel prep consisting of clear liquids the evening before (2 days in older children), and a cathartic the day before works well. Alternatively (although most children do not tolerate the volume well), Go-Lytely (Braintree Laboratories, Inc., Braintree, MA) can be administered by mouth in a dose of 4 cc/kg/hour for four hours the day preceding the examination, to be accompanied by a clear liquid diet to follow. The patient should be NPO for the examination.

3. First introduce a finger into the rectum to be certain that no obstructing lesions are present.

4. Next, insert the colonoscope and advance in the direction of the lumen. The general technique is similar to that used in adults (see Chapter 56).

5. It may be helpful to have an assistant hold the scope at the anus and advance the scope as necessary while the endoscopist manipulates the scope.

6. Redirect the scope by palpating the patient's abdomen, or by repositioning the patient as necessary. Sometimes it is useful to jiggle the endoscope to aid in its advancement into the colon.

7. Occasionally, the endoscope will be difficult to advance, or remain in the same location despite insertion of significant additional length of scope. The scope may have formed a loop or the bowel may have telescoped on itself. Withdraw the body of the scope until the end of the scope retracts. It should then be possible to continue to advance the scope. Advance the colonoscope to the cecum, and inspect 360° of the mucosal circumference for each length of bowel as the scope is withdrawn.

8. **Biopsy** is best performed with a cup biopsy forceps to minimize tissue destruction. It may be advisable to send specimens for cultures or special studies in addition to routine histology.

9. Before performing **polypectomy**, carefully assess the nature of the polyp. Pedunculated polyps may be removed by snare with electrocautery. Sessile polyps may be biopsied for histology, but removal may require operative resection.

10. **Sigmoid volvulus** may sometimes be reduced endoscopically (sigmoidoscope or colonoscope).

    a. Suspect the diagnosis from clinical presentation and abdominal x-rays, especially in mentally impaired patients or those with chronic constipation.

    b. If the passage of the sigmoidoscope fails to reduce the volvulus, flexible colonoscopy or operative reduction may be required.

11. **Severe constipation** occurs in some pediatric patients. Mechanical disimpaction under anesthesia may be required. This is particularly likely in the mentally impaired, in patients with undiagnosed Hirschsprung's disease, or following corrective surgery for Hirschsprung's disease or imperforate anus. Digital disimpaction accompanied by irrigation may be necessary to make room for the sigmoidoscope, which is of limited use in the evaluation of this problem.

12. The **complications** of pediatric colonoscopy include bleeding and perforation. Prevention, recognition, and management are similar to the adult.

Appendix: SAGES Publications

SAGES issues and periodically revises **guidelines, statements, and standards** on a variety of subjects related to endoscopy, laparoscopy, and education. **Patient education information** brochures are also available for selected laparoscopic procedures. A list of materials available at press time for this manual is given below. Documents may be viewed or downloaded from the World Wide Web at **www.sages.org**. They are also available from:

Society of American Gastrointestinal Endoscopic Surgeons
2716 Ocean Park Blvd., Suite 3000
Santa Monica, CA 90405
Phone: (310) 314-2404
FAX: (310) 314-2585
email: SAGESMail@aol.com

A. SAGES Guidelines, Statements, and Standards

1. Statement on Concentration in General Surgery Residency
2. Position Statement on Advanced Laparoscopic Training
3. Integrating Advanced Laparoscopy into Surgical Residency Training
4. Video Production Guidelines
5. Guidelines for the Surgical Practice of Telemedicine
6. Statement on First Assistants
7. Global Statement on New Procedures
8. Granting of Ultrasonography Privileges for Surgeons
9. Guidelines for Laparoscopic Surgery During Pregnancy
10. Guidelines for Diagnostic Laparoscopy, Clinical Application
11. Guidelines for the Clinical Application of Laparoscopic Biliary Tract Surgery
12. Guidelines for Surgical Treatment of Gastroesophageal Reflux Disease (GERD)
13. Statement on Policy, Laparoscopic Appendectomy
14. Guidelines for Collaborative Practice in Endoscopic/Thoracoscopic Spinal Surgery for the General Surgeon
15. Guidelines for Granting of Privileges for Laparoscopic and/or Thoracoscopic General Surgery
16. Framework for Post-Residency Surgical Education and Training

17. Granting of Privileges for Gastrointestinal Endoscopy by Surgeons
18. Summary Statement on Surgical Endoscopic Training and Practice
19. Guidelines for Office Endoscopic Services
20. Guidelines for General Surgery Resident Education in Gastrointestinal Endoscopy
21. Guidelines for Training in Diagnostic and Therapeutic Endoscopic Retrograde Cholangiopancreatography (ERCP)

B. Patient Information Brochures

1. Laparoscopic Gallbladder Removal
2. Laparoscopic Anti-Reflux Surgery (GERD)
3. Laparoscopic Colon Resection
4. Laparoscopic Hernia Repair

C. SAGES Laparoscopic Equipment Troubleshooting Guide

This is a laminated single-sheet guide suitable for attachment to a laparoscopic video cart.

Index

Abdomen, access to, 22–35
    pediatric, 387–388
Abdomen puncture sites, 29
Abdominal pain, 110–111
    diagnostic laparoscopy for, 111–112
Abdominal surgery, previous,
    laparoscopy in, 104–108
Abdominal tumors, laparoscopic
    staging of, 115
Abdominal wall, bleeding from, 33–34
Abdominal wall crepitus, 399
Abdominal wall hemorrhage, 399
Abdominal wall lift devices, 43–50
    planar, 46
    technique for, 47–50
    types of, 43–47
Abdominoperineal resection, *see also*
    Segmental colectomies, anterior
    resection, and abdominoperineal
    resection, laparoscopic
    performing, 296–297
Abscess
    intra-abdominal, 110
    subphrenic, 334
    at surgical site, 192
Acalculous cholecystitis, 110
    acute, 128
Achalasia, 213
Acid–base balance, 39
Adenocarcinomas of pancreas, 126
Adhesion lysis, 106
Adhesions, managing, with previous
    abdominal surgery, 105–106
Adrenalectomy, laparoscopic, 353–362
    complications of, 362
    indications and choice of operative
        approach for, 353–354
    retroperitoneal, 360–362
    transabdominal, 354–360
Air embolism, 37
Ampulla of Vater, 483
Anastomosis, 79–80
Anastomotic leak, 262–263
Anastomotic strictures, 263–264
    dilatation of, 544
Anesthesia
    monitoring and, 15–20
    topical, 423

Anesthetic, choice of, 16–17
Angled lens laparoscope, 106
Anorectal trauma, 546
Antecolic loop
    cholecystojejunostomy,
        performing, 317–319
Anterior resection, *see also* Segmental
    colectomies, anterior resection,
    and abdominoperineal resection,
    laparoscopic
    performing, 296
Antibiotic prophylaxis for endoscopic
    procedures, 472
Appendectomy, laparoscopic, 275–280
    complications of, 279–280
    incomplete, 280
    indications for, 275
    patient positioning and room setup
        for, 275
    pediatric complications of, 400
    performing, 276–279
    trocar position and choice of
        laparoscope for, 275–276
Appendicitis, acute, in pregnancy, 98–99
Argon, 40–41
Argon beam coagulator, 64
Argon plasma coagulator, 455
Arm position, patient, 13
Arterial air embolism, 37
Ascending colon, 557–558
Aspiration cytology, fine-needle, 436
Aspirin, 472

Babcock clamp, 208
Balloon dissection, 54–55
Balloon stone extraction, 510
Balloon techniques, 171
Bare fiber systems, 66
Bariatric surgery, laparoscopic, 247–252
    vertical banded gastroplasty
        technique, 247–250
    vertical Roux–en–Y gastric bypass
        technique, 250–252
Basket stone removal, 510
Basket techniques, 171–173
BICAP (bipolar circumactive probe),
    452
Bile duct cannulation, 504

Bile duct injury
    after laparoscopic cholecystectomy,
        141
    management of, 188–191
Bile leakage, 188, 191–192
    as complication of choledo-
        choscopy, 530–531
Biliary balloon catheter, 181
Biliary sphincterotomy, 508–509
Biliary stenting, 512–513
Biliary tract disease, 99
Biliary tract stone removal, 510–511
Biliary tree, definition and drainage
    of, 190
Billroth gastrectomies, 241–242
Billroth II anastomoses, 496–499
Biopsy, 116
    colonoscopic, 559
Biopsy forceps, 541
Biopsy techniques, 434–436
    cholangioscope, 528
Bipolar circumactive probe (BICAP),
    452
Bipolar electrosurgery, 59
Blade configuration, 64–65
Bleeding, *see also* Hemorrhage
    from abdominal wall, 33–34
    in Calot's triangle, 137
    as complication of choledo-
        choscopy, 531
    as complication of colonoscopy,
        571
    control of, 544
    diffuse, from peritoneal biopsy site,
        349–350
    from liver biopsy, 350
    with previous abdominal surgery,
        107
    from trocar site, 34
    upper gastrointestinal, nonvariceal,
        see Nonvariceal upper
        gastrointestinal bleeding
    variceal, sclerotherapy of, *see*
        Sclerotherapy of variceal
        bleeding
Bleeding diatheses, medications
    causing, 472
Blunt trauma, 112
Body mass index, 94
Botulinum toxin injection, 213
Bowel injury, remote, 399–400
Bowel preparation, 552–553
Bowel trauma, 305
Bradycardia, 471
Bronchus intubations, main stem, 19
Brush cytology, 434–435

Brush cytology technique,
    cholangioscope, 528
Bupivacaine, 20
Buried bumper syndrome, 477–478

Calculous biliary tract disease, 128
Calot's triangle, 133
    bleeding in, 137
Cancer staging
    elective diagnostic laparoscopy
        and, 115–127
    pediatric, diagnostic laparoscopy
        and, 396
    pediatric complications of, 405–
        406
Cannulation
    cholangiopancreatography and,
        502–507
    multiple attempts at, 507
Capacitive coupling, 63–64
Carbon dioxide (CO), 38–39
    advantages of, 38, 41
    disadvantages of, 38–39, 41
    increased, 38–39
Carbon dioxide cylinders, 5–6
Carbon dioxide embolism, 18
Carcinoma
    esophageal, 118–121
    of gallbladder, 139–140
    pancreatic, 122–123
Cardia, 431
Cardiac depression, 41
Cardiomyotomy, laparoscopic, 213–
    220
    complications of, 219–220
    diagnostic workup for, 213
    indications and patient preparation
        for, 213–214
    myotomy in, 216–218
    patient positioning and room setup
        for, 214
    performing, 215–219
    trocar position and choice of
        laparoscope for, 215
Cardiopulmonary complications of
    upper gastrointestinal
    endoscopy, 471–472
Cardiopulmonary function,
    deteriorating, 18
Catheter, dislodgment of, 273
Cautery tool, 106
CCD (charge–coupled device), 88
Cecal volvulus, 567
Cecum, 557–558
Celiac axis, nodes in, 127
Celiac disease, 480

Charge-coupled device (CCD), 88
Checklist, equipment, 1–3
Cholangiocatheters, 152
Cholangiogram, 143–147
Cholangiography
  alternative methods of, 159
  cystic duct, 151–156
  routine intraoperative (RIOC),
      143–160
Cholangiograsper, 144
Cholangiopancreatography,
    cannulation and, 502–507
Cholangioscopy, peroral, 526–527
Cholangitis, 194
  as complication of ERCP, 518
Cholecystectomy, laparoscopic, 128–
    136
  avoiding complications during,
      137–141
  complications of, 188–194
  indications for, 128–129
  patient preparation, position and
      room setup for, 129–130
  pediatric, complications of, 401
  performing, 132–136
  in small operating room, 5
  trocar position and choice of
      laparoscope for, 130–132
  ultrasound and Doppler for, 162–
      165
Cholecystitis acalculous, see
    Acalculous cholecystitis
  acute, 128
Cholecystocholangiography, 159, 160
Cholecystojejunostomy, performing,
    317–319
Cholecystojejunostomy and
    gastrojejunostomy, laparoscopic,
    314–324
  complications of, 322–324
  indications for, 314
  leakage of, 322–323
  patient positioning and room setup
      for, 314–315
  trocar position and choice of
      laparoscope for, 315– 316
Choledochoduodenostomy, 499–500
Choledochojejunostomy, 500
Choledochoscope, damaging, 533
Choledochoscopic techniques, 173–
    175
Choledochoscopy
  completion check, 181
  complications of, 530–533
  diagnostic, see Diagnostic
    choledochoscopy

postoperative, 525–528
  therapeutic, 529–530
  transhepatic, 528
Choledochotomy, laparoscopic
  closure of, 181–185
  common bile duct exploration via,
      178–187
  complications of, 193–194
  indications and patient preparation
      for, 178
  patient position and room setup for,
      179
  performing, 179–180
  postoperative management for,
      186–187
  stone extraction through, 180
  trocar position and choice of
      laparoscope for, 179
Cholelithiasis, symptomatic, 128
Chromoscopy, 436
Chylous ascites, 350
Clip appliers, endoscopic, 57
"Closed" technique with Veress
    needle, 24–30
CO, see Carbon dioxide
Coagulating current, 60
Coagulation, 61
Colitis, glutaraldehyde-induced, 549
Colonoscopic biopsies, 559
Colonoscopy
  complications of, 570–575
  decompressive, see Decompressive
    colonoscopy
  diagnostic, see Diagnostic
    colonoscopy
  pediatric, 584–585
  therapeutic, 565–570
Color Doppler, 162
Colostomy, laparoscopic, 281–285
  complications of, 284–285
  indications for, 281
  patient positioning and room setup
      for, 281
  technique of, 283–284
  trocar position and choice of
      laparoscope for, 282
Common bile duct, 163, 164
  free cannulation of, 504
  stricture of, 532–533
Common bile duct exploration,
    laparoscopic (LCDE)
  complications of, 188–194
  indications, contraindications, and
      choice of approach, 167–168

Common bile duct exploration, laparoscopic (LCDE) (*cont.*)
  patient positioning, equipment needed, and room setup for, 168–169
  preparation for, 170
  techniques for, 171–176
  transcystic duct approach, 167–176
  trocar position and choice of laparoscope and choledochoscope for, 169–170
  via laparoscopic choledochotomy, 178–187
Common bile duct injury, 192–193
Completion check choledochoscopy, 181
Completion fluorocholangiogram, 186
Complications
  avoiding, recognizing, and managing, 33–35
  with previous abdominal surgery, 107
Connections on rear panel, 7
Conscious sedation of patients, 419–420
Constipation, severe, 585
Contact-type fibers, 66
Continuous suturing, 79
Contralateral groin exploration during herniorrhaphy, 397
Control panel, fluoroscopy, close-up view of, 150
Crohn's disease, 480
Crural closure, 205–206
Crural dissection, 202–204
Current density, 60–61
Cuschieri transcystic biliary decompression set, 182
Cutting current, 60
Cyanoacrylate, 445
Cystic duct, 143
Cystic duct cholangiography, 151–156
Cytology, 434
  brush, 434–435
  fine-needle aspiration, 436

Danger signs, radiographic, 157–158
Decompression by T-tube, 185
Decompressive colonoscopy
  for Ogilvie's syndrome, 565–567
  for sigmoid volvulus, 567–568
Delayed gastric emptying, 232
Dentures, dislodgment of, 475

Descending colon, 557
Desiccation, 61
Diagnostic choledochoscopy, 523–528
  intraoperative, 523–525
Diagnostic colonoscopy, 551–563
  general principles of, 555–556
  indications for, 551–552
  patient positioning and room setup for, 552–554
  performing, 556–558
Diagnostic laparoscopy, 109, 115–117
  for abdominal pain, 111–112
  elective, cancer staging and, 115–127
  indications for, 115–116
  pediatric cancer staging and, 396
  technique of, 116–117
  for trauma, 112–114
Diagnostic upper gastrointestinal endoscopy, 422–436
  indications for, 422
  patient preparation for, 423
  performance of, 423–432
Diathermy snare, 457
Digital fluorocholangiography, 165
Digital recording, 90–91
Dilatation, 458–459
  of anastomotic strictures, 544
  of strictures, 476
Dipyridamole (Persantine), 473
Direct coupling effect, 63
Dissection, circumferential, of esophagus, 204–205
Distal pancreatectomy, 307–313
  complications of, 312–313
  indications for, 307
  initial dissection and mobilization of pancreas for, 309
  patient positioning and room setup for, 307
  performing, 307, 309–311
  with splenic salvage, 311
  trocar position and choice of laparoscope for, 308
Dither-torquing, intubation by, 539–541
Documentation, 88–92
  of findings with endoscopes, 418
Doppler
  Color, 162
  for laparoscopic cholecystectomy, 162–165
Dor procedure, 219
Dulocq technique, 53–54

Duodenal bulb, 429
Duodenal diverticula, 506
Duodenoscope, 497
Dysphagia, 219–220

EES (extraperitoneal endoscopic
    surgery), 52
EGD (esophagogastroduodenoscopy),
    see Diagnostic upper
    gastrointestinal endoscopy
Electrocautery, avoiding, 541
Electrosurgery, 59–64
    monopolar, see Monopolar
        electrosurgery
Emergency laparoscopy, 109–114
Endocarditis, 471–472
Endoluminal gastric resections, 237–
    240
Endoluminal gastric surgery, 457–458
Endoscopes
    documentation of findings with,
        418
    flexible, see Flexible endoscopes
    handling, 415–418
    manipulation of, 415–417
    room setup for, 415
Endoscopic band ligation treatment of
    internal hemorrhoids, 569–570
Endoscopic clip appliers, 57
Endoscopic drainage of pancreatic
    pseudocysts, 514
Endoscopic foreign body removal,
    460–461
Endoscopic gastrostomy,
    percutaneous, see Percutaneous
    endoscopic gastrostomy
Endoscopic hemorrhoid ligation,
    complications of, 574–575
Endoscopic mucosal resection, 435
Endoscopic palliation, 459–460
Endoscopic placement of jejunal
    feeding tubes, 468
Endoscopic polypectomy, 457–458
Endoscopic procedures, antibiotic
    prophylaxis for, 472
Endoscopic retrograde
    cholangiopancreatography
    (ERCP), 140, 485–494
    complications of, 516–521
    facilities and equipment for, 489–
        490
    indications for, 485–488
    patient preparation for, 491
    performing, 491–494
    therapeutic, 508–514
Endoscopic ultrasound (EUS), 436

rectal, 560–563
Endoscopic variceal band ligation, see
    Variceal band ligation,
    endoscopic
Endoscopy
    diagnostic upper gastrointestinal,
        see Diagnostic upper
        gastrointestinal endoscopy
    gastrointestinal, pediatric, 577–585
    of postoperative stomach, 432–434
    with surgically altered anatomy,
        496–500
    upper gastrointestinal, see Upper
        gastrointestinal endoscopy
Endotracheal intubation, 438
Endotracheal (ET) tube, 16
End-to-end anastomosis, 79–80
Energy induced hemostasis, 58–59
Energy sources used in hemostasis,
    59–67
Enteroenterostomy, see also Small
    bowel resection, enterolysis, and
    enteroenterostomy
    technique of, 261
Enterolysis, see also Small bowel
    resection, enterolysis, and
    enteroenterostomy
    technique of, 260–261
Enteroscopy, small bowel, see Small
    bowel enteroscopy
Enterotomy, inadvertent, 266
Epinephrine injection, 453–455
Epistaxis, 483
Equipment checklist, 1–3
Equipment position, laparoscopic, 1–3
Equipment setup, laparoscopic, 3–8
ERCP, see Endoscopic retrograde
    cholangiopancreatography
Esophageal carcinoma, 118–121
Esophageal hiatus, approach to, 119
Esophageal opening, 424
Esophageal perforation, 231–232, 474
Esophageal sphincter, lower, 426
Esophageal stents, 476
Esophagitis, 477
Esophagogastroduodenoscopy (EGD),
    see Diagnostic upper
    gastrointestinal endoscopy
Esophagoscopy, pediatric, 577–580
Esophagus, circumferential dissection
    of, 204–205
Ethanolamine oleate, 443
Ethanol injection, 453–455
ET (endotracheal) tube, 16
EUS, see Endoscopic ultrasound
Extracorporeal knot, 78

Extracorporeal tying, 73
Extraperitoneal endoscopic surgery
    (EES), 52
Extraperitoneal exposure, 49–50
Extraperitoneal space, 52–56
    access to, 53–54
    anatomic considerations, 53
    dissection of, 54–55
    maintenance of, 55
    potential problems in, 56
Eye–hand coordination, 71

Falciform lift device, 43–44
Fecalith, lost, 400
Feedings, leakage of, 478
Feeding tube placement, percutaneous
    endoscopic, 462–468
Feeding tubes, jejunal, endoscopic
    placement of, 468
Feldene (Piroxicam), 472
Fetal monitoring, intraoperative, 101–
    102
Fever of unknown origin, 111
Fiberoptic endoscopes, 407–408
Fine-needle aspiration cytology, 436
Fire prevention, 17
Fitz–Hughes–Curtis syndrome, 110
Flaccid sphincter, 154
Flexible endoscopes
    care of, 413
    characteristics of, 407–409
    equipment setup for, 410–412
    troubleshooting, 412–413
Flexible sigmoidoscopy, 534–541
    approaches to, 537–541
    complications of, 541, 545–549
    indications for, 534
    patient preparation for, 535
    technique of, 535–541
    therapeutic, 543–549
Flumazenil, 420–421, 474
Fluorocholangiogram, completion,
    186
Fluorocholangiography, digital, 165
Fluoroscopy, 148–149
Forceps biopsy, 435
Foreign body removal, 545
    endoscopic, 460–461
    pediatric, 579
Fragmentation, specimen, 86
Fulguration, 63
Fundic mobilization, 206
Fundoplication, laparoscopic, 196
    complications of, 211–212
    indications and preoperative
        evaluation of, 196–198

Nissen, technique of, 202–209
partial, 210
patient position and room setup for,
    198–199
pediatric complications of, 402–
    403
postoperative considerations for,
    211
short and loose, creating, 206–209
trocar position and principles of
    exposure for, 199–201

Gallbladder, carcinoma of, 139–140
Gallbladder problems, during
    laparoscopic cholecystectomy,
    138–140
Gallstone pancreatitis, 129
Gallstones, 99
Gasless lift devices, 45
Gastrectomies
    Billroth, 241–242
    distal partial, laparoscopic,
        241–242
Gastric bypass, vertical roux–en–Y,
    laparoscopic, 250–252
Gastric cancers, 121, 236
Gastric cannula, Innerdyne, 239
Gastric emptying, delayed, 232
Gastric lymphoma, 236
Gastric perforation, 226, 231–232
Gastric resections, 236–246
    approaches to, 236–237
    complications of, 245–246
    endoluminal, 237–240
    indications for, 236
    laparoscopic, 240–245
    patient positioning and room setup
        for, 237
Gastric surgery, endoluminal, 457–
    458
Gastrocolic fistula, 478
Gastroduodenoscopy, pediatric, 581–
    583
Gastroesophageal reflux, laparoscopic
    treatment of, 196–212
Gastroesophageal reflux disease, 197
Gastrohepatic omentum, 120, 121
Gastrointestinal endoscopy, pediatric,
    577–585
Gastrojejunostomy, see also
    Cholecystojejunostomy and
    gastrojejunostomy, laparoscopic
    leakage of, 323
    performing, 319–322

Gastroplasty, vertical banded, laparoscopic, technique of, 247–250

Gastrostomy, laparoscopic, 221–226
cannula position and choice of laparoscope for, 221–222
complications of, 225–226
indications for, 221
leakage of, 225–226
with mucosa-lined tube, 224–225
patient positioning and room setup for, 221
performing, 222–225
percutaneous endoscopic, see Percutaneous endoscopic gastrostomy

General anesthesia, 16
Gluing, tissue, 80
Glutaraldehyde-induced colitis, 549
Gold probe, 452
Grading system for hemoperitoneum, 113
Groin exploration during herniorrhaphy contralateral, 397
Guidelines, statements, and standards, SAGES, 586–587
Gunshot wounds, 113

Hashimoto's subcutaneous lift method, 45
Hasson cannula, 23
"open" technique with, 31–33
Heater probe, 450–452
Helium, 40, 41
Heller myotomy, see Cardiomyotomy, laparoscopic
Hematomas, 35
Hemicolectomy, laparoscopic-assisted
left, 290–295
right, 287–290
Hemoclips, 455
Hemoperitoneum, grading system for, 113
Hemorrhage, see also Bleeding
abdominal wall, 399
as complication of ERCP, 519–520
intra-abdominal, 265
during laparoscopic cholecystectomy, 137–138
management of, 67–68
Hemorrhoid ligation, endoscopic, complications of, 574–575
Hemorrhoids, internal, endoscopic band ligation treatment of, 569–570

Hemostasis, laparoscopic, 57–68
energy induced, 58–59
energy sources used in, 59–67
mechanical methods of, 57–58
Hepatic flexure, 557
Hepatic tumors, 121
Hepatocellular cancer, 121–122
Hepatoduodenal ligament, nodes in, 127
Hernia, recurrence of, 377
Hernia repair, 104, 379–385
Herniorrhaphy, contralateral groin exploration during, 397
Hiatal dissection, 216
Hiatal hernia, laparoscopic treatment of, 196–212
Hodgkin's disease, 123–124
laparoscopic staging for, 344–345
Hopkins rod lens system, 88
Hydrostatic balloons, 459
Hyperamylasemia, 516
Hypercapnia, 18
Hypertension, 18
Hypotension, 471
Hypoxemia, 471
Hypoxia, 18

Ileal-pouch–anal anastomosis, laparoscopic-assisted proctocolectomy with, see Proctocolectomy with ileal-pouch–anal anastomosis, laparoscopic- assisted
Ileocecal valve, 557–558
Ileocolic resection, laparoscopic-assisted, 287–290
Ileus, postoperative, 264–265
Iliac dissection, 346–349
Infection as complication
of colonoscopy, 573
of upper gastrointestinal endoscopy, 473
Inguinal hernia repair, laparoscopic, 364–377
complications of, 374–377
indications for, 364
patient positioning and room setup for, 365
totally extraperitoneal approach, 372–374
transabdominal preperitoneal approach, 365–372
Injection therapy, 453–455
Innerdyne gastric cannula, 239
Instrumentation, laparoscopic, 2

Instrument considerations with
   previous abdominal surgery, 106
Instruments, laparoscopic, 2
Insufflating agent
   choice of, 37–38
   ideal, 37
Insufflator, 22–24
Insufflator testing, 22, 23
Insulation failure, 63
Internal hemorrhoids, endoscopic
   band ligation treatment of, 569–
      570
Interrupted suturing, 79
Intestinal loop, malrotation of, 285
Intra-abdominal abscess, 110
Intra-abdominal hemorrhage, 265
Intracorporeal knots, 73
Intracorporeal knot tying, 69–71
Intrahepatic stones, 511
Intraoperative considerations, 18–19
Intraoperative diagnostic
   choledochoscopy, 523–525
Intraoperative enteroscopy, 482
Intraoperative fetal monitoring, 101–
   102
Intraperitoneal exposure, 47–49, 50
Intravariceal injection, 444–446
Intubation, endotracheal, 438
Irrigation techniques, 171

Jejunal feeding tubes, endoscopic
   placement of, 468
Jejunostomy, complications of, 477–
   479
Jejunostomy tube placement, 267–273
   complications of, 272–273
   indications for, 267
   patient positioning and room setup
      for, 267
   technique of, 268–272
   trocar position and choice of
      laparoscope for, 267–268

Ketoralac, 20
Knot-tying, 73–78
   intracorporeal, 69–71

Laparoscopic adrenalectomy, see
   Adrenalectomy, laparoscopic
Laparoscopic antegrade
   sphincterotomy, 175–176
Laparoscopic-assisted ileocolic
   resection, 287–290
Laparoscopic-assisted left
   hemicolectomy, 290–295

Laparoscopic-assisted
   proctocolectomy with ileal-
   pouch–anal anastomosis, see
   Proctocolectomy with ileal-
   pouch–anal anastomosis,
   laparoscopic-assisted
Laparoscopic-assisted sigmoid colon
   resection, 290–295
Laparoscopic bariatric surgery, see
   Bariatric surgery, laparoscopic
Laparoscopic cardiomyotomy, see
   Cardiomyotomy, laparoscopic
Laparoscopic cholecystectomy, see
   Cholecystectomy, laparoscopic
Laparoscopic choledochotomy, see
   Choledochotomy, laparoscopic
Laparoscopic colostomy, see
   colostomy, laparoscopic
Laparoscopic common bile duct
   exploration, see Common bile
   duct exploration, laparoscopic
Laparoscopic distal partial
   gastrectomy, 241–242
Laparoscopic equipment position, 1–3
Laparoscopic equipment setup, 3–8
Laparoscopic equipment
   troubleshooting guide, SAGES,
   587
Laparoscopic fundoplication, see
   Fundoplication, laparoscopic
Laparoscopic gastric resections, 240–
   245
Laparoscopic gastrostomy, see
   Gastrostomy, laparoscopic
Laparoscopic hemostasis, see
   Hemostasis, laparoscopic
Laparoscopic inguinal hernia repair,
   see Inguinal hernia repair,
   laparoscopic
Laparoscopic instrumentation, 2
Laparoscopic instruments, 2
Laparoscopic patient preparation, 12–
   13
Laparoscopic plication of perforated
   ulcer, 233–235
Laparoscopic procedures,
   troubleshooting, 8–11
Laparoscopic repair of ventral hernia,
   see Ventral hernia, laparoscopic
   repair of
Laparoscopic room layout, 1–8
Laparoscopic small bowel resection,
   see Small bowel resection,
   enterolysis, and
   enteroenterostomy

Laparoscopic splenectomy, *see*
    Splenectomy, laparoscopic
Laparoscopic staging
    of abdominal tumors, 115
    for Hodgkin's disease, 344–345
Laparoscopic suturing, 69–71
Laparoscopic total gastrectomy, 242–245
Laparoscopic treatment of
    gastroesophageal reflux and
    hiatal hernia, 196–212
Laparoscopic ultrasound (LUS), 124
    in cancer staging, 124–127
    for laparoscopic cholecystectomy,
    162–165
Laparoscopic vagotomy, *see*
    vagotomy, laparoscopic
Laparoscopic vertical banded
    gastroplasty, technique of, 247–250
Laparoscopic vertical Roux–en–Y
    gastric bypass, 250–252
Laparoscopy, diagnostic, *see*
    Diagnostic laparoscopy
    emergency, 109–114
    in massive obesity, 94–97
    pediatric, *see* Pediatric laparoscopy
    during pregnancy, *see* Pregnancy,
    laparoscopy during
    with previous abdominal surgery,
    104–107
Laser energy, 65–67
Laser photocoagulation, 453
Laser types, 66
LCDE, *see* Common bile duct
    exploration, laparoscopic
Left hemicolectomy, laparoscopic-
    assisted, 290–295
Lens-tipped trocar, 53
Lift devices, abdominal wall, *see*
    Abdominal wall lift devices
Ligatures, 58
Linear stapling devices, 58
Lithotomy–Trendelenburg position,
    13
Lithotripsy, 175, 511
Lithotriptors, 529–530
Liver biopsy, 117
    bleeding from, 350
Local anesthesia, 17
Lower abdomen puncture sites, 29
Lower esophageal sphincter, 426
Low-pressure pneumoperitoneum, 43
Lugol's solution, 436
Lumbar retroperitoneal space, 53
LUS, *see* Laparoscopic ultrasound

Lymph node biopsy, dissection, and
    staging laparoscopy, 336–351
    complications of, 349–351
    indications for, 336
    instruments for, 341
    patient positioning and room setup
    for, 337–340
    technique of, 341–343
    trocar placement for, 342
Lymph nodes, 126–127
Lymphocele, 351

Main stem bronchus intubations, 19
Malrotation of intestinal loop, 286
Management
    of bile duct injury, 188–191
    of hemorrhage, 67–68
    of transcystic drainage catheter,
    186
Mayo Clinic sonde technique, 481–482
Meckel's diverticulum, 111
Meperidine, 20
Mercury-filled rubber bougies, 458
Mesenteric ischemia, 110
Methylene blue, 436
Midline scar, 29
Monitoring
    anesthesia and, 15–20
    of patients, 419
    safety considerations and, 17–18
Monopolar electrosurgery, 59
    complications of, 63–64
Morcellation, specimen, 86
Motor skill, 71
Mucosal perforation, 219
Mucosal resection, endoscopic, 435
Muscle relaxation, 16
Myotomy, Heller, *see*
    Cardiomyotomy, laparoscopic

Narcan, 474
National Television Systems
    Committee (NTSC) format, 89
Needle biopsy, 116
Needle handling and passage, 72–73
Needle tips, 71
Neoplastic seeding, 479
Nerve injury, 375–376
Nissen fundoplication, technique of,
    202–209
Nitrous oxide, 16, 39, 41
Nonsteroidal antiinflammatory drugs
    (NSAIDs), 472–473
Nonvariceal upper gastrointestinal
    bleeding

complications with, 455
control of, 448–455
diagnosis of, 448
indications of, 448–450
methods and results of controlling,
450–455
NSAIDs (nonsteroidal anti-
inflammatory drugs), 472–473
N staging, 563
NTSC (National Television Systems
Committee) format, 89

Obesity
massive, laparoscopy in, 94–97
thromboembolic complications in,
95–96
Ogilvie's syndrome
conditions associated with, 566
decompressive colonoscopy for,
565–567
"Open" technique with Hasson
cannula, 31–33
Operating room, 1
patient preparation in, 13
small, laparoscopic
cholecystectomy in, 5
Operating table, 1
Opioids, 20
Opposing flat knot, 75
Oral sodium phosphate, 552
Overhand flat knot, 73–75
Overtube complications, 441

Pain management, 20
PAL (Phase Alternating Line) format,
89
Pancreas
adenocarcinomas of, 126
initial dissection and mobilization
of, for distal pancreatectomy,
309
Pancreatectomy, distal, *see* Distal
pancreatectomy
Pancreatic carcinoma, 122–123
Pancreatic duct stenting, 513
Pancreatic duct stone removal, 512
Pancreatic leak, 312
Pancreatic pseudocysts, endoscopic
drainage of, 514
Pancreatic sphincterotomy, 509–510
Pancreatitis
as complication of
choledochoscopy, 532
as complication of ERCP, 516–518
as complication of transcystic duct
exploration, 193

gallstone, 129
Papillotomy, precut, 507–508
Para-aortic lymph nodes, 124
Para-aortic node dissections, 337,
345–346
Patient information brochures,
SAGES, 587
Patient monitoring, 419
Patient preparation
laparoscopic, 12–13
in operating room, 13
Patient recovery, 420–421
Patients, conscious sedation of, 419–
420
Pediatric colonoscopy, 584–585
Pediatric esophagoscopy, 577–580
Pediatric foreign body removal, 579
Pediatric gastroduodenoscopy, 581–
583
Pediatric gastrointestinal endoscopy,
577–585
Pediatric laparoscopy, 386–388
complications of, 399–406
complications of specific surgical
procedures, 400–406
contraindications for, 386
contralateral groin exploration
during herniorrhaphy, 397
diagnostic laparoscopy and cancer
staging, 396
general considerations, 386–388
general laparoscopic complications,
399–400
indications for, 386
instruments for, 387
patient positioning and room setup
for, 386–387
pyloromyotomy, 397
specific surgical procedures, 389–
406
Pediatric sigmoidoscopy, 583
PEG, *see* Percutaneous endoscopic
gastrostomy
Pelvic fluid collections and abscesses,
postoperative pediatric, 400
Penetrating trauma, 112
Peptic ulceration, intractable, 236
Percutaneous endoscopic gastrostomy
(PEG), 462–468
complications of, 477–479
indications for, 462–463
"pull" technique for placement of,
465–468
"push" technique for placement of,
463–465

Perforated ulcer, laparoscopic plication of, 233–235
Perforation
  as complication of choledochoscopy, 531
  as complication of colonoscopy, 571–572
  as complication of ERCP, 520–521
Periampullary tumors, 506–507
Peripancreatic nodes, 122
Peritoneal biopsy site, diffuse bleeding from, 349–350
Peritoneal cavity, 25
  access to, with previous abdominal surgery, 105
Peritoneum, retractors exposing, 32
Peritonitis, 110
Peroral cholangioscopy, 526–527
Persantine (dipyridamole), 473
Phase Alternating Line (PAL) format, 89
Photocoagulation, laser, 453
Physiologic changes associated with pneumoperitoneum, 19
Piroxicam (Feldene), 472
Plication, laparoscopic, of perforated ulcer, 233–235
Pneumoperitoneum, 37–41
  low-pressure, 43
  physiologic changes associated with, 19
Pneumothorax, 19, 219
Polyethylene glycol-electrolyte, 552
Polypectomy, 543–544
  endoscopic, 457–458
  incomplete, 548
PONV (postoperative nausea and vomiting), 15
Postoperative bile leakage after laparoscopic chole-cystectomy, 140
Postoperative choledochoscopy, 525–528
Postoperative ileus, 264–265
Postoperative nausea and vomiting (PONV), 15
Postoperative stomach, endoscopy of, 432–434
Postsplenectomy sepsis, 333
Precut papillotomy, 507
Precut sphincterotomy, 509
Pregnancy, laparoscopy during, 98–99
  advantages and feasibility of, 99–100
  disadvantages and concerns about, 100–101
  guidelines for, 101–102
  indications for, 98–99
Preoperative analysis and planning with previous abdominal surgery, 104
Preoperative considerations, 15
Pressure injuries, 306
Pretied suture loops, 58
Proctocolectomy with ileal-pouch–anal anastomosis, laparoscopic-assisted, 300–306
  completion of operation for, 305
  complications of, 305–306
  indications for, 300
  patient positioning and room setup for, 300
  performing, 302–304
  trocar position and choice of laparoscope for, 301
Propulcid, 12
Pseudocysts, pancreatic, endoscopic drainage of, 514
"Pull" technique for PEG placement, 465–468
Puncture, umbilical, 24–28
Puncture sites, alternate, 29
Push enteroscopy, 480–481
"Push" technique for PEG placement, 463–465
Pyloromyotomy, 397
  pediatric complications of, 401–402
Pylorus
  opening, 428
  view of, 492

Radiographic equipment, 148–151
Radiographic danger signs, 157–158
Rear panel, connections on, 7
Recording media, 91–92
Recovery of patients, 420–421
Rectal endoscopic ultrasound, 560–563
Rectum, 556
Regional anesthesia, 16–17
Respiratory acidosis, 100
Retractors
  conventional, 46–47
  exposing peritoneum, 32
  U-shaped, 43
Retrieval bags, 84–85
Retrogastric dissections, technique of, 341–343
Retroperitoneal laparoscopic adrenalectomy, 360–362
Retroperitoneum spaces, 53

Retropubic space, 53
Return electrode, 59
RGB signal, 89
Right hemicolectomy, laparoscopic-
    assisted, 287–290
RIOC, *see* Cholangiography, routine
    intraoperative
Roeder knot, 78
Room layout, laparoscopic, 1–8
Routine intraoperative
        cholangiography, *see*
        Cholangiography, routine
        intraoperative
Roux–en–Y gastric bypass, vertical,
    laparoscopic, 250–252
Rubber bougies, mercury-filled, 458

Safety considerations, monitoring and,
    17–18
SAGES guidelines, statements, and
    standards, 586–587
SAGES laparoscopic equipment
    troubleshooting guide, 587
SAGES patient information brochures,
    587
SAGES publications, 586–587
Sclerosing agents, 443
Sclerotherapy of variceal bleeding,
    442–446
    complications of, 446
    contraindications, 442
    indications and results, 442
    performing, 444–446
    technical considerations, 442–444
SECAM format, 89
Segmental colectomies, anterior
        resection, and abdominoperineal
        resection, laparoscopic, 286–
        298
    complications of, 297–298
    indications for, 286
    patient position and room setup,
        286–287
Seldinger technique, 182, 270
Semi-lithotomy position, 13
Shaft advancement, 536
Shaft torquing, 536
Sheathed videoendoscope system, 534
Shock, unexplained, 110
Side-to-side anastomosis, 80
Sigmoid colon, 556–557
Sigmoid colon resection,
    laparoscopic-assisted, 290–295
Sigmoidoscopy
    flexible, *see* Flexible
        sigmoidoscopy

pediatric, 583
Sigmoid volvulus, decompressive
    colonoscopy for, 567–568
Slip knot, 76–77
Small bowel enteroscopy, 480–484
    complications of, 483–484
    indications for, 480
    technique of, 480–483
Small bowel obstruction, 110, 264
    postoperative, 298
Small bowel resection, enterolysis,
        and enteroenterostomy, 254–266
    complications of, 262–266
    indications for, 254
    patient positioning and room setup
        for, 254–255
    technique of, 256–260
    trocar position and choice of
        laparoscope for, 255–256
Smooth muscle tumors of stomach,
    236
Snare, diathermy, 457
Snare polypectomy, 543
Sodium morrhuate, 443
Sodium phosphate, oral, 552
Sodium tetradecyl sulfate, 443
Sonde enteroscopy, 481
Space of Bogros, 53
Space of Retzius, 53
Specimen entrapment, 85
Specimen fragmentation, 86
Specimen morcellation, 86
Specimen removal
    principles of, 82–86
    routes of, 82–84
Specimen retrieval, complications of,
    86
Specimen retrieval bags, 84–85
Specimen rupture, 86
Sphincter, flaccid, 154
Sphincterotomy
    biliary, 508–509
    laparoscopic antegrade, 175–176
    pancreatic, 509–510
    precut, 509
    technique of, 498
    transhepatic-guided, 508
Splenectomy, 124
    distal pancreatectomy with, 307,
        309–311
    laparoscopic, 326–334
        complications of, 332–334
        disorders treated by, 326
        indications for, 326–327
        patient positioning and room
            setup for, 327–328

pediatric complications of, 403–405

performing, 330–332

trocar position and choice of laparoscope for, 329–330

Splenic flexure, 557

Splenic hilar lymph nodes, 124

Splenic salvage, distal pancreatectomy with, 311

Square knot, 73–77

Staging

  cancer, *see* Cancer staging,

    laparoscopic, *see* laparoscopic staging

Stapling, 80

Stapling devices, linear, 58

Stenting

  biliary, 512–513

  pancreatic duct, 513

Stomach

  postoperative, endoscopy of, 432–434

  smooth muscle tumors of, 236

Stone basket, 174

Stone extraction through laparoscopic choledochotomy, 180–181

Stone removal

  biliary tract, 510–511

  pancreatic duct, 512

Stone retrieval, 529–530

Structural Balloon, 55

Subphrenic abscess, 334

Sump syndrome, 499

Surgeon's knot, 73–77

Surgery, preparation for, 12–13

Surgically altered anatomy, endoscopy with, 496–500

Suture choice, 79

Suture loops, pretied, 58

Suture material, 72

Suturing, 58

  continuous, 79

  interrupted, 79

  laparoscopic, 69–71

Suturing instruments, 71–73

Suturing techniques, 79–80

Tachycardia, 18

TAPP (transabdominal preperitoneal) laparoscopic inguinal herniorrhaphy, 365–372

Teeth, dislodgment of, 475

TEP (totally extraperitoneal) laparoscopic inguinal herniorrhaphy, 372–374

Testicular complications, 376

Therapeutic choledochoscopy, 529–530

Therapeutic colonoscopy, 565–570

Therapeutic endoscopic retrograde cholangiopancreatography, 508–514

Therapeutic flexible sigmoidoscopy, 543–549

Thermal therapy, 450–453

Thermal tissue destruction, 59

Thoracoscopic vagotomy, 231

Three-trocar technique, 121

Thromboembolic complications in obesity, 95

Ticlopidine (Ticlid), 473

Tip deflection, controlling, 409, 536

Tissue approximation, principles of, 69–80

Tissue destruction, thermal, 59

Tissue gluing, 80

Tissue sampling techniques, 434–436

Topical anesthesia, 423

Totally extraperitoneal (TEP) laparoscopic inguinal herniorrhaphy, 372–374

Toupet procedure, 218

  modified, 210

Transabdominal laparoscopic adrenalectomy, 354–360

Transabdominal preperitoneal (TAPP) laparoscopic inguinal herniorrhaphy, 365–372

Transanal specimen extraction, 84

Transcystic drainage catheter, management of, 186

Transcystic duct approach, 167–168

Transcystic duct exploration, complications of, 191–193

Transhepatic choledochoscopy, 528

Transhepatic-guided sphincterotomy, 508

Transvaginal specimen extraction, 84

Transverse colon, 557

Trauma, diagnostic laparoscopy for, 112–114

Triangle of Calot, *see* Calot's triangle

Trocars, 71

  lens-tipped, 53

  placement of, 29–30

Trocar site bleeding, 34

  during laparoscopic cholecystectomy, 137

Troubleshooting

  flexible endoscopes, 412–413

  laparoscopic procedures, 8–11

T staging, 562–563

T-tube, decompression by, 185

Ulcer, perforated, laparoscopic
    plication of, 233–235
Ultrasonic aspirator, cavitational, 64
Ultrasonic coagulating shears, 65
Ultrasonic energy, 64–65
Ultrasonic scalpel, 64
Ultrasound, endoscopic, see
        Endoscopic ultrasound
    laparoscopic, see Laparoscopic
        ultrasound
Umbilical puncture, 24–28
Unexplained shock, 110
Upper abdomen puncture sites, 29
Upper gastrointestinal bleeding,
        nonvariceal, see nonvariceal
        upper gastrointestinal bleeding
Upper gastrointestinal endoscopy
    complications of, 470–479
    diagnostic, see Diagnostic upper
        gastrointestinal endoscopy
    therapeutic, 457–461
Upper gastrointestinal malignancies
    palliation of, 459–460
Ureteral injury, 305–306
Urinary tract complications, 375
U-shaped retractors, 43

Vagotomy, laparoscopic, 227–232
    complications of, 231–232
    indications for, 227
    patient positioning and room setup
        for, 227
    performing, 228–231
    trocar position and choice of
        laparoscope for, 227–228
    types of, 228–231
Variceal band ligation, endoscopic,
        438–441
    complications of, 441
    indications for, 438
    patient positioning and room setup
        for, 438
    technique of, 438–440

Variceal bleeding, sclerotherapy of,
        see Sclerotherapy of variceal
        bleeding
Variceal injection, 444–446
Vascular injury, 374–375
    major, 35
Vas deferens complications, 376
Vater, ampulla of, 483
Venous air embolism, 37
Ventral hernia, laparoscopic repair of,
        379–385
    complications of, 385
    indications and contraindications
        for, 379
    patient positioning and room setup
        for, 379–380
    technique of, 381–385
    trocar position and choice of
        laparoscope for, 380–381
Veress needle, 23–24
    "closed" technique with, 24–30
Vertical banded gastroplasty,
        laparoscopic, technique of, 247–
        250
Vertical Roux–en–Y gastric bypass,
        laparoscopic, 250–252
Video-endoscopy, 408–409
Video imaging, components of, 88–89
Videoscope, 534
Video signals, types of, 89–91
Videotapes, 91
Visceral injury, 35, 86
    with previous abdominal surgery,
        107
Volvulus, 567

Warfarin, 473
Wire-guided dilators, 458–459
Working space, generation of, 52–56
Wound infection, 86
Wounds, gunshot, 113

Yankauer suction, 473